Blueprints

PEDIATRICS

FOURTH EDITION

Blueprints
PEDIATRICS

FOURTH EDITION

Bradley S. Marino, MD, MPP, MSCE
Assistant Professor of Anesthesia
Department of Anesthesiology and Critical Care
Assistant Professor of Pediatrics
Department of Pediatrics
University of Pennsylvania
Divisions of Cardiology and Critical Care Medicine
The Children's Hospital of Philadelphia
Philadelphia, Pennsylvania

Katie S. Fine, MD
Private Pediatrician
Charlotte, North Carolina

Lippincott Williams & Wilkins
a Wolters Kluwer business
Philadelphia · Baltimore · New York · London
Buenos Aires · Hong Kong · Sydney · Tokyo

Acquisitions Editor: Nancy Anastasi Duffy
Managing Editor: Kelly Horvath
Marketing Manager: Jennifer Kuklinski
Associate Production Manager: Kevin P. Johnson
Creative Director: Doug Smock
Compositor: International Typesetting and Composition
Printer: Quebecor World Dubuque

First Edition, Blackwell 1997
Second Edition, Blackwell 2001
Third Edition, Blackwell 2004

Library of Congress Cataloging-in-Publication Data

Marino, Bradley S.
  Blueprints pediatrics / Bradley S. Marino, Katie S. Fine.—4th ed.
    p. ; cm.—(Blueprints)
  Includes index.
  ISBN 1-4051-0501-1
  1. Pediatrics—Outlines, syllabi, etc. I. Fine, Katie S. (Katie Snead)
II. Title. III. Series.
  [DNLM: 1. Pediatrics—Examination Questions. WS 18.2 M339b 2007]
RJ48.3.M37 2007
618.92'00076—dc22   2006004933

To purchase additional copies of this book, call our customer service department at **(800) 638-3030** or fax orders to **(301) 223-2320**. International customers should call **(301) 223-2300**.

Visit Lippincott Williams & Wilkins on the Internet: *http://www.LWW.com*.
Lippincott Williams & Wilkins customer service representatives are available from 8:30 am to 6:00 pm, EST.

06 07 08 09 10
1 2 3 4 5 6 7 8 9 10

Preface

*B*lueprints Pediatrics was first published almost 10 years ago as part of a series of books designed to help medical students prepare for USMLE Steps 2 and 3. This examination preparation remains the core mission of the series. To that end, the authors review the subject parameters posted by the testing board before each edition. Our goal is integration of the material into a complete yet concise review guide that is well organized, straightforward, and factually current. However, we have been pleased to hear from our readers that the book is utilized by many students during third year and senior rotations. Residents in emergency medicine and family practice, as well as nurse practitioners and physicians' assistants have found *Blueprints* helpful during the pediatric portion of their training. We believe this continued usefulness is because the book covers a broad range of basic yet important topics that must be mastered in order to treat children.

Each chapter in the book contains a single subject for review. Most can be read in under an hour. The topics contained in each chapter are grouped in an orderly fashion, each followed by a "Key Points" section that allows for immediate review and highlights the concepts most frequently tested. The 75 questions found at the end of the book are written in the "clinical vignette" style used on USMLE and Pediatric Board examinations. Thus readers not only can evaluate their grasp of the material but also begin to acclimate themselves to the expected testing environment.

The fourth edition of *Blueprints Pediatrics* is the strongest to date. It incorporates many of the suggestions we have received from medical students and faculty with regard to content and organization. For example, the cardiology chapter has been edited to better reflect USMLE testing requirements, with clearer figures and more targeted information. In addition, the authors' dual backgrounds in academic medicine and private practice allow us to keep abreast of emerging research and its effect on the understanding of pathology and patient care. The development chapter tackles aberrant development as well as development delay. New guidelines regarding the febrile infant and treatment of urinary tract infections have been added to their respective chapters. Gene loci linked to specific diseases are listed whenever known. The oncology chapter has been updated to reflect the rapid evolution of treatment regimens. Infectious diseases, such as SARS and human metapneumovirus, which were unheard of 10 years ago, are included. Finally, the new edition contains an adolescent medicine chapter, given that this is now a recognized specialty field with topic-specific questions of its own.

We hope you find *Blueprints Pediatrics* to be a beneficial investment, regardless of how you use it.

Bradley S. Marino, MD, MPP, MSCE, and Katie S. Fine, MD

Acknowledgments

This book is a tribute to our patients. Each day we are reminded how truly precious children are and what an honor it is to care for them. We are forever grateful to our colleagues (residents, fellows, and faculty) whose limitless understanding and support allow us to pursue projects such as this. We would specifically like to thank the faculty of The Children's Hospital of Philadelphia, whose editorial comments in the following chapters made sure that the fourth edition of *Blueprints Pediatrics* represented the latest knowledge in pediatric medicine: Dermatology (Albert C. Yan, MD), Endocrinology (Sogol Mostoufi-moab, MD), Gastroenterology (Kathy Loomes, MD), Genetics (Sulagna Saitta, MD, PhD), Hematology (Leslie Raffini, MD), Immunology, Allergy, and Rheumatology (Erin E. McGintee, MD, and David Sherry, MD), Infectious Disease (Theoklis Zaoutis, MD), Neonatology (David Munson, MD), Nephrology and Urology (Kevin Meyers, MD), Neurology (Sabrina Smith, MD), Nutrition (Monica Nagle, RD, CNSD, LDN), Oncology (Michael Fisher, MD, Leslie S. Kersun, MD, Yael Mosse, MD, Susan Rheingold, MD, Jeff Skolnick, MD), and Pulmonology (Samuel Goldfarb, MD).

We would like to dedicate this edition of *Blueprints Pediatrics* to our friend and colleague, Dr. Brian Stidham. He was a brilliant caring physician and a loving, devoted father and husband. His compassion and commitment to his patients and family was an example to us all.

Finally, we would like to thank our families, without whose support, patience, and encouragement none of this would be possible.

B.M.
K.F.

Contents

Abbreviations

ABG	arterial blood gas	G6PD	glucose-6-phosphate dehydrogenase
ACTH	adrenocorticotropic hormone	GI	gastrointestinal
AIDS	acquired immunodeficiency syndrome	Hb	hemoglobin
ALL	acute lymphocytic leukemia	Hib	*Haemophilus influenzae* type b
ALT	alanine transaminase	HIV	human immunodeficiency virus
AMP	adenosine monophosphate	HLA	human leukocyte antigen
ANA	antinuclear antibody	IFA	immunofluorescent antibody
AP	anteroposterior	Ig	immunoglobulin
ARDS	adult respiratory distress syndrome	IM	intramuscular
ASD	atrial septal defect	INH	isoniazid
ASO	anti-streptolysin O	IVC	inferior vena cava
AST	aspartate transaminase	IVIG	intravenous immunoglobulin
AZT	zidovudine	JRA	juvenile rheumatoid arthritis
BUN	blood urea nitrogen	JVP	jugular venous pressure
CAVV	common atrioventricular valve	KUB	kidneys/ureter/bladder
CBC	complete blood count	LDH	lactate dehydrogenase
CDC	Centers for Disease Control and Prevention	LFTs	liver function tests
		LP	lumbar puncture
CF	cystic fibrosis	L/S	lecithin-to-sphingomyelin (ratio)
CHF	congestive heart failure	LV	left ventricle
CK	creatine kinase	LVH	left ventricular hypertrophy
CNS	central nervous system	MMR	measles-mumps-rubella
CSF	cerebrospinal fluid	MRI	magnetic resonance imaging
CT	computed tomography	NG	nasogastric
DIC	disseminated intravascular coagulation	NPO	nil per os (nothing by mouth)
DMD	Duchenne-type muscular dystrophy	NSAID	nonsteroidal anti-inflammatory drug
DTP	diphtheria/tetanus/pertussis	PCR	polymerase chain reaction
DTRs	deep tendon reflexes	PDA	patent ductus arteriosus
DVT	deep venous thrombosis	PFTs	pulmonary function tests
EBV	Epstein-Barr virus	PMI	point of maximal intensity
ECG	electrocardiography	PPD	purified protein derivative
ECMO	extracorporeal membrane oxygenation	PT	prothrombin time
EEG	electroencephalography	PTT	partial thromboplastin time
ELISA	enzyme-linked immunosorbent assay	RBC	red blood cell
EMG	electromyography	RF	rheumatoid factor
ESR	erythrocyte sedimentation rate	RPR	rapid plasma reagent (test)
FEV	forced expiratory volume	RSV	respiratory syncytial virus
FTA-ABS	fluorescent treponemal antibody absorption	RV	right ventricle
		RVH	right ventricular hypertrophy
FVC	forced vital capacity	SIDS	sudden infant death syndrome

s/p	status post	US	ultrasound
T_3RU	triiodothyronine resin uptake	VMA	vanillylmandelic acid
T_4	thyroxine	VSD	ventricular septal defect
TSH	thyroid-stimulating hormone	vWF	von Willebrand factor
UA	urinalysis	WBC	white blood cell
URI	upper respiratory infection		

Emergency Management: Evaluation of the Critically Ill or Injured Child

The critically ill or injured child must be evaluated rapidly to minimize morbidity and mortality. Whether presenting to the physician's office, local clinic, community hospital, or tertiary care center, the patient is stabilized by administering basic life support and pediatric advanced life support measures recommended by the American Heart Association. Once the patient is clinically stable, a problem list can be generated and the cause of the child's symptoms can be determined.

DIFFERENTIAL DIAGNOSIS

Of the causes of pediatric cardiorespiratory arrest, respiratory etiologies (45%), cardiac etiologies (25%), and primary central nervous system disorders (20%) account for 90% of all cases. Table 1-1 lists the differential diagnosis for children with cardiopulmonary arrest, excluding neonates.

CLINICAL MANIFESTATIONS AND TREATMENT

PRIMARY SURVEY

The **primary survey** (Fig. 1-1) involves assessment of Airway, Breathing, Circulation, Disability, and Exposure.

The aim is identification of life-threatening conditions. Figure 1-2 outlines resuscitative measures.

The goals of **airway** management are to recognize and relieve obstruction, prevent aspiration of gastric contents, and promote adequate gas exchange. The airway is assessed and, if necessary, secured as follows:

- Immobilization of the cervical spine if there is a possibility of spinal cord injury.
- Clearing the oropharynx with a Yankauer suction catheter (blind finger sweep is contraindicated because a foreign body may be forced further down the oropharynx).
- Opening the airway via the jaw-thrust or chin-lift maneuver and relieving any obstruction caused by the tongue or soft tissues of the neck.
- Placing the head in the midline "sniffing position," often via a rolled-up towel beneath the occiput (hyperextension of the neck may result in obstruction of the airway).
- Provision of 100% oxygen via face mask.
- If indicated, placement of an oral or a nasopharyngeal airway.

Once an airway is established, air exchange **(breathing)** should be evaluated. Examination of chest wall movement reveals the presence and effectiveness of spontaneous respirations. If spontaneous respiration is present with adequate oxygenation,

TABLE 1-1 The Differential Diagnosis of Cardiopulmonary Arrest in Children

Respiratory	Metabolic
Upper airway obstruction	Diabetic ketoacidosis
Lower airway obstruction	Addison disease
Restrictive lung disease	Hyperthyroidism
Insufficient gas transfer	Hypoglycemia
Inadequate gas exchange	Hyperkalemia
	Hypocalcemia
	Hyponatremia
Cardiac	**Multisystem**
Congenital heart disease	Sudden infant death syndrome
Primary arrhythmia	Drug intoxication[a]
Myocarditis	Multiple traumas
Pericarditis	Anaphylaxis
Cardiac tamponade	Hypothermia
Congestive heart failure	Septic shock
Central Nervous System	**Renal**
Meningitis	Acute and chronic renal failure
Encephalitis	
Acute hydrocephalus	
Head trauma	
Tumor	
Hypoxic-ischemic injury	
Gastrointestinal	
Abdominal trauma	
Bowel perforation or obstruction	
Peritonitis	
Dehydration	

[a]Narcotics, tricyclic antidepressants, barbiturates, and benzodiazepines.

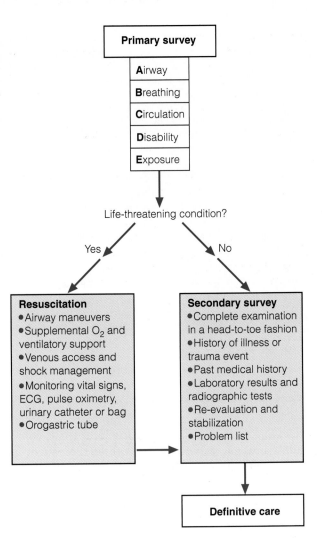

Figure 1-1 • Algorithm of the initial assessment of the pediatric patient.

and provides the seal for the uncuffed tube.) The size of the endotracheal tube chosen should be

$$= 4\left(\frac{Age\ in\ Year}{4}\right)$$

intubation is not indicated. If chest wall excursion is not adequate, endotracheal tube placement is indicated (if not already in place to secure the airway). If the child is younger than 8 years, an uncuffed tube should be used to reduce the risk of subglottic edema and stenosis. (Note: In children younger than 8 years, the cricoid ring is the narrowest part of the airway

Blood oxygenation (via pulse oximetry or arterial blood gas measurement) and blood carbon dioxide (CO_2) level (by arterial or venous blood gas measurement) should be assessed and will help guide respiratory management.

Neonatal intubation is traditionally performed without premedication, but intubation of the infant

Infant	Older Child
Airway	
Determine unresponsiveness	
Call for help	
Position patient supine	
Support head and neck	
Head tilt/chin lift or jaw thrust	
No blind finger sweeps	
Breathing	
2 initial breaths	
Then: 20 breaths/min	
"Mouth to nose"	"Mouth to mouth"
Circulation	
Check brachial pulse	Check carotid pulse
Activate EMS System	
Compression location: 1 finger breadth below intermammary line on sternum	Compression location: lower 1/3 of sternum
Compression method: Hands encircle chest or 2 fingers on sternum	Compression method: 1 or 2 hands on sternum
Compression depth: 0.5–1″	Compression depth: 1–1.5″
Compression rate: 100/min	Compression rate: 80–100/min
One rescuer—Compression:ventilation ratio = 30:2 Two rescuer—Compression:ventilation ratio = 15:2 Reassessment: Palpate pulse every 5 cycles	

Figure 1-2 • Basic CPR in infants and children. (Modified from Nichols DG, Yaster M, Lappe DG, et al. *Golden Hour: The Handbook of Advanced Pediatric Life Support.* 2nd ed. St. Louis: Mosby–Yearbook; 1991:128.)

In the hypotensive, hemodynamically unstable, or unconscious patient, premedication is not indicated. Cricoid pressure should be applied, and the patient should be intubated. Rarely, a patient cannot be intubated or ventilated with a bag and mask, and an emergency needle cricothyrotomy is required to establish an airway.

Circulation may be assessed by evaluating pulses (central and peripheral), capillary refill, and blood pressure. The absence of a pulse in the large arteries of an unconscious patient who is not breathing defines a cardiorespiratory arrest. *In children, heart rate is the most sensitive measure of intravascular volume status.* Capillary refill is the most sensitive measure of adequate circulation. Blood pressure fluctuations are an insensitive indicator because hypotension is a late finding in hypovolemia. Cardiorespiratory monitors are helpful for specifying the electrical activity of the heart.

If pulselessness is noted on examination of the brachial pulse in the infant or the carotid pulse in the child, chest compressions should be started. Figure 1-3 outlines vascular access management during cardiopulmonary resuscitation. Once access has been established, initial fluid resuscitation with lactated Ringer solution or normal saline should be given as a 20 mL per kg bolus as quickly as possible. If necessary, these boluses should be repeated. However, if there is no response or the patient has suffered acute blood loss, consider a

or child is done with premedication in the following **rapid-sequence** fashion:

1. Preoxygenation with 100% oxygen.
2. Administration of a vagolytic drug (e.g., atropine).
3. Administration of a sedative, hypnotic, and/or opioid drug (e.g., thiopental, Versed, fentanyl).
4. Application of cricoid pressure.
5. Administration of a paralyzing dose of a neuromuscular blocking agent (e.g., pancuronium or vecuronium, a nondepolarizing agent; or succinylcholine, a depolarizing agent).

If succinylcholine is used, a defasciculating dose of a neuromuscular blocking agent should be given before administration of succinylcholine (e.g., pancuronium or vecuronium).

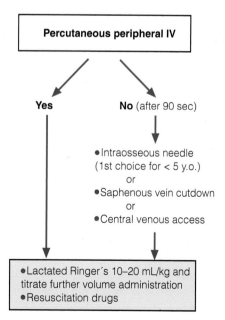

Figure 1-3 • Vascular access management during cardiopulmonary resuscitation.

10 mL per kg infusion of albumin, crystalloid, or type O-negative whole blood. If hypotension caused by hemorrhage is suspected, gaining proximal control of the hemorrhage is critical.

Optimally, a full set of screening tests (including complete blood count, arterial and/or venous blood gas, electrolyte and chemistry panel, and blood glucose) is obtained at the time of vascular access. If ingestion is a possibility, serum and urine toxicology and an acetaminophen and salicylate level may be obtained.

In the patient with tachyarrhythmias (subventricular tachycardia [SVT], ventricular tachycardia [VT]), therapeutic decisions are based on whether the patient is hemodynamically stable or unstable.

Supraventricular Tachycardia

- *Hemodynamically stable:* Vagal maneuvers, adenosine (AV [atrioventricular] reciprocating tachycardia), Diagoxin, esmolol, or procainamide amiodarone (automatic tachycardia).
- *Hemodynamically unstable or SVT refractory to medications:* Synchronized cardioversion 0.50 to 1.0 J per kg; increased to 2 J per kg if initial cardioversion is unsuccessful.

Ventricular Tachycardia

- *Hemodynamically stable:* Amiodarone or procainamide, and treatment of hypomagnesemia and/or hypokalemia. Amiodarone and procainamide should not be used together because they both prolong the QT interval, and both may cause hypotension.
- *Hemodynamically unstable or VT refractory to medications:* Synchronized cardioversion 0.50 to 1.0 J per kg; increased to 2 J per kg if initial cardioversion is unsuccessful.
- *Pulseless VT or VF:* Nonsynchronized defibrillation (2 J per kg, followed by 4 J per kg if unsuccessful) is indicated. Epinephrine is administered if resuscitation is unsuccessful after two electrical shocks, followed by shock again, 4 J per kg. Subsequent defibrillation attempts should be preceded with intravenous lidocaine, amiodarone, or epinephrine.

For a full discussion of drug physiology, indications, dosage, route of administration, effects, and side effects, see *The Harriet Lane Handbook* or *Golden Hour: The Handbook of Advanced Pediatric Life Support*. Table 1-2 describes the indications and effects of each drug.

For **disability,** a rapid screening neurologic examination is performed to note pupillary response, level of consciousness, and localizing findings.

SECONDARY SURVEY

The **secondary survey** includes a head-to-toe physical examination to determine the extent of injury and further prioritize treatment. The patient's level of consciousness is assessed using the Glasgow Coma Scale (see Table 15-5). In preparation for the secondary survey, the patient should be undressed. Because of children's large surface-to-body mass ratio, they cool rapidly, and passive heat loss can be problematic. **Exposure** (hypo- or hyperthermia) must be detected and dealt with promptly.

1-1 KEY POINTS

1. No matter what the cause of cardiorespiratory arrest, the algorithms outlined for pediatric basic and advanced cardiac life support should be followed. A primary survey (**A**irway, **B**reathing, **C**irculation, **D**isability, and **E**xposure) is followed by a secondary survey.
2. Approximately half of the causes of pediatric arrest are caused by respiratory arrest, which can be brought about by upper airway obstruction, lower airway obstruction, restrictive lung disease, or any etiology that results in inadequate gas exchange.
3. Figure 1-4 summarizes the cardiopulmonary resuscitation (CPR) algorithm.
4. If resuscitation does not establish cardiac output, the following mechanical or metabolic causes should be investigated: hypothermia, tension pneumothorax, hemothorax, cardiac tamponade, profound hypovolemia, profound metabolic imbalance, toxin ingestion, and closed head injury.

SHOCK

Shock is a syndrome characterized by the inability of the circulatory system to provide adequate nutrients to meet the body's metabolic demands. Children, especially neonates, will initially try to compensate by becoming tachycardic. Hypotension, a late finding, leads to cellular hypoperfusion, metabolic acidosis, and cellular death. Three relationships explain hypotension in shock:

- **Blood pressure** (cardiac output × systemic vascular resistance).
- **Cardiac output** (stroke volume × heart rate).
- **Stroke volume** (determined by preload [ventricular

TABLE 1-2 Drugs Used in Pediatric Cardiorespiratory Resuscitation		
Drug	**Indication**	**Effect**
Atropine	Bradycardia and atrioventricular block	Increases heart rate and conduction through the atrioventricular node by decreasing vagal tone
Bicarbonate	Severe refractory metabolic acidosis and/or hyperkalemia	Increases blood pH
Elemental calcium (calcium gluconate or calcium chloride)	Hypocalcemia, hyperkalemia, hypermagnesemia, and calcium channel blocker overdose	Increases myocardial contractility, increases ventricular excitability, and increases conduction velocity through the myocardium
Dextrose	Hypoglycemia	Increases blood glucose level
Epinephrine (1:10,000)	Asystole, bradycardia, pulseless VT, VF	Increases systemic vascular resistance, chronotropy, and inotropy, thereby increasing cardiac output and blood pressure (increasing diastolic blood pressure increases coronary artery perfusion pressure)
Epinephrine (1:1,000)	Pulseless arrest after above dose or as first dose down endotracheal tube if no vascular access available	Same as above
Lidocaine	Ventricular ectopy, VT, VF	Helps make refractory pulseless VT and VF more susceptible to cardioversion, may suppress hemodynamically stable VT, and decreases the likelihood of recurrence of ventricular ectopy
Amiodarone	Atrial (refractory SVT) and ventricular arrhythmias (refractory pulseless VT, refractory VF, hemodynamically stable VT)	Blocks Na, K, and Ca channels and β-receptors in the myocardium as well as α- and β-receptors in the vascular periphery
Naloxone	Presumed or known opiate intoxication	Rapid reversal of opiate effect

NOTE: Drugs that can be given by endotracheal tube include lidocaine, atropine, naloxone hydrochloride, and epinephrine (high dose).
VT, ventricular tachycardia; VF, ventricular fibrillation; SVT, supraventricular tachycardia.

end-diastolic volume], afterload [systemic vascular resistance], and myocardial contractility)

The three stages of shock are compensated, uncompensated, and irreversible. In the **compensated stage,** homeostatic mechanisms maintain essential organ perfusion. Blood pressure, urine output, and cardiac function all seem to be normal. In the **uncompensated stage,** homeostatic mechanisms fail because of ischemia, endothelial injury, and the elaboration of toxic materials. Cellular function eventually deteriorates, and multiorgan system organ dysfunction results. When this process has caused irreparable functional loss in essential organs, the terminal, or **irreversible stage,** of shock is reached.

The types of shock include hypovolemic, cardiogenic, distributive, and septic (Table 1-3). **Hypovolemic shock** results from decreased intravascular volume, which results in decreased venous return and myocardial preload. Because of the reduction in myocardial preload, there is a resultant decrease in stroke volume, cardiac output, and blood

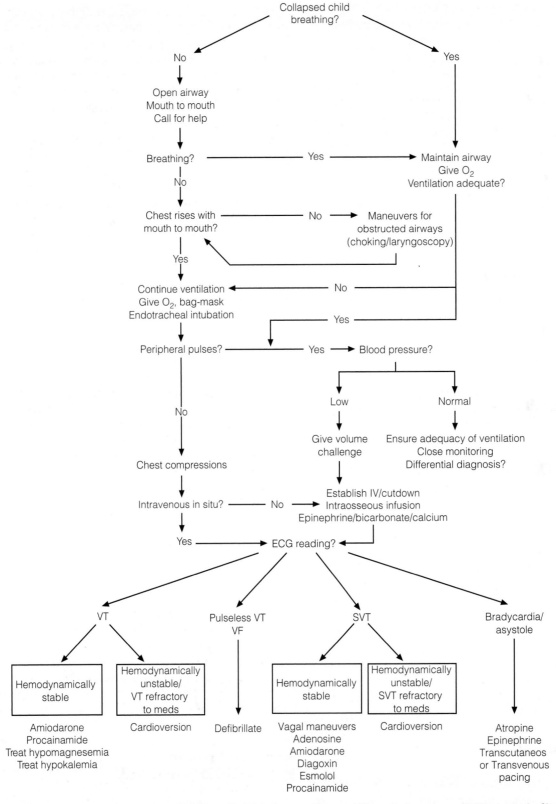

Figure 1-4 • Cardiopulmonary resuscitation algorithm. ECG, electrocardiogram; VT, ventricular tachycardia; VF, ventricular fibrillation; SVT, supraventricular tachycardia.

■ **TABLE 1-3** The Etiologies of Shock	
Hypovolemic	**Distributive**
Water and electrolyte losses	Anaphylaxis
Hemorrhage	Neurologic injury (head or spinal cord)
Plasma losses (third spacing)	Drug toxicity
Cardiogenic	**Septic**
Congenital heart disease	Infection
Ischemic heart disease	
Cardiomyopathies	
Arrhythmias	
Infections	
Miscellaneous	
Pulmonary embolism	
Adrenal insufficiency	

pressure. This is the most common etiology of shock in children.

Cardiogenic shock is the result of "pump failure." Inadequate stroke volume results in diminished cardiac output and hypotension.

Distributive shock results from an abnormality in vasomotor tone that leads to maldistribution of a normal circulatory volume and a state of relative hypovolemia. Because of peripheral pooling, preload is reduced, causing a decrease in stroke volume, cardiac output, and blood pressure. Systemic vascular resistance is also decreased because of vasomotor dysfunction. Because both systemic vascular resistance and cardiac output are reduced, severe hypotension results.

Septic shock results when certain pathogens infect the blood. The early compensated stage of septic shock is characterized by decreased vascular resistance (distributive shock), whereas in the late uncompensated phase, hypovolemia from third spacing and pump failure caused by myocardial depression becomes more apparent. Compensated septic shock is called "warm" septic shock; uncompensated septic shock is referred to as "cold" septic shock.

CLINICAL MANIFESTATIONS

History and Physical Examination

The history should focus on potential causes. Hypovolemic shock is likely if there is a history of

vomiting, diarrhea, polyuria, burns, trauma, surgery, gastrointestinal bleeding, intestinal obstruction, long periods in the sun, or pancreatitis. A history of congenital heart disease, arrhythmias, or chemotherapy (doxorubicin) administration may indicate cardiogenic shock. Distributive shock should be contemplated when there is a history of toxic ingestion, anaphylaxis, or head or spinal cord injury. In addition, any immunocompromised patient who presents with a history of fever and is ill-appearing may be in septic shock.

Serial vital signs are critical in the diagnosis and management of children with shock. In early "warm" compensated septic shock, vasodilation, warm extremities, tachycardia, a widened pulse pressure, and adequate urine output are seen. In contrast, symptoms of hypovolemic, cardiogenic, and late "cold" uncompensated septic shock include vasoconstriction, tachycardia, cold extremities, poor peripheral pulses, altered consciousness, pallor, sweating, ileus, and oliguria.

DIAGNOSTIC EVALUATION

During the stabilization period, the clinician must determine into which category of shock the patient's illness falls. Any patient with shock should be placed on a cardiac monitor. The level of tachycardia is the best determinant of the level of intravascular depletion or vasomotor abnormality. Hypotension is a late finding and occurs only after 40% of the intravascular volume has been depleted. Diagnostic tests are determined on the basis of the specific causes suspected.

TREATMENT

The treatment of shock is aimed at ensuring perfusion of critical vascular beds (coronary, cerebral, hepatic, and renal) and preventing or correcting metabolic abnormalities arising from cellular hypoperfusion. Management of hypoxia reduces the level of metabolic acidosis. Correcting metabolic acidosis results in both better cellular function and myocardial performance and decreased systemic and pulmonary vascular resistance.

Hypovolemic shock is treated with normal saline or lactated Ringer solution (see Chapter 7 for details). If hemorrhage is the cause of the hypovolemia, type O-negative, cross-matched whole blood or packed red cells may be given. In cardiogenic shock resulting from a congenital heart defect, surgery, balloon angioplasty, or valvuloplasty and/or inotropic support may be indicated. Children with severe ischemic injury to the heart, dilated cardiomyopathy, or myocarditis may need heart transplantion. In distributive shock caused by anaphylaxis, intravenous steroids, diphenhydramine, subcutaneous epinephrine, and albuterol nebulizers are used. Sometimes intubation for laryngospasm and vasopressors for intractable hypotension are needed. Septic shock is treated with vasopressors, fluids, and broad-spectrum antibiotics. Antibiotics are considered a resuscitation medication for septic shock.

🔑 1-2 KEY POINTS

1. Determine the category of shock and whether the patient has early or late manifestations.
2. Hypovolemic shock accounts for most cases of shock.
3. In hypovolemic shock, blood pressure depression is a late finding, and the level of tachycardia is the most sensitive measure of intravascular fluid status.
4. In septic shock, antibiotics are a resuscitation medication, and their administration should not be delayed.

Suggested Additional Reading

Pediatric basic and advanced life support. In: 2005 International Consensus Conference on Cardiopulmonary Resuscitation and Emergency Cardiovascular Care Science with Treatment Recommendations. *Circulation* 2005;112(22 Suppl): II173–90.

2005 American Heart Association Guidelines for Cardiopulmonary Resuscitation and Emergency Cardiovascular Care. Part 11: Pediatric Basic Life Support *Circulation*. 2005;112:IV-156–IV-166.

2005 American Heart Association Guidlines for Cardiopulmonary Resuscitation and Emergency Cardiovascular Care. Part 12: Pediatric Advanced Life Support *Circulation*. 2005;112:IV-167–IV-187.

Poisoning, Burns, and Injury Prevention

Nowhere does the old adage "an ounce of prevention is worth a pound of cure" resonate more true than in pediatrics. Together, accidents and injuries are the largest cause of morbidity and mortality in children. When an untoward event occurs, timely evaluation and treatment may limit disability and preserve quality of life.

ACUTE POISONING

Poisoning is one of the more common pediatric medical emergencies, resulting in more than 2 million emergency visits a year. Approximately 85% of childhood poisonings occur in children *younger than 5 years.* These are more likely to involve only one substance and may denote either **accidental** ingestion or (more rarely) abuse by caretakers. Adolescents account for the remaining 15%; such ingestions are usually **intentional**, represent a suicide attempt or gesture, and may involve multiple substances. Intentional ingestions are more likely to require intervention and result in death. Recreational drug use in this older population can result in unintentional but fatal overdoses.

CLINICAL MANIFESTATIONS

History and Physical Examination

The history should include the substance ingested, when, how much, early symptoms, subsequent behavior, and any attempts at treatment. The physical examination begins with the primary survey to evaluate the need for emergency cardiopulmonary support. Other findings on physical examination include temperature and vitals, odors on the breath/ skin/clothing, pupil size and reactivity, and skin color and feel. Table 2-1 lists the characteristic clinical manifestations and treatment of the most common poisonings in children.

DIFFERENTIAL DIAGNOSIS

The possibility of toxicologic ingestion should be considered in any patient presenting with acute-onset illness involving multiple organ systems, including altered mental status, acute behavior changes, respiratory compromise, seizures, arrhythmias, or coma.

DIAGNOSTIC EVALUATION

Screening studies should include a pulse oxygenation check, dextrose stick, electrocardiogram, serum electrolytes and osmolarity, and a venous blood gas to determine pH. Blood and urine toxicology screens are variably helpful; most routine drug screens do not detect iron, clonidine, organophosphates, and digitalis.

TREATMENT

Parents should be instructed to immediately call 911 to be connected with their local poison center. *A policy statement (2003) by the American Academy of Pediatrics recommends that syrup of ipecac no longer be routinely kept in the home or used by parents in acute poisonings.* The administration of ipecac in the home does not appear to improve patient outcome.

Patients who present in unstable condition must be evaluated and treated according to the ABCDEs discussed in Chapter 1. In regard to ingestions, the

TABLE 2-1 Signs, Symptoms, and Treatment of Specific Pediatric Poisonings

Substance[a]	Clinical Manifestations	Suggested Laboratory Studies[b]	Antidote (A)/Treatment (T)
Acetaminophen	Nausea/vomiting, anorexia; may progress over days to jaundice, abdominal pain, liver failure	Serum acetaminophen level 4–24 hr after ingestion,[c] (late) serum hepatic transaminases ($\uparrow$), prothrombin time ($\uparrow$)	A: Oral N-acetyl cysteine (most effective within 8 hr of ingestion) T: Gastric emptying (within 1 hr); activated charcoal (within 4 hr)
Antihistamines (anticholinergic toxicity)	"Mad as a hatter, red as a beet, blind as a bat, hot as a hare, dry as a bone"; drowsiness, delirium, hallucinations, seizure; skin flushing; fused dilated pupils; fever, cardiac dysrhythmias; dry mouth, speech and swallowing difficulties, nausea, vomiting	Drug screen	A: Physostigmine in select cases of severe anticholinergic signs and symptoms T: Gastric emptying (early); activated charcoal; whole bowel irrigation for sustained-release preparations; cardiorespiratory support, seizure control
Aspirin	Hypernea/tachypnea (respiratory alkalosis/metabolic acidosis), fever, nausea, vomiting, dehydration, tinnitus, agitation, seizures	Blood gas ($\uparrow$ pH, $\downarrow$ P_{CO_2}, $\downarrow$ bicarbonate), glucose ($\uparrow$), electrolytes ($\downarrow$ potassium), PT and PTT (prolonged), serum salicylate level	A: None T: Gastric emptying/activated charcoal,[d] fluid and electrolyte management,[e] hemodialysis in severe cases
Ethanol (in cold preparations and mouthwash)	Lethargy, CNS depression, nausea/vomiting, ataxia, respiratory depression, coma, hypotension, hypothermia (in young children)	Serum ethanol level, blood glucose ($\downarrow$), electrolytes ($\downarrow$ potassium), blood pH ($\downarrow$)	A: None T: Supportive care, glucose if needed, correction of electrolytes, parenteral fluids
Hydrocarbons (in fuels, household cleaners, polishes, and other solvents)	Tachypnea, coughing, respiratory distress, cyanosis, fever (aspiration); nausea/vomiting, gastrointestinal discomfort (oral ingestion); mental status changes	Arterial blood gas monitoring, chest radiograph (initial and 4–6 hr after exposure)	A: None T: Prevent aspiration (resulting in chemical pneumonitis); Avoid gastric emptying;[f] supportive respiratory care
Iron	Nausea/vomiting, diarrhea, gastrointestinal blood loss, acute liver failure, seizures, shock, coma	Serum iron level (3–5 hr postingestion), serum pH ($\downarrow$), glucose ($\uparrow$), bilirubin and liver function tests ($\uparrow$), PT (prolonged), WBC ($\uparrow$)	A: Deferoxamine chelation T: Gastric lavage (early); whole bowel irrigation; dialysis (late, severe)
Organophosphates (insecticides)	SLUDGE (salivation, lacrimation, urination, defecation, gastric cramping, emesis); small but reactive pupils; sweating; muscle fasciculations; confusion; coma	Plasma or red blood cell cholinesterase activity ($\downarrow$)	A: Atropine sulfate followed by pralidoxime chloride T: Gastric lavage (early); activated charcoal (if ingested)

(Continued)

TABLE 2-1 Signs, Symptoms, and Treatment of Specific Pediatric Poisonings (*continued*)

Substance[a]	Clinical Manifestations	Suggested Laboratory Studies[b]	Antidote (A)/Treatment (T)
Opiates	Bradycardia, hypotension, decreased respiratory rate, pinpoint pupils, somnolence, coma	Toxicologic screen (urine and serum)	A: Naloxone[g] T: Gastrointestinal decontamination if appropriate; respiratory support
Sympathomimetics (decongestants; also amphetamines, cocaine)	Tachycardia, hypertension, fever, large but reactive pupils, sweating, agitation, delirium/psychosis, seizures	Electrolytes (↓ potassium), blood glucose (↑), ECG	A: None T: Gastric lavage/activated charcoal/cathartics; sedatives for severe agitation; cardiorespiratory support
Theophylline	Tachycardia, hypotension, tachypnea, vomiting, agitation, seizures	Serum theophylline level (q2–4h), blood glucose (↑), potassium (↓), pH (↓), calcium (↑), phosphate (↓), ECG	A: None T: Activated charcoal/whole bowel decontamination; hemodialysis in severe ingestions
Tricyclic antidepressants	Tachycardia, hypertension progressing to hypotension, confusion, drowsiness, dry mucous membranes, dilated but responsive pupils, agitation, seizures, coma, dysrhythmias	ECG (widened QRS complex, ventricular arrhythmias)	A: None[h] T: Gastric lavage/activated charcoal,[i] sodium bicarbonate (blood alkalinization) for conduction abnormalities

[a]Substances in bold type represent the most common pediatric toxicologic emergencies.
[b]All patients with suspected ingestions should receive serum and urine toxicology screens because ingestion of multiple substances is common, especially in intentional poisonings.
[c]An accepted nomogram exists for predicting the severity of the toxicity based on a blood acetaminophen measurement taken at least 4 hr after ingestion.
[d]Aspirin ingestions causes delayed gastric emptying, so gastrointestinal (GI) decontamination plays a significant role.
[e]Alkalinization of serum increases renal excretion of salicylates and prevents salicylate entry into CNS; corrects hypokalemia, which inhibits salicylate excretion.
[f]Some specific exceptions.
[g]Naloxone administration may result in withdrawal symptoms (tachypnea, tachycardia, sweating, agitation, seizures) in chronic users.
[h]Despite the anticholinergic effects of tricyclic antidepressants, physostigmine is *contraindicated* in these ingestions.
[i]Tricyclic antidepressant ingestions cause delayed gastric emptying, so GI decontamination plays a significant role.
PT, prothrombin time; PTT, partial thromboplastin time; CNS, central nervous system; WBC, white blood count; ECG, electrocardiogram.

"D" in the mnemonic may stand for **d**extrose (because several common agents ingested result in hypoglycemia); empirical **d**rug treatment (relating to possible antidotes, cardiac stabilizers, etc.); and appropriate **d**econtamination. Treatment decisions should be based on the estimated maximal potential dose ingested.

Gastric lavage both removes and dilutes stomach contents. It is generally only effective if performed in the first hour or when the compound ingested slows gastric emptying (aspirin, tricyclic antidepressants). Pill fragments recovered may aid in diagnosis. **Activated charcoal** by mouth or nasogastric tube minimizes absorption by binding the substance and hastening its elimination; however, activated charcoal is ineffective in ingestions with alcohol, hydrocarbons, iron, and lithium. **Whole bowel irrigation** is an option for ingestions with iron or following activated charcoal in cases of ingestions with extended-release preparations. Hemodialysis is a late option in some life-threatening circumstances.

PREVENTION

Pediatricians have played a major role in decreasing the number and severity of poisonings, including lobbying for child-resistant medicine bottle and household cleaner caps and incorporating anticipatory guidance into well-child visits. Specific topics include "childproofing" the home, keeping medicines in a lock box, and securing cleaning products from children's reach.

🔑 2-1 KEY POINTS

1. Information gleaned from the vitals, physical examination, and early laboratory data may suggest the substance ingested by conforming to a specific toxidrome.
2. Syrup of ipecac is no longer recommended for parent use in an acute ingestion. Parents should be instructed to call 911 or their local poison center for guidance.

LEAD POISONING

Lead poisoning is one of the most important preventable health problems in primary care pediatrics. The elimination of lead in house paint (in 1977) and gasoline (in 1988) has decreased the average blood level of lead by 75%. The primary source of lead today is lead-containing paint present in buildings constructed before 1950. Children breathe in lead dust, ingest paint chips, and play in lead-contaminated soil. Other sources of exposure include ingredients used in some cultural customs and folk remedies (e.g., kohl, greta, pay-loo-ah) and industrial materials/emissions.

Although there is no direct correlation between blood levels and morbidity, levels of 10 to 19 μg per dL are considered borderline, and the term *lead poisoning* is reserved for levels of **20 μg per dL** or greater. Lead poisoning disproportionately affects lower socioeconomic populations.

CLINICAL MANIFESTATIONS

The great majority of affected children exhibit nonspecific or no symptoms. Early symptoms of lead poisoning include irritability, hyperactivity, apathy, decreased play, anorexia, *intermittent abdominal pain*, *constipation*, and *intermittent vomiting*. Children with chronically elevated lead levels may manifest developmental delay, behavioral problems, attention disorders, and poor school performance. **Acute encephalopathy**, the most serious complication of lead poisoning, is characterized by increased intracranial pressure, vomiting, ataxia, confusion, seizures, and coma.

TREATMENT

The most effective therapy involves **removing the poison** from the child's environment. Leaded paint should be stripped and surfaces cleaned with high-phosphate detergent and a special high-efficiency particle accumulator vacuum. Such an overhaul invariably increases the amount of lead dust in the air, so the inhabitants must be temporarily housed elsewhere. Although the direct benefits in lead poisoning are unproven, many treatment centers recommend optimizing the patient's iron and calcium intake through diet and/or multivitamins. All children with elevated blood lead levels should receive developmental screening.

All elevated screening (capillary) blood tests should be confirmed with a venous sample before treatment is initiated unless the child is acutely symptomatic. **Asymptomatic** children with levels less than 45 μg per dL should be retested at 1- to 3-month intervals. Intervention involves environmental education related to eliminating exposure. **Symptomatic** children should be immediately removed to a lead-free environment and treated with chelation. Children with levels between 45 and 69 μg per dL may be treated with inpatient intravenous **edetate calcium-disodium** (EDTA) or outpatient **oral succimer** (DMSA). Intramuscular **dimercaprol** (BAL) is added to EDTA for the inpatient (required) treatment of children with levels exceeding 70 μg per dL. *Chelation must be administered in a lead-free environment.* A rebound increase in blood lead levels occurs even in the absence of lead exposure because of the release of lead from bone stores.

PREVENTION

Targeted screening is based on risk assessment information gathered during well-child visits. The Centers for Disease Control and Prevention (CDC) recommends lead screening at 12 and 24 months for patients living in areas with many pre-1950 homes and unusually high percentages of elevated blood lead levels. Siblings of affected children should also be screened.

🔑 2-2 KEY POINTS

1. Patients with blood lead levels of 20 µg per dL or greater have lead poisoning.
2. The great majority of children with lead poisoning have nonspecific or no symptoms.
3. Treatment varies based on the patient's blood level and whether the patient is symptomatic.
4. Chelation must only be given when the patient is in a lead-free environment.

TRAFFIC AND MOTOR VEHICLE ACCIDENTS

Motor vehicle injuries remain the leading cause of accidental death in children older than 1 year and adolescents. Most infants and adolescents sustain trauma as vehicle occupants, whereas school-age children tend to be injured as pedestrians or bike riders. Factors associated with an increased risk of automobile injury and death include male gender, age of 13 to 18 years, warm or inclement weather, night or weekend driving, and alcohol intoxication.

The routine use of **seat belts** and **child car seats** is highly effective in reducing the incidence of severe injury and death. All states require car seat restraint of passengers weighing less than 40 pounds. Children 20 pounds or heavier *and* 1 year or older may ride facing forward, whereas lighter/younger infants must face the rear. When a child passenger has reached the height/weight limit for his or her car seat (usually up to 40 pounds), a booster seat should be employed. The child should be restrained in a booster seat until the standard lap belt fits correctly (across the chest and thighs) and the child is tall enough for the legs to bend at the knees with the feet hanging down. This usually does not occur until the child is 8 to 12 years of age or at least 57 inches tall. Older children should remain belted with lap and shoulder straps at all times. Because air bags are designed primarily for adults, children should always ride belted in the back seat. *No evidence indicates that driver education programs are an effective deterrent to accidents involving teenage drivers.*

Head trauma is the accidental injury most associated with death in children. **Bike helmets** decrease the risk of significant closed head trauma caused by traffic accidents involving bicycles. In many jurisdictions, laws mandate their use by children. Children younger than 10 years should be supervised while walking or playing near streets.

DROWNING

Drowning is a frequent cause of morbidity and mortality in the pediatric population. Incidence peaks in the older infant/toddler age group and again in adolescence. Rates are twice as high in blacks and three times higher in boys. **Bathtubs** are the most common site of drowning in the first year of life. Large buckets and residential pools are particularly dangerous for toddlers, whereas natural water sources account for most adolescent injuries.

Reliable predictors of outcome include water temperature, time of submersion, presence of aspiration (and pulmonary damage), and effectiveness of early resuscitation efforts. Submersion for more than 5 minutes in warm water associated with significant aspiration and minimal response to initial cardiopulmonary resuscitation (CPR) virtually always results in major disability or death.

All patients with a history of near drowning should be evaluated with serial chest radiographs and blood gas measurements for 24 hours. Those with hypoxemia and mental status changes require aggressive respiratory and circulatory support.

Toddlers and young children must be supervised at all times while in the bathtub or around pools or other bodies of water. Residential and commercial swimming pools should be fenced in and have locked gates. CPR training is available to parents through the American Heart Association and many area hospitals. Learning to swim is an important preventive measure but does not take the place of close supervision.

FOREIGN BODY ASPIRATION

The natural curiosity of children coupled with the toddler's tendency to put everything in the mouth make **foreign body aspiration** a frequent occurrence in the pediatric population. Most objects and foodstuffs are immediately expelled from the trachea by coughing. Unfortunately, foreign bodies that lodge in the upper or lower respiratory tract are more problematic.

EPIDEMIOLOGY

The highest incidence is noted in children 6 to 30 months of age. Aspiration into the lower airways is much more common than tracheal obstruction. Although the angle of the right main stem bronchus in adults favors right-sided aspiration, no such propensity exists in children given the symmetric bronchial angles in this age group. Inadequate supervision results in increased risk. Many children do not have fully erupted second molars until 30 months of age; inappropriate food choices include nuts, popcorn, hot dogs, hard vegetables, meat with bones, and seeds. **Nuts** account for more than 50% of foreign body aspirations.

DIFFERENTIAL DIAGNOSIS

Patients who do not acutely obstruct their airways may present up to a week after the initial event with no witnessed episode of choking. Wheezing and respiratory distress may be mistaken for asthma; pneumonia is a consideration when breath sounds are decreased. Of note, findings on auscultation in cases of foreign body aspiration are localized to one side of the chest only. Chronic foreign body aspiration should be considered in patients with recurrent focal pneumonias and/or lung abscesses.

CLINICAL MANIFESTATIONS

Following an initial episode of choking and coughing, many children may be asymptomatic for a time. When symptoms occur, presentation varies depending on where the foreign body lodges in the respiratory tree (Table 2-2). If the obstruction is **complete**,

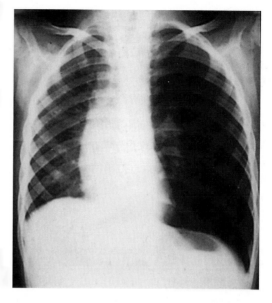

Figure 2-1 • Expiratory film in foreign body aspiration with partial obstruction. The obstructed left lung is hyperinflated; the heart and mediastinum are shifted to the right.

the chest radiograph shows significant one-sided atelectasis and the heart is drawn toward the affected lung throughout the entire respiratory cycle. However, a **partial** obstruction allows air to enter during inspiration, and it becomes trapped (ball-valve obstruction). In these cases, the inspiratory film may appear normal, but the radiograph after expiration shows a hyperinflated obstructed lung with mediastinal shift away from the blockage (Fig. 2-1).

Decubitus films may be helpful in infants and young children. Chest radiographs should include the entire neck area as well.

TREATMENT

In the field, a child who is actively coughing, crying, or speaking should not be directly interfered with. If the airway is compromised, the choking response protocol (abdominal thrusts) is the same for children as for adults, with the exception that the blind oropharyngeal sweep is omitted in children. For infants, back thumps and chest thrusts are alternated, with the infant's body angled slightly head-down.

Foreign bodies must be removed from the airway to alleviate symptoms. **Rigid bronchoscopy** is the treatment of choice. Thereafter, prognosis depends on the degree of lung damage, which is directly related to

TABLE 2-2 Signs and Symptoms of Foreign Body Aspiration	
Location of Obstruction	**Associated Signs and Symptoms**
Trachea	
Total obstruction	Acute asphyxia, severe retractions with poor chest wall movement
Extrathoracic, partial	Inspiratory and expiratory stridor, retractions
Intrathoracic, partial	Expiratory wheeze; frequently inspiratory stridor as well
Main stem bronchus	Cough and expiratory wheeze; may be blood-tinged sputum
Lobar/segmental bronchus	Decreased breath sounds over affected lobe, wheezing, bronchi

time interval to diagnosis. Most patients recover quickly with minimal sequelae.

PREVENTION

Infants are not developmentally prepared to protect their airways from small morsels of food, including hard candy, nuts, and popcorn. Small toys, coins, buttons, and balloons should be kept out of the toddler's reach. Federal legislation requires toys with small parts to be labeled as inappropriate for children younger than 3 years.

🔑 2-3 KEY POINTS

1. Nuts are the most frequently aspirated foreign body in children.
2. After and initial episode of coughing and/or choking, the patient may be asymptomatic for up to several days.
3. Physical examination findings in a patient with foreign body aspiration are localized to one side of the chest.
4. Rigid bronchoscopy is the treatment of choice for pediatric foreign body aspiration.

BURNS

Burns are the third leading cause of injury in children, behind motor vehicle accidents and drowning, and they are the second most frequent cause of accidental death. An estimated 15% to 25% of burns are the result of **abuse**. Fortunately, the great majority of burns are not life-threatening. Patients who survive severe burns are often left with significant scarring and disability.

EPIDEMIOLOGY

The great majority of burns are **scald** injuries, resulting from contact with hot liquids. These may occur in association with spillage of hot food or drinks or be related to bathing injuries. Scald burns that end in straight lines without associated splash marks suggest abuse. **Contact** burns are the next most common and result from direct contact with

a hot surface (iron, stove). Contact burns caused by cigarettes are the most common burn injury in abused children. **Flame** burns are less frequent but result in a high mortality rate because of associated smoke inhalation injury. Typical scenarios for an **electrical** burn involve a young child putting conductive material into a wall socket or an infant sucking on the connected end of an extension cord. **Chemical** burns result from exposure to strong acidic or alkaline material.

RISK FACTORS

Boys and children younger than 4 years, particularly those with disabilities, are at the greatest risk for burn injury.

CLINICAL MANIFESTATIONS

Clinical severity is based on affected body surface area and depth. Partial-thickness burns are divided into first-degree and second-degree burns. **First-degree** burns involve only the epidermis; the skin is red, dry, and tender but does not blister. First-degree burns usually heal within a week with no residual scarring. **Second-degree** burns may be superficial (less than half the depth of the dermis) or deep (involving most of the dermis but leaving appendages such as sweat glands and hair follicles intact). Superficial partial-thickness burns are often caused by scald injuries. They are painful and exhibit blisters and/or weeping but generally resolve in a few weeks with little scarring. Deep second-degree injuries may or may not be painful. They result in significant scarring and may require skin grafting. **Third-degree** burns extend into the subcutaneous tissue and are nontender because of sensory nervous tissue loss. Specific injury sites and patterns are characteristic of abuse (Fig. 2-2).

TREATMENT

Burned areas should be placed immediately in lukewarm water or covered with wet gauze or cloth. Minor burns (superficial burns involving 10% of the total body surface area or less) respond to gentle cleansing, **silver sulfadiazine** (an antimicrobial agent),

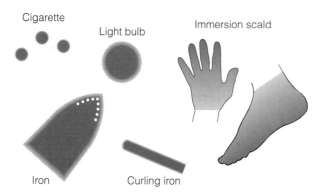

Figure 2-2 • Burn injury patterns consistent with abuse.

and daily dressing changes until re-epithelialization occurs. Burns that are severe, circumferential, extensive (more than 10% to 15% of the body), or that involve the face, hands, perineum, or feet require more specialized care. Treatment includes appropriate management of airway, breathing, and circulation issues; effective electrolyte and fluid therapy to account for increased fluid loss; specialized nutritional support; prevention of infection; pain management; excision and skin grafting; optimization of cosmetic recovery; and early mobility and rehabilitation.

PREVENTION

Installing and maintaining **smoke detectors** and decreasing **water heater thermostat** settings are the two most successful preventive measures for avoiding burn injury. All sleepwear for children should be constructed of flame-retardant material. Smoking cessation decreases the likelihood that matches or lighters will be left where children can experiment with them. Parents should be counseled to practice escape routes and reinforce the "stop, drop, and roll" technique for extinguishing fire.

CHILD ABUSE AND NEGLECT

Injuries intentionally perpetrated by a caretaker that result in morbidity or mortality constitute **physical abuse. Sexual abuse** is defined as the involvement of a child in any activity meant to provide sexual gratification to an adult. Failure to provide a child with

appropriate food, clothing, medical care, schooling, and a safe environment constitutes **neglect**.

EPIDEMIOLOGY

Almost half the children who are brought for medical attention as a result of physical abuse are younger than 1 year; the great majority of them are preschoolers. An estimated 10% of emergency room visits that involve children younger than 5 years are a result of abuse. Parents, the mother's boyfriend, and stepparents are the most frequent perpetrators. Reports of abuse that increase in number and severity of injury over time are highly correlated with increased mortality.

Reports of sexual abuse have skyrocketed over the past few decades. The abuse may occur at any age. Relatives and family acquaintances account for most cases; molestation by strangers is uncommon. In 80% of reports, the victims are girls; most are abused by stepfathers, fathers, or other male family members. Male sexual abuse is probably underrecognized.

Neglect results in more deaths than physical and sexual abuse combined. It is the most common cause of failure to thrive in developed nations.

RISK FACTORS

Abuse and neglect occur at all socioeconomic levels but are more prevalent among the poor. Children with special needs (mental retardation, cerebral palsy, prematurity, chronic illness) are at particular risk. Caretakers who themselves have suffered abuse, who are alcohol or substance abusers, or who are under extreme stress are more likely to abuse or neglect.

DIFFERENTIAL DIAGNOSIS

Most cases of suspected abuse are subsequently substantiated by child protective services. Care should be taken to differentiate bruises from mongolian spots, which commonly occur in the buttocks area. Osteogenesis imperfecta occasionally has been mistaken for abuse. Skin conditions such as bullous impetigo may mimic cigarette burns or other forms of abuse. Children with extensive bruising should undergo coagulation studies to rule out hematologic abnormalities.

CLINICAL MANIFESTATIONS

History

An injury **inconsistent with the stated history** or a **history that changes over time**, coupled with **delay in obtaining appropriate medical care**, strongly suggests abuse. Age-inappropriate sexual behavior and knowledge are consistent with sexual abuse. Victims of physical or sexual abuse may act out by abusing others, attempting suicide, running away, or engaging in high-risk behaviors. Abuse places children at an increased risk for poor school performance, low self-esteem, and depression.

Physical Examination

Growth parameters are often stunted in abused children. As with burns, the location and pattern of injury may strongly suggest abuse (Fig. 2-3). Bruises, burns, or lacerations in different stages of healing occur in chronic or repeated abuse. Bruises associated with normal play are generally limited to the shins and elbows. Bruises on the chest, head, neck, or abdomen and bruises on a nonambulatory child are extremely suspicious. Vigorous shaking may lead to **shaken baby syndrome (SBS)**, which results from acceleration/deceleration forces to the head. Virtually pathognomic injuries include intracranial (subdural) hemorrhage, diffuse axonal injury, and widespread retinal hemorrhages, which may result in permanent vision loss. SBS has the highest mortality rate of any reported form of child abuse. Falls from beds, changing tables, cribs, counters, or toilet seats do not cause the injuries seen in SBS.

DIAGNOSTIC EVALUATION

A skeletal survey and bone scan reveal areas of past injury that may not be evident on physical examination. Fractures that are highly specific for abuse include bilateral fractures, bucket-handle fractures, metaphyseal chip fractures, and fractures of the (especially posterior) ribs, scapula, sternum, or spinous processes. (Note: Spiral fractures were once thought to be singularly indicative of abuse; it is now recognized that nonabusive twisting forces may also cause spiral fractures.) Fractures that occur before ambulation are usually inflicted. CT scans reveal **intracranial injuries,** *which in infants are highly suggestive of abuse;* 95% of intracranial injuries and 66%

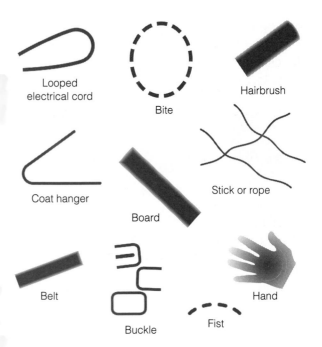

Figure 2-3 • Body marks consistent with abuse.

of all head injuries in infants are caused by abuse. When sexual abuse is suspected, rectal, oral, vaginal, and urethral specimens should be examined for *Neisseria gonorrhoeae*, *Chlamydia trachomatis*, and other sexually transmitted diseases. Other studies include blood tests for syphilis and human immunodeficiency virus (HIV).

TREATMENT/PREVENTION

Health care workers are **required by law** to report any suspicion of child abuse or neglect to state protection agencies. Victims should be immediately removed from their homes and placed in protective custody at a hospital or a state facility. Many family intervention programs that focus on social support, nursing staff visits, and parenting skills are being evaluated across the United States in an attempt to provide children with safer home environments. Pediatricians can aid in preventing child abuse by providing parents with realistic expectations for their child's behavior at each well-child visit. It is also important to recognize when the family and/or caregiver experiences acute crisis or social isolation; referral for supportive services may make a significant difference in the home environment of the child.

🔑 2-4 KEY POINTS

1. Child neglect is the most common cause of failure to thrive in developed countries.
2. An injury inconsistent with the history, a history that changes over time, and a delay in seeking appropriate medical care all strongly suggest abuse.
3. Shaken baby syndrome (SBS) includes intracranial bleeding, diffuse axonal injury, and retinal hemorrhages.
4. Intracranial injuries in the absence of substantiated major trauma are virtually pathognomonic of abuse in infants.
5. Health care workers are required by law to report any suspicion of child abuse or neglect to state protection agencies.

SUDDEN INFANT DEATH SYNDROME

By definition, **sudden infant death syndrome (SIDS)** consists of the unexpected death of an infant younger than 1 year for which the etiology remains unclear despite a thorough history and postmortem evaluation. The cause of SIDS remains unknown but is thought to be related to delayed maturation of brainstem respiratory or cardiovascular control and arousal mechanisms.

RISK FACTORS

Although multiple factors have been associated with an increased risk for SIDS, none has proven prognostic value (Table 2-3). More cases are reported during the winter months.

DIFFERENTIAL DIAGNOSIS

Cases that initially appear to be SIDS may in fact result from infection, congenital heart disease, metabolic disorders, seizures, accidental trauma, or abuse.

Apparent life-threatening events (ALTEs) are characterized by choking, gagging, or apnea in combination with changes in color (cyanosis) and muscle tone. They understandably are extremely frightening to the caregiver. Table 2-4 lists the differential diagnoses.

TABLE 2-3 Sudden Infant Death Syndrome (SIDS): Risk Factors

Prone Sleeping Position[a]
Child/Birth Factors
Male gender
Low birth weight/intrauterine growth restriction[a]
Prematurity[a]
Multiple gestation
African American or Native American
Maternal Factors
Maternal smoking during pregnancy[a]
Young maternal age
Lower socioeconomic status
Higher parity
Single parenthood
Fewer years of maternal education
Environmental Factors
Soft bedding
Potentially obstructive materials in the bed

[a]Factors with highest risk.

PREVENTION

Since the "Back to Sleep" campaign was initiated by the National Institutes of Health, the incidence of SIDS has decreased by 43%. Infants should be placed

TABLE 2-4 Differential Diagnosis of Apparent Life-Threatening Events (ALTEs)

Infection
Respiratory syncytial virus
Pertussis
Aspiration
Gastroesophageal reflux
Cardiac dysrhythmias
Metabolic disease
Neurologic abnormalities/seizures
Abuse

on their backs while sleeping. Contrary to popular belief, 24-hour home apnea monitoring does not decrease the likelihood of SIDS. Their use should be reserved for infants with documented episodes of apnea, bradycardia, or desaturation.

🔑 2-5 KEY POINTS

1. Babies should be put to bed on their backs.
2. Home apnea monitors do not decrease the likelihood of sudden infant death syndrome (SIDS).

Additional Suggested Reading

American Academy of Pediatrics Committee on Drugs. Treatment guidelines for lead exposure in children. *Pediatrics.* 1995;96:155.

Dubowitz H, Giardino A, Gustavson E. Child neglect: guidance for pediatricians. *Pediatr Rev.* 2000; 21:111–116.

Farrell PA, Weiner GM, Lemons JA. SIDS, ALTE, apnea, and the use of home monitors. *Pediatr Rev.* 2002;23:3–9.

Feingold M, Anderson RL. Lessons and tactics to lead the charge against lead poisoning. *Contemp Pediatr.* 2004;21:49–68.

Klein GL, Herndon DN. Burns. *Pediatr Rev.* 2004;25:411–417.

Markowitz M. Lead poisoning. *Pediatr Rev.* 2000;21:327–335.

McGuigan ME. Poisoning potpourri. *Pediatr Rev.* 2001;22:295–302.

Rovin JD, Rodgers BM. Pediatric foreign body aspiration. *Pediatr Rev.* 2000;21:86–89.

Sirotnak AP, Grigsby T, Krugman RD. Physical abuse of children. *Pediatr Rev.* 2004;25:264–277.

Cardiology

The field of pediatric cardiology has experienced a remarkable evolution over the past half century because of advances in diagnostic techniques, interventional cardiac catheterization and cardiac surgical procedures, pediatric anesthesia, neonatal medicine, and intensive care. **Functional heart murmurs** are very common in childhood and do not signify disease. The incidence of structural heart disease is approximately 8 in 1,000 live births. Critical **congenital heart disease (CHD)**, requiring surgery or an interventional cardiac catheterization procedure in the neonatal period, occurs in approximately 1 in 400 live births. Children may acquire **structural heart disease** later in life, or they may suffer from **functional heart disease** (i.e., myocarditis or cardiomyopathy) or **arrhythmias**.

HEART MURMURS

Heart murmurs are very common in children; they are heard on routine physical exams in approximately a third of patients. **Functional (*"innocent"*) heart murmurs** are the result of normal physiologic flow turbulence. Each of these murmurs has specific characteristics that usually allow it to be confidently diagnosed by physical examination alone (Table 3-1). It is equally important to recognize the signs and symptoms of potentially pathologic murmurs to facilitate rapid diagnosis and intervention, if necessary (Table 3-2).

CLINICAL MANIFESTATIONS

History

Infants with heart disease may have a history of difficulty feeding, with tachypnea, irritability, diaphoresis, cyanosis, and/or failure to thrive. Significant symptoms in older patients include shortness of breath,

dyspnea on exertion, exercise intolerance, palpitations, paroxysmal nocturnal dyspnea, orthopnea, and syncope. Chest pain is a frequent complaint in older children and adolescents; however, it is rarely cardiac in origin. Children who have syndromes often associated with heart disease (e.g., Turner, Down, William, Noonan, DiGeorge/Velocardiofacial) are at a higher risk for a pathologic murmur. The family history should include questions regarding syncope, sudden death, heart attacks, or stroke before 50 years of age, connective tissue disorders (Marfan's syndrome), hyperlipidemia, hypercholesterolemia, arrhythmia, valvular disease, cardiomyopathy, and CHD.

Physical Examination

The physical examination includes a comparison of the child's weight and height to normal values for age and sex and to previous measurements on a growth curve. Careful attention should be paid to vital signs, including heart rate, respiratory rate, and blood pressure. The examiner should assess for cyanosis and digital clubbing (indicating a right-to-left shunt), as well as signs of congestive heart failure (extremity edema and hepatomegaly). Pulses should be palpated in both upper and lower extremities and compared. The examiner should inspect and palpate the chest for placement of the apical impulse and any heaves or thrills. Auscultation allows detection and characterization of heart sounds (normal and extra) and murmurs. Murmurs may be systolic, diastolic, or continuous and should be graded according to their intensity.

DIAGNOSTIC EVALUATION

Pulse oximetry assesses for decreased oxygen saturation in the blood. The chest radiograph evaluates heart size

■ TABLE 3-1 Functional Heart Murmurs

Murmur	Typical Age at Presentation	Characteristics	Source
Vibratory (Still murmur)	2–8 yr	Grade II–III midsystolic musical or vibratory murmur heard best near the left lower sternal border and apex	Vibrations in ventricular or mitral structures caused by flow in the left ventricle
Venous hum	3–7 yr	Continuous, soft humming murmur heard at the neck or right upper chest that disappears in the supine position	Turbulent flow in the jugular venous/superior vena cava systems
Pulmonary flow murmur	6 yr–adolescence	Systolic ejection murmur best heard at the left upper sternal border	Turbulence of flow where the main pulmonary artery connects to the right ventricle (across the pulmonary valve)
Carotid bruit	3–8 yr	Systolic ejection murmur heard best at the neck	Turbulence of flow where the brachiocephalic vessels attach to the aorta
Peripheral pulmonary stenosis (PPS)	Neonate (birth–2 mo)	Medium-pitched systolic ejection murmur best heard at the left upper sternal border, radiating through to the back	Turbulence of flow where the main pulmonary artery branches into left and right arteries

■ TABLE 3-2 Concerning Signs on Cardiac Examination

Heaves, thrills, or other abnormal or increased precordial activity

Brachiofemoral delay and/or decreased femoral pulses

Abnormal first or second heart sound (abnormal splitting)

Extra heart sounds

   Gallop rhythms (S_3, S_4, or summation gallop)

   Ejection click

   Opening snap

   Pericardial rub

Murmurs

   Very loud, harsh, or blowing

   Does not change in intensity relative to patient positioning

and pulmonary vascularity. All patients with suspected pathologic murmurs should receive an electrocardiogram (ECG) and echocardiogram (ECHO).

TREATMENT

The treatment of heart disease may be medical, surgical, interventional in the cardiac catheterization laboratory, or a combination of these, depending on the specific abnormality.

EVALUATION OF THE CYANOTIC NEONATE

Cyanosis is a physical sign characterized by a bluish tinge of the mucous membranes, skin, and nail beds. Cyanosis results from hypoxemia (decreased arterial oxygen saturation). Cyanosis does not become clinically evident until the absolute concentration of deoxygenated hemoglobin is at least 3.0 g per dL. Factors that influence the degree of cyanosis include the total hemoglobin concentration (related to the hematocrit) *and* factors that affect the O_2 dissociation curve (pH, P_{CO_2}, temperature, and ratio of adult to fetal hemoglobin). Cyanosis will be evident sooner (and more pronounced) under the following conditions: (a) high hemoglobin concentration (polycythemic patient), (b) decreased pH (acidosis), (c) increased P_{CO_2} (decreased respiratory rate), (d) increased temperature, and (e) increased ratio of adult to fetal hemoglobin.) Cyanosis should not be confused with **acrocyanosis** (blueness of the *distal* extremities *only*). Acrocyanosis is caused by peripheral vasoconstriction and is a normal finding during the first 24 to 48 hours of life.

DIFFERENTIAL DIAGNOSIS

Cyanosis in the newborn may be cardiac, pulmonary, neurologic, or hematologic in origin (Table 3-3). Cyanosis is one of the most common presentations of CHD. Pulmonary's disorders may lead to cyanosis as a result of primary lung disease, airway obstruction, or extrinsic compression of the lung. Neurologic causes of cyanosis include central nervous system dysfunction and respiratory neuromuscular dysfunction.

CLINICAL MANIFESTATIONS

History and Physical Examination

A complete birth history that includes maternal history; prenatal, perinatal, and postnatal complications; history of labor and delivery; and neonatal course should be obtained. Exactly when the child developed cyanosis is critical because certain congenital heart defects present at birth, whereas others may take as long as 1 month to become evident.

The initial physical examination should focus on the vital signs and the cardiac and respiratory examinations, assessing for evidence of right, left, or biventricular congestive heart failure and respiratory distress. Blue or dusky mucous membranes are consistent with cyanosis. Rales, stridor, grunting, flaring, retractions, and evidence of consolidation or effusion should be evaluated on pulmonary examination. On cardiovascular examination, the precordial impulse is palpated, and the clinician should evaluate for systolic or diastolic murmurs, the intensity of S_1, S_2 splitting abnormalities, and the presence of an S_3 or S_4 gallop, ejection click, opening snap, or rub. Examination of the extremities should focus on the

■ **TABLE 3-3** Differential Diagnosis of Cyanosis in the Neonate

Cardiac

Ductal-independent mixing lesions

    Truncus arteriosus

    Total anomalous pulmonary venous return without obstruction

    D-transportation of the great arteries[a]

Lesions with ductal-dependent PBF

    Tetralogy of Fallot with pulmonary atresia[b]

    Ebstein anomaly[b]

    Critical pulmonic stenosis

    Tricuspid valve atresia[b] with normally related great arteries[b]

    Pulmonic valve atresia with intact ventricular septum

    Heterotaxy[b]

Lesions with ductal-dependent SBF

    Hypoplastic left heart syndrome

    Interrupted aortic arch

    Critical coarctation of the aorta

    Critical aortic stenosis

    Tricuspid valve atresia with transportation of the great arteries[b]

Pulmonary

    Primary lung disease

    Respiratory distress syndrome

    Meconium aspiration

    Pneumonia

    Persistent pulmonary hypertension of the newborn

Airway obstruction

    Choanal atresia

    Vocal cord paralysis

    Laryngotracheomalacia

Extrinsic compression of the lungs

    Pneumothorax

    Chylothorax

    Hemothorax

Neurologic

    CNS dysfunction

    Drug-induced depression of respiratory drive

(Continued)

■ TABLE 3-3 Differential Diagnosis of Cyanosis in the Neonate *(continued)*

Postasphyxial cerebral dysfunction

Central apnea

Respiratory neuromuscular dysfunction

　Spinal muscular atrophy

　Infant botulism

　Neonatal myasthenia gravis

Hematologic

　Methemoglobinemia

　Polycythemia

ᵃA patent ductus arteriosus may improve mixing, especially with an intact ventricular septum.
ᵇMost forms.
PBF, pulmonary blood flow; SBF, systemic blood flow.

strength and symmetry of the pulses in the upper and lower extremities, evidence of edema, and cyanosis of the nail beds. Hepatosplenomegaly may be consistent with right ventricular or biventricular heart failure.

DIAGNOSTIC EVALUATION

The goal of the initial evaluation of the cyanotic neonate is to determine whether the cyanosis is cardiac or noncardiac in origin. Preductal and postductal oxygen saturation and four extremity blood pressures should be documented. An ECG, chest radiograph, and hyperoxia test should be performed.

Preductal (right upper extremity) **and postductal** (lower extremity) **oxygen saturation measurements** allow evaluation for *differential* cyanosis and *reverse differential* cyanosis. When preductal saturation is higher than postductal measurement (differential cyanosis), possible diagnoses include persistent pulmonary hypertension of the newborn (PPHN; see Chapter 13) and lesions with left ventricular outflow tract obstruction such as interrupted aortic arch, critical coarctation of the aorta, and critical aortic stenosis. Deoxygenated blood from the pulmonary circulation enters the descending aorta through a patent ductus arteriosus (PDA), decreasing the postductal oxygen saturation. When preductal saturation is lower than the postductal saturation (reverse differential cyanosis), possible diagnoses include transposition of the great arteries with PPHN or left ventricular outflow obstruction (i.e., critical coarctation of the aorta, interrupted aortic

arch, critical aortic stenosis). Oxygenated blood from the pulmonary circulation enters the descending aorta through a PDA, increasing the postductal oxygen saturation.

Four extremity blood pressure measurements, which show a systolic blood pressure in the upper extremities greater than 10 mm Hg higher than that in the lower extremities, is consistent with arch hypoplasia, coarctation of the aorta, or other lesions with ductal-dependent systemic blood flow with a restrictive ductus arteriosus. The **chest radiograph** is obtained to determine the size of the heart and whether the pulmonary vascularity is increased or decreased. The **ECG** evaluates the heart rate, rhythm, axis, intervals, forces (atrial dilatation, ventricular hypertrophy), and repolarization (abnormal Q-wave pattern, ST/T waves, and corrected QT interval).

A **hyperoxia test** should be carried out in all neonates with a resting pulse oximetry reading less than 95%, visible cyanosis, or circulatory collapse. The hyperoxia test consists of obtaining a baseline right radial (preductal) arterial blood gas measurement with the child breathing room air ($F_{IO_2} = 0.21$), and then repeating the measurement with the child inspiring 100% oxygen ($F_{IO_2} = 1.00$). PaO_2 should be measured directly via arterial puncture, although properly acquired transcutaneous oxygen monitor (TCOM) values are also acceptable. **Pulse oximetry measurements are not appropriate for interpretation of the hyperoxia test.** A PaO_2 greater than 250 mm Hg on 100% oxygen essentially rules out cardiac disease. These patients are more likely to have a pulmonary cause for their cyanosis. A PaO_2 between 50 mm Hg and 150 mm Hg on 100% oxygen suggests a cardiac lesion characterized by complete mixing *without* restricted pulmonary blood flow (Table 3-4). A PaO_2 less than 50 mm Hg on 100% oxygen indicates a cardiac lesion with parallel circulation *or* a mixing lesion *with* restricted pulmonary blood flow.

The combined results of the tests just described will point the clinician in the right direction as to the source of the cyanosis, and may also suggest a likely diagnosis. If a cardiac cause is deemed likely, an echocardiogram **(ECHO)** and cardiology consultation should be obtained.

TREATMENT

Cyanotic infants require immediate assessment of the ABCs (Chapter 1) and stabilization. **Prostaglandin E1**

■ **TABLE 3-4** Cyanotic Congenital Heart Diseases (grouped by hyperoxia test results)

Pao$_2$ between 50 and 150 mmHg on 100% oxygen (suggesting a cardiac lesion with complete mixing *without* restricted pulmonary blood flow):

Truncus arteriosus

Total anomalous pulmonary venous connection without obstruction

Hypoplastic left heart syndrome (HLHS) and HLHS variants

Pao$_2$ less than 50 mm Hg on 100% oxygen (suggesting a cardiac lesion with parallel circulation or a mixing lesion *with* restricted pulmonary blood flow):

D-transposition of the great arteries with or without ventricular septal defect

Ebstein anomaly

Tricuspid atresia with normally related great arteries and critical pulmonary valve stenosis or atresia

Tetralogy of Fallot with critical pulmonary valve stenosis or atresia

Pulmonary atresia with intact ventricular septum

Critical pulmonary valve stenosis

🔧 3-1 KEY POINTS

1. The absolute concentration of deoxygenated hemoglobin determines the presence of cyanosis.
2. Cyanosis in the newborn may be cardiac, pulmonary, neurologic, or hematologic in origin.
3. Following stabilization of a cyanotic infant, the goal of the preliminary workup (chest radiograph, electrocardiogram, and hyperoxia test) is to determine whether the lesion is cardiac or noncardiac in origin.
4. Comparison of preductal to postductal measurements of oxygen saturation allows the clinician to evaluate for differential cyanosis.
5. The results of the hyperoxia test may indicate whether the cyanosis is cardiac in origin.
6. Pulse oximetry measurements are not acceptable for interpretation of the hyperoxia test.
7. Prostaglandin E1 (PGE1) therapy should be started in all unstable infants with suspected congenital heart disease (CHD).

CYANOTIC CONGENITAL HEART DISEASE: DUCTAL-INDEPENDENT MIXING LESIONS

TRUNCUS ARTERIOSUS

Truncus arteriosus (Fig. 3-1) is a rare form of cyanotic CHD that consists of a single arterial vessel arising from the base of the heart, which gives way to the coronary, systemic, and pulmonary arteries. A ventricular septal defect (VSD) is almost always present. There is complete mixing of systemic and pulmonary venous blood in the truncal vessel. This lesion, along with other conotruncal anomalies (tetralogy of Fallot, interrupted aortic arch, VSD, isolated arch anomalies, and vascular rings), is associated with 22q11 microdeletion (i.e., **DiGeorge's syndrome and velocardiofacial syndrome**).

Clinical Manifestations

A nonspecific murmur and minimal cyanosis may be present at birth. Congestive heart failure develops in a matter of weeks as the pulmonary vascular resistance falls and pulmonary blood flow increases at the expense of systemic blood flow. On examination,

(PGE1) administration, via continuous intravenous infusion, should be started in any unstable infant with a strong suspicion of CHD. In newborns with mixing lesions or defects that have ductal-dependent pulmonary or systemic blood flow, PGE1 acts to maintain patency of the ductus arteriosus until definitive surgical treatment can be accomplished. Rarely, the patient with CHD may become progressively more unstable after the institution of PGE1 therapy, indicating a defect that has obstructed blood flow out of the pulmonary veins or left atrium. These lesions include hypoplastic left heart syndrome with restrictive or intact foramen ovale; other variants of mitral atresia with restrictive foramen ovale; transposition of the great arteries with an intact ventricular septum and restrictive foramen ovale; and total anomalous pulmonary venous return with obstruction.

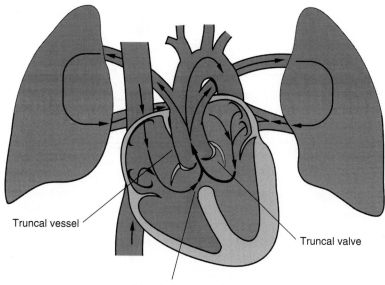

Figure 3-1 • Truncus arteriosus. Typical anatomic findings include **(A)** a single truncal vessel arising from the heart giving off the coronary arteries (not shown), pulmonary arteries, and aortic vessels; **(B)** abnormal truncal valve (quadricuspid) with stenosis and/or regurgitation, which is common; **(C)** left aortic arch shown (right aortic arch occurs in 30% of cases); **(D)** large conoventricular ventricular septal defect; **(E)** complete mixing (of the systemic and pulmonary venous return), which occurs at the great vessel level. From LifeART image copyright © 2006 Lippincott Williams & Wilkins. All rights reserved.

a systolic ejection murmur is heard at the left sternal border, there is a single second heart sound (S_2), pulse pressure is widened, and bounding arterial pulses are palpated. A chest radiograph reveals marked cardiomegaly, increased pulmonary vascularity, and occasionally a right aortic arch. Seventy percent of children with truncus arteriosus have biventricular hypertrophy on ECG. Hypocalcemia and absence of the thymic shadow (on chest radiograph) will occur if the truncus is associated with DiGeorge's syndrome.

Treatment

At most centers, surgical repair is performed in the neonatal period. This involves closing the VSD, separation of the pulmonary arteries from the truncal vessel, and placing a conduit between the right ventricle and the pulmonary arteries.

D-TRANSPOSITION OF GREAT ARTERIES

D-transposition of great arteries (D-TGA) (Fig. 3-2) accounts for 5% of congenital heart defects and is the most common form of cyanotic CHD presenting in the neonatal period. There is a 3:1 male predominance. In this defect, the aorta arises anteriorly from the morphologic right ventricle, and the pulmonary artery arises posteriorly from the left ventricle. The pulmonary and systemic circuits thus are in parallel rather than in series; the systemic circuit (deoxygenated blood) is recirculated through the body, whereas the pulmonary circuit (oxygenated blood) recirculates through the lungs. The three basic variants are D-TGA with intact ventricular septum (60%), D-TGA with VSD (20%), and D-TGA with VSD and pulmonic stenosis (20%).

A lesion that allows mixing of the systemic and pulmonary circulations is necessary for survival. Mixing in newborns occurs at a patent foramen ovale (PFO) and the ductus arteriosis, or through other addition defects (atrial septal defects [ASDs] or VSDs). Balanced bidirectional shunting must be present or one of the parallel circuits would become depleted of blood.

Clinical Manifestations

Severe cyanosis is present from birth; the degree varies according to how much mixing is taking place. The infant

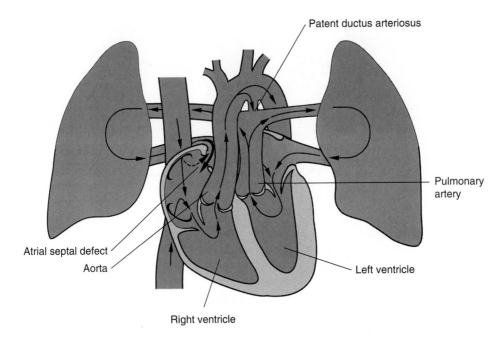

Figure 3-2 • Transposition of the great arteries with an intact ventricular septum, a large patent ductus arteriosus (on PGE1), and atrial septal defect (status post balloon atrial septostomy). Note the following: **(A)** The aorta arises from the morphologic right ventricle and the pulmonary artery from the morphologic left ventricle; **(B)** "mixing" between the parallel circulations (see text) at the atrial (after balloon atrial septostomy) and ductal levels; **(C)** shunting from the left atrium to the right atrium via the atrial septal defect with equalization of atrial pressures; **(D)** shunting from the aorta to the pulmonary artery via the ductus arteriosus.
From LifeART image copyright © 2006 Lippincott Williams & Wilkins. All rights reserved.

may also be tachypneic. On cardiac examination, a loud, single S_2 is appreciated. A systolic murmur indicates the presence of a VSD and/or pulmonic stenosis. The chest radiograph usually reveals cardiomegaly and increased pulmonary vascular markings. (Note: If pulmonary stenosis is present and severe, vascular markings may be decreased.) An "egg-shaped silhouette" is characteristic and results from the anterior aorta being superimposed on the posterior pulmonary artery, thereby narrowing the mediastinum. The ECG generally reveals right axis deviation and right ventricular hypertrophy because the right ventricle is the systemic ventricle.

Treatment

Immediate PGE1 administration is necessary to keep the ductus arteriosus open and increase aorta (deoxygenated) to pulmonary artery (oxygenated) shunting. A balloon atrial septostomy (Rashkind procedure) may be performed in the cardiac catheterization laboratory to increase atrial level mixing. The arterial switch procedure, which restores the left ventricle as the systemic ventricle, is generally performed during the first week of life.

TOTAL ANOMALOUS PULMONARY VENOUS CONNECTION

Total anomalous pulmonary venous connection (TAPVC) (Fig. 3-3) is a rare lesion (1% to 2% of CHDs) in which the pulmonary veins are not connected to the left atrium and drain anomalously directly into the right atrium either directly or indirectly through other systemic pathways.

There are four variants:

- **Supracardiac** (50% of cases): Blood drains via a vertical vein into the innominate vein or into the superior vena cava.
- **Cardiac** (20% of cases): Blood drains into the coronary sinus or directly into the right atrium.
- **Infradiaphragmatic** (20% of cases): Blood drains via a vertical vein into the portal or hepatic veins.
- **Mixed** (10% of cases): Blood returns to the heart via a combination of the routes just described.

TAPVC can occur *with or without obstruction*. Pulmonary venous flow is obstructed when the anomalous vein enters a vessel at an acute angle or courses between or through other mediastinal structures. The

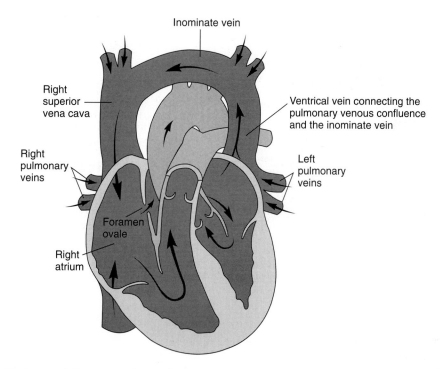

Figure 3-3 • Supradiaphragmatic total anomalous pulmonary venous connection. Note the following: **(A)** Pulmonary venous confluence does not connect with the left atrium but ascends to connect via a vertical vein with the innominate vein. This connection is frequently obstructed between the left pulmonary artery and left main stem bronchus; **(B)** all systemic blood flow must be derived via a right-to-left shunt at the PFO.
From Pillitteri A. *Maternal and Child Nursing.* 4th ed. Philadelphia: Lippincott Williams & Wilkins, 2003.

presence or absence of obstruction determines whether there is pulmonary venous hypertension and severe cyanosis (obstruction) or increased pulmonary blood flow and mild cyanosis (no obstruction). Because there is no pulmonary venous return to the left side of the heart, shunting of blood from right to left, through an ASD or PFO, is necessary for blood flow to the systemic vascular bed.

Clinical Manifestations

The infant without obstruction may present with mild cyanosis at birth and progressive congestive heart failure. There is an active precordium with a right ventricular heave, a wide and fixed split S_2 with a loud pulmonary component, and a systolic ejection murmur at the left upper sternal border. On chest radiograph, cardiomegaly (particularly right sided) is noted with increased pulmonary vascularity. On ECG, right-axis deviation and right ventricular hypertrophy are seen.

Infants with pulmonary venous obstruction display marked cyanosis and respiratory distress. A loud, single (or narrowly split) S_2 is heard on cardiac examination, and other signs of congestive heart failure may be present. The chest radiograph generally shows normal heart size with markedly increased pulmonary vascular markings and diffuse pulmonary edema. Right ventricular hypertrophy is seen on ECG.

Treatment

Corrective surgery is performed emergently in the newborn period if pulmonary venous obstruction is present. If the anomalous pulmonary veins are unobstructed (typically cardiac subtype), repair is accomplished electively prior to the child exhibiting symptoms of congestive heart failure during infancy. *PGE1 is generally not given* because a PDA will add more blood volume to an already flooded pulmonary circuit.

CYANOTIC CONGENITAL HEART DISEASE: LESIONS WITH DUCTAL-DEPENDENT PULMONARY BLOOD FLOW

TRICUSPID ATRESIA

Tricuspid atresia with normally related great arteries (NRGA) (Fig. 3-4) is a rare defect (1% of CHD) that consists of complete absence of right atrioventricular connection, which leads to severe hypoplasia or absence of the right ventricle (i.e., hypoplastic right heart syndrome). Ninety percent of cases of tricuspid atresia have an associated VSD. The systemic venous return is shunted from the right atrium to the left atrium through the PFO or an ASD, and the left atrium and left ventricle handle both systemic and pulmonary venous return. Oxygenated and deoxygenated blood is mixed in the left atrium. The VSD allows blood to pass from the left ventricle to the right ventricular outflow chamber and pulmonary arteries. The vast majority of patients with tricuspid atresia with NRGA also have pulmonary stenosis. Cyanosis is severe in the neonatal period and proportionally related to the amount of pulmonary blood flow.

In 30% of cases, tricuspid atresia is also present, which results in blood passing from the left ventricle through the VSD to the right ventricular outflow and the ascending aorta. Tricuspid atresia with TGA is often associated with coarctation of the aorta and/or aortic arch hypoplasia. Unlike tricuspid atresia with NRGA, tricuspid atresia with TGA is a cyanotic lesion with ductal-dependent systemic blood flow.

Clinical Manifestations

Neonates with tricuspid atresia and NRGA with pulmonary stenosis present with progressive cyanosis, poor feeding, and tachypnea during the first 2 weeks of life. If pulmonary atresia is present, severe cyanosis is noted when the ductus arteriosus becomes restrictive or closes. On cardiac examination, abnormalities include the holosystolic murmur of a ventricular septal defect at the left lower sternal border and (possibly) the continuous murmur of a PDA. On ECG, there is superior axis deviation and left ventricular hypertrophy. Findings on chest radiograph include normal heart size and decreased pulmonary vascular markings.

Neonates with tricuspid atresia and TGA also present with cyanosis, poor feeding, and tachypnea. If severe arch hypoplasia or coarctation of the aorta is

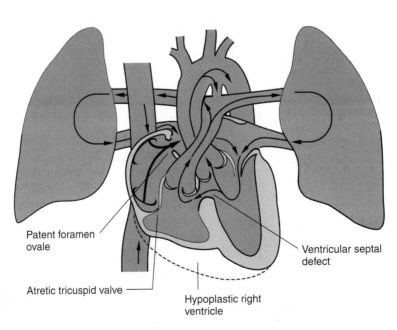

Patent foramen ovale

Ventricular septal defect

Atretic tricuspid valve

Hypoplastic right ventricle

Figure 3-4 • Tricuspid atresia with normally related great arteries and a small patent ductus arteriosus. Typical anatomic findings include **(A)** atresia of the tricuspid valve; **(B)** hypoplasia of the right ventricle; **(C)** restriction to pulmonary blood flow at two levels: a small ventricular septal defect and a stenotic pulmonary valve. Note: All systemic venous return must pass through the PFO to reach the left atrium and left ventricle.

present, the patient may present with shock after closure of the ductus arteriosus. Clinical severity depends on the degree of arch obstruction. The chest radiograph may reveal cardiomegaly and increased pulmonary vascular markings as the pulmonary vascular resistance falls and the child's pulmonary blood flow increases, resulting in congestive heart failure.

Treatment

A child with tricuspid atresia with NRGA should have PGE1 started to maintain ductal patency and pulmonary blood flow, and a balloon atrial septostomy or surgical atrial septectomy should be performed if the atrial connection is not adequate. Surgical management for tricuspid atresia may involve placing a modified Blalock-Taussig shunt to maintain pulmonary blood flow. The modified Blalock-Taussig shunt is a Gore-Tex tube placed between the subclavian artery and the pulmonary artery. Sometimes a generous VSD is present with minimal pulmonary valve stenosis and no surgery is required during the neonatal period. Ultimately, a cavopulmonary anastomosis (hemi-Fontan or bidirectional Glenn) is performed to provide stable pulmonary blood flow. In most centers, a modified Fontan procedure is performed to redirect the inferior vena cava and hepatic vein flow into the pulmonary circulation.

A child with tricuspid atresia with TGA should have PGE1 started to maintain ductal patency and systemic blood flow, and a balloon atrial septostomy or surgical atrial septectomy should be performed if the atrial connection is not adequate. Surgical management for tricuspid atresia with TGA depends on the degree of arch obstruction and pulmonary stenosis. Patients with hemodynamically significant arch obstruction require Damus-Kaye-Stansel or Stage 1 reconstruction with Blalock-Taussig shunt or Right ventricle to pulmonary artery shunt with or without atrial septectomy. If there is no arch obstruction and no pulmonary artery stenosis, a pulmonary artery band may be necessary. If there is no arch obstruction with severe pulmonary stenosis or atresia, a modified Blalock-Taussig shunt to maintain adequate pulmonary blood flow is necessary. Some children have no arch obstruction and have just enough pulmonary stenosis and do not require any neonatal intervention. Staged palliation progresses as noted earlier for patients with tricuspid atresia with NRGA.

TETRALOGY OF FALLOT

Tetralogy of Fallot (TOF) (Fig. 3-5) is the most common CHD (7%) presenting in childhood. Fifteen percent of

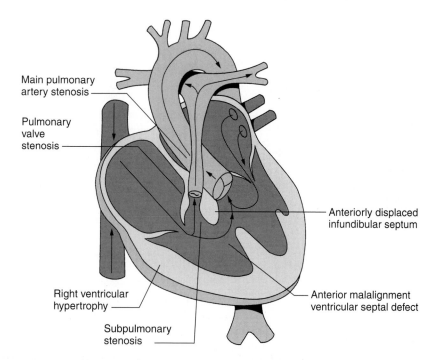

Figure 3-5 • Tetralogy of Fallot. Typical anatomic findings include (**A**) an anteriorly displaced infundibular septum, resulting in subpulmonary stenosis, a large anterior malalignment VSD and overriding of the aorta over the muscular septum; (**B**) hypoplasia of the pulmonary valve, main, and branch pulmonary arteries, resulting in right ventricular hypertrophy; (**C**) a right-to-left shunt at the ventricular level.

all patients with TOF have 22q11 microdeletion; 50% of patients with 22q11 microdeletion have TOF. The four defects include an anterior malalignment VSD, which results in valvar and subvalvar pulmonary valve stenosis, right ventricular hypertrophy, and an "overriding" large ascending aorta. Infants with TOF are cyanotic because of right-to-left shunting across the VSD and decreased pulmonary blood flow. The degree of right ventricular outflow obstruction determines the timing and severity of the cyanosis. In neonates, blood shunted from the aorta to the pulmonary artery through the PDA provides additional pulmonary blood flow. Infants with severe obstruction and ductus-dependent blood flow present within hours of birth. Cyanosis may not develop in children with mild obstruction until later in the infant period. Associated lesions include other VSDs, right aortic arch, left anterior descending (LAD) coronary artery from the right coronary artery coursing across the right ventricular outflow tract, and aortopulmonary collateral arteries.

Clinical Manifestations

Infants present with cyanosis and tachypnea of varying severity. They may have characteristic periodic episodes of cyanosis, rapid and deep breathing, and agitation known as "**tet spells**," caused by an increase in right ventricular outflow tract resistance, which leads to increased right-to-left shunting across the VSD. Such spells may last minutes to hours and may resolve spontaneously or lead to progressive hypoxia, metabolic acidosis, and death.

On cardiac examination, a right ventricular heave may be palpable, and a loud systolic ejection murmur is heard in the left upper sternal border. The heart size is generally normal on chest radiograph, with decreased pulmonary vascular markings. The heart may be "boot shaped." Twenty-five percent of children with TOF have a right-sided aortic arch. The ECG reveals right axis deviation and right ventricular hypertrophy.

Treatment

The treatment of tet spells is aimed at diminishing right-to-left shunting by increasing systemic vascular resistance and decreasing pulmonary vascular resistance. Initial measures include calming the patient and vagal maneuvers (holding the child in a knee-chest position), the administration of supplemental oxygen, and morphine sulfate to diminish the agitation and hyperpnea and minimize oxygen consumption. If these measures are not successful, volume expansion and vasoconstrictors may be given to increase systemic blood pressure and systemic vascular resistance. In addition, β-blockers may be given to reduce infundibular spasm, and sodium bicarbonate may be given to reduce acidosis and decrease pulmonary vascular resistance. In most institutions, surgical repair is performed during the first 3 to 6 months of life or after the first hypercyanotic episode ("tetspell"). Neonates with TOF with critical pulmonary valve stenosis are generally repaired at presentation. In some cases of TOF with multiple VSDs, LAD from the right coronary artery coursing across the right ventricular outflow tract, or pulmonary atresia, a modified Blalock-Taussig shunt may be placed during the neonatal period prior to definitive repair later.

EBSTEIN ANOMALY

Ebstein anomaly (Fig. 3-6) is an extremely rare anomaly in which the septal leaflet of the tricuspid valve is displaced into the right ventricular cavity and the anterior leaflet of the tricuspid valve is sail-like and redundant. This results in a portion of the right ventricle being incorporated into the right atrium. Functional hypoplasia of the right ventricle results, as well as tricuspid regurgitation. In severe cases of Ebstein anomaly, the majority of the pulmonary blood flow comes from the PDA and not the right ventricle. A PFO is present in 80% of neonates with the anomaly, and there is a right-to-left shunt at the atrial level. The right atrium is massively dilated, which may result in supraventricular tachycardia (SVT). Wolff-Parkinson-White (WPW) syndrome is associated with Ebstein anomaly.

Clinical Manifestations

Neonates with severe disease present with cyanosis and congestive heart failure in the first few days of life. The cardiac examination reveals a widely fixed split S_2 and a gallop rhythm. A tricuspid regurgitant blowing holosystolic murmur is heard at the left lower sternal border. Chest radiograph shows extreme cardiomegaly with notable right atrial enlargement and decreased pulmonary vascular markings. Characteristic

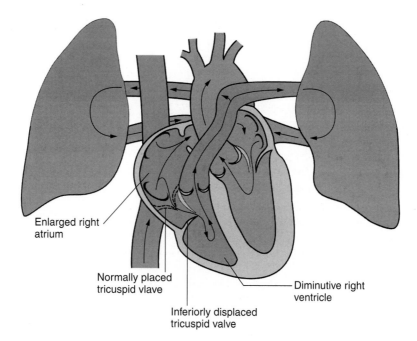

Figure 3-6 • Ebstein anomaly. Typical anatomic findings include **(A)** inferior displacement of the tricuspid valve into the right ventricle (the normal placement of the tricuspid valve is noted in dashed lines); **(B)** diminutive right ventricle; **(C)** marked enlargement of the right atrium because of "atrialized" portion of right ventricle as well as tricuspid regurgitation; **(D)** right-to-left shunting at the atrial level.

ECG findings include right bundle branch block with right atrial enlargement. SVT may be present. WPW syndrome is indicated by a delta wave and a short PR interval.

Children with milder forms of the disease may present later in childhood with fatigue, exercise intolerance, palpitations, and/or mild cyanosis with clubbing.

Treatment

Severely cyanotic newborns require PGE1 infusion to maintain pulmonary blood flow through a PDA. Congestive heart failure may be treated with digoxin, diuretics, and an angiotensin-converting enzyme (ACE) inhibitor. If WPW is present, propranolol may be used to prevent SVT. If WPW is not present, adenosine may be used to treat SVT, and digoxin may be used to prevent SVT.

In general, all attempts are made to avoid surgical intervention. Surgery on the abnormal tricuspid valve has yielded poor results. Patients with the most severe forms of Ebstein anomaly may require either heart transplantation or staged palliation to a Fontan circulation.

CYANOTIC CONGENITAL HEART DISEASE: LESIONS WITH DUCTAL-DEPENDENT SYSTEMIC BLOOD FLOW

HYPOPLASTIC LEFT HEART SYNDROME

Hypoplastic left heart syndrome (HLHS) (Fig. 3-7) is the second most common congenital cardiac lesion presenting in the first week of life and the most common cause of death from CHD in the first month of life. In this syndrome, there is hypoplasia of the left ventricle, aortic valve stenosis or atresia, mitral valve stenosis or atresia, and hypoplasia of the ascending aorta with discrete coarctation of the aorta. These lesions reduce or eliminate blood flow through the left side of the heart. Oxygenated blood from the pulmonary veins is shunted left to right through an atrial defect. Right ventricular cardiac output goes to both the pulmonary arteries and through the ductus arteriosus to the descending aorta. Systemic blood flow is completely ductal dependent, and coronary

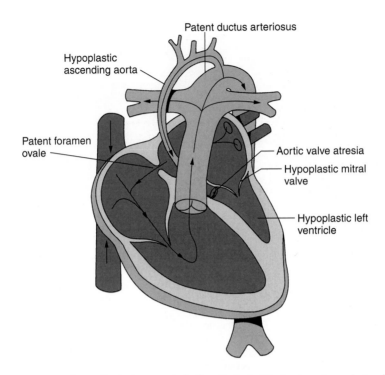

Figure 3-7 • Hypoplastic left heart syndrome. Typical anatomic findings include **(A)** atresia or hypoplasia of the left ventricle and the mitral and aortic valves; **(B)** a diminutive ascending aorta and transverse aortic arch (associated with coarctation of the aorta if the PDA becomes restrictive or closes); **(C)** coronary blood flow, which is usually retrograde from the PDA through the tiny ascending aorta.

perfusion is retrograde when aortic atresia or critical aortic stenosis is present.

Clinical Manifestations

As the ductus arteriosus closes, neonates with HLHS have severely diminished systemic blood flow and present in shock. They manifest signs of congestive heart failure with moderate cyanosis, tachycardia, tachypnea, pulmonary rales, and hepatomegaly. Peripheral pulses are poor or absent. A right ventricular heave may be present. A single S_2 and a systolic ejection murmur are heard at the left lower sternal border if mitral stenosis and aortic stenosis is present. The chest radiograph reveals pulmonary edema and progressive cardiac enlargement. The ECG is consistent with right ventricular hypertrophy, and there is poor R wave progression across the precordial leads.

Treatment

PGE1 should be started to maintain ductal-dependent systemic blood flow. No corrective surgery is available. The stage I (or Norwood) palliation, which is performed in the first week of life, allows the majority of neonates to survive infancy. The stage I procedure involves amalgamation of the pulmonary artery and aorta to provide unobstructed systemic blood flow, atrial septectomy, and modified Blalock-Taussig shunt to provide restrictive pulmonary blood flow. After the stage I procedure, a cavopulmonary anastomosis is performed at 4 to 6 months of age, and a modified Fontan completion procedure is generally performed at 2 years of age. Some centers do not perform the stage I palliation and proceed directly to heart transplantation.

INTERRUPTED AORTIC ARCH

Interrupted aortic arch is essentially an extreme form of coarctation of the aorta (Fig. 3-8). There are three types of interrupted aortic arch: Type A is interruption beyond the left subclavian artery, type B is interruption between the left subclavian and left common carotid arteries, and type C is interruption between the left common carotid and the brachiocephalic arteries. Systemic blood flow depends on patency of the ductus arteriosus, which shunts blood from the pulmonary artery to the aorta. Interrupted aortic arch is often associated with DiGeorge's syndrome because of the 22q11 microdeletion.

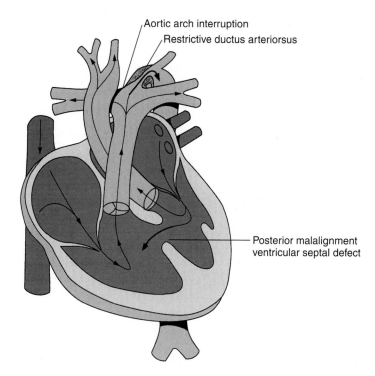

Figure 3-8 • Interrupted aortic arch with restrictive PDA. Typical anatomic findings include **(A)** atresia of a segment of the aortic arch between the left subclavian artery and the left common carotid (the most common type of interrupted aortic arch—"type B"); **(B)** posterior malalignment of the infundibular septum resulting in a large VSD and a narrow subaortic area; **(C)** a bicuspid aortic valve, which occurs in 60% of patients.

Clinical Manifestations

Neonates with interrupted aortic arch have ductal-dependent systemic blood flow and present with circulatory collapse as the ductus closes. Pulmonary edema occurs early, closely followed by congestive heart failure. The clinical presentation is similar to that of HLHS after the ductus arteriosus closes.

Treatment

PGE1 therapy should begin immediately to maintain systemic blood flow via right-to-left shunting at the PDA. Surgical treatment involves end-to-end anastomosis of the interrupted aortic segments.

ACYANOTIC CONGENITAL HEART DISEASE

Acyanotic cardiac defects that result in *increased pulmonary blood flow* (left-to-right shunts) include ASD, VSD, PDA, and common atrioventricular canal. Acyanotic lesions that result in *pulmonary venous*

hypertension include coarctation of the aorta and aortic valve stenosis. The acyanotic structural anomaly that results in *normal or decreased pulmonary blood flow* is pulmonary valve stenosis.

ATRIAL SEPTAL DEFECTS

Atrial septal defects account for 8% of CHD and have a 2:1 female-to-male predominance. There are three types of atrial septal defects:

- Ostium secundum defect, seen in the midportion of the atrial septum.
- Ostium primum defect, located in the lower portion of the atrial septum.
- Sinus venosus defect, found at the junction of the right atrium and the superior or inferior vena cava.

The degree of atrial shunting depends on the size of the ASD and the relative compliance of the ventricles in diastole. Because right ventricular diastolic compliance is usually greater than left ventricular diastolic compliance, left-to-right shunting occurs at the atrial level and results in right atrial and right ventricular enlargement and increased pulmonary blood flow.

Clinical Manifestations

Atrial septal defects are usually asymptomatic, although exercise intolerance may be noted in older children. Paradoxical embolism may occur. Supraventricular tachycardia from atrial enlargement may also occur. On examination, a right ventricular heave is often present. A systolic ejection murmur in the pulmonic (left upper sternal border) area and a mid-diastolic rumble in the lower right sternal border reflect the increased flow across the pulmonary and tricuspid valves. S_1 is loud, and S_2 is widely split on both inspiration and expiration ("fixed" splitting). The chest radiograph reveals enlargement of the heart and main pulmonary artery with increased pulmonary vascularity. The ECG often shows right ventricular enlargement. Right-axis deviation is seen in secundum defects, whereas primum defects have characteristic extreme left-axis deviation.

Treatment

Spontaneous closure of small secundum ASDs (the most common type) often occurs in the first year of life. Congestive symptoms may be treated with digoxin and diuretics. In asymptomatic children with suitable secundum ASDs, transcatheter device closure may be undertaken after 2 years of age. Moderate- to large-size secundum ASDs that have not spontaneously closed and are not candidates for device closure must be addressed surgically. Ostium primum and sinus venosus ASDs will not close spontaneously and must be addressed surgically. Any symptomatic ASD should be closed as soon as possible. Surgical closure involves pericardial patch or suture closure. *Subacute bacterial endocarditis prophylaxis* is indicated in primum and sinus venosus ASDs; patients with secundum defects do not require such precautions.

VENTRICULAR SEPTAL DEFECTS

The VSD is the most common congenital heart defect, accounting for 25% of all congenital heart defects. The five types of VSD are as follows:

- Muscular
- Inlet
- Conoseptal hypoplasia
- Conoventricular
- Malalignment

Muscular and conoventricular VSDs are the most common types. Muscular ventricular septal defects occur in the muscular portion of the septum and may be single or multiple and located in the posterior, apical, or anterior portion of the septum. The inlet VSD is an endocardial cushion defect and occurs in the inlet portion of the septum beneath the septal leaflet of the tricuspid valve. Conoseptal hypoplasia VSDs are positioned in the outflow tract of the right ventricle (RV) beneath the pulmonary valve. The conoventricular VSD occurs in the membranous portion of the ventricular septum. Malalignment VSDs result from malalignment of the infundibular septum. Anterior malalignment results in TOF, and posterior malalignment results in aortic stenosis or subaortic stenosis with arch hypoplasia or interruption.

When the VSD is small (restrictive), shunt flow is left to right from the high pressure LV to the lower pressure RV. Small shunts result in relatively normal pulmonary blood flow and pulmonary vascular resistance (PVR). When the VSD is large (nonrestrictive), LV and RV pressure are equal and PVR and systemic vascular resistance (SVR) determine shunt flow. When the PVR is less than the SVR, the shunt flow is left to right. The amount of LV and left atrial dilatation is directly proportional to the size of the left-to-right shunt. Right ventricular hypertrophy occurs when PVR increases. If left untreated, the large VSD may result in elevated pulmonary arterial pressures and may lead to pulmonary vascular obstructive disease, pulmonary hypertension, and **Eisenmenger's syndrome**. In severe cases of Eisenmenger's syndrome, the VSD shunt reverses right to left when the PVR exceeds the SVR.

Clinical Manifestations

Clinical symptoms are related to the size of the shunt. A small shunt produces no symptoms, whereas a large shunt gives rise to signs of congestive heart failure and growth failure. The smaller the defect, the louder the harsh systolic murmur, heard best at the mid- to-lower left sternal border. As the PVR increases in patients with nonrestrictive VSDs, shunting from left-to-right decreases, the murmur shortens, and the pulmonary (late) component of S_2 increases in intensity. Eisenmenger's syndrome results in a right ventricular heave, pulmonary valve ejection click, short systolic ejection murmur, diastolic murmur of pulmonary valve insufficiency, and a loud, single S_2.

Small VSDs have a normal chest radiograph and electrocardiogram. Moderate-size VSDs may show mild cardiomegaly and slightly increased pulmonary vascularity on chest radiograph. Large left-to-right shunts result in cardiomegaly, increased pulmonary vascularity, and enlargement of the left atrium and left ventricle. The ECG is consistent with left atrial, left ventricular, or biventricular hypertrophy. Right ventricular hypertrophy predominates when pulmonary vascular resistance is high.

Treatment

Most small VSDs close without intervention (40% by 3 years, 75% by 10 years); in cases which do not, surgery is unnecessary. Muscular VSDs are the most likely to close spontaneously. The treatment for large VSDs, with significant left-to-right shunting and variable levels of congestive heart failure, is surgical closure before pulmonary vascular changes become irreversible. Surgical closure usually involves Dacron patch closure. In some cases, transcatheter device placement in the interventricular septum may be used for VSD closure. Congestive heart failure is treated with digoxin, diuretics, and an ACE inhibitor. Patients with unrepaired VSDs require bacterial endocarditis prophylaxis.

COMMON ATRIOVENTRICULAR CANAL

The common atrioventricular canal defect (Fig. 3-9) results from deficiency of the endocardial cushions and results in an ostium primum ASD and inlet VSD with lack of septation of the mitral and tricuspid valves (common atrioventricular valve [CAVV]). The various forms of atrioventricular canal defects account for 5% of all CHD. In an **incomplete atrioventricular canal** defect, the CAVV leaflets attach directly to the top of the muscular portion of the ventricular septum. As a result, there is no communication beneath the atrioventricular valves between the right and left ventricles. The communication at the atrial level is an ostium primum ASD. The mitral valve is cleft, and there may be some degree of mitral regurgitation. In **complete common atrioventricular canal**, there is a CAVV that is not attached to the muscular ventricular septum. As a result, there is a large inlet VSD located between the CAVV and the top of the muscular ventricular septum. In this defect, there is a left-to-right shunting at the ostium primum ASD and inlet VSD. Because of the increase in pulmonary blood flow, pulmonary hypertension and pulmonary vascular disease may develop over time. In untreated cases, Eisenmenger's syndrome may develop.

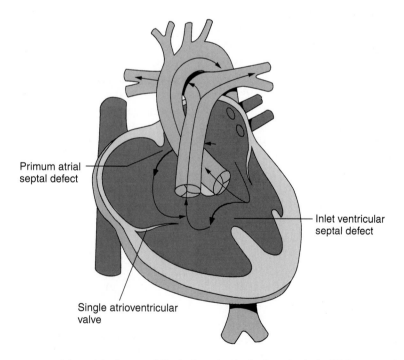

Primum atrial septal defect

Inlet ventricular septal defect

Single atrioventricular valve

Figure 3-9 • Complete common atrioventricular canal. Typical anatomic findings include **(A)** large atrial and ventricular septal defects of the endocardial cushion type; **(B)** single atrioventricular valve; **(C)** left-to-right shunting, which is noted at the atrial and ventricular level when pulmonary vascular resistance falls during the neonatal period.

Clinical Manifestations

The clinical manifestations and treatment of incomplete common atrioventricular canal are the same as those described for an ASD. There may be a blowing systolic murmur heard best at the left lower sternal border and apex, consistent with mitral regurgitation through the mitral valve cleft.

In complete common atrioventricular canal, the degree of congestive heart failure depends on the magnitude of the left-to-right shunting and the amount of CAVV regurgitation. If shunting or valve regurgitation is significant, congestive heart failure is seen early in infancy, with tachypnea, dyspnea, and failure to thrive. On examination, a blowing holosystolic murmur is heard at the left lower sternal border, and S_2 is widely split and fixed. Cardiac enlargement and increased pulmonary vascularity are visible on the chest radiograph. The ECG reveals a superior axis, which is characteristic of a canal defect and dilatation of both right and left atria.

Treatment

Prior to surgical repair, congestive heart failure is treated with digoxin, diuretics, and an ACE inhibitor. The symptomatic patient with complete common atrioventricular valve (CAVV) is generally repaired during infancy. The asymptomatic child with incomplete canal without pulmonary hypertension may undergo elective repair within the first few years of life. Infants with a large VSD component should be repaired by 6 months to decrease the risk of pulmonary artery hypertension and pulmonary vascular obstructive disease. The ASD and VSD portions are patch-closed by a one- or two-patch technique to divide the CAVV into a LV inflow and an RV inflow and close the septal defects resulting from the endocardial cushion defects. Suture closure of the cleft leaflets of the septated left-sided atrioventricular inflow is performed to make the LV inflow as competent as possible. Complete heart block occurs in 5% of patients undergoing repair, and residual mitral insufficiency often persists.

PATENT DUCTUS ARTERIOSUS

Persistent patency of the ductus arteriosus accounts for 10% of CHD. The incidence is higher in premature neonates. The ductus arteriosus connects the underside of the aorta and the left pulmonary artery just distal to the takeoff of the left subclavian artery

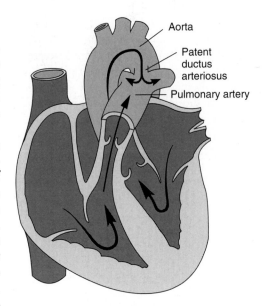

Figure 3-10 • Patent ductus arteriosus. The ductal arteriosus connects the underside of the aorta to the takeoff of the left pulmonary artery. When pulmonary vascular resistance falls, blood flows from left-to-right from aorta to pulmonary artery. From Pillitteri A. *Maternal and Child Nursing.* 4th ed. Philadelphia: Lippincott Williams & Wilkins, 2003.

from the aorta (Fig. 3-10). The direction of blood flow through a PDA depends on the relative resistances in the pulmonary and systemic circuits. In the *nonrestrictive* (large) PDA, a left-to-right shunt is present as long as the systemic vascular resistance is greater than the pulmonary vascular resistance. If pulmonary vascular resistance rises above systemic vascular resistance, a right-to-left shunt develops.

Clinical Manifestations

Symptoms are related to the *size* of the defect and the *direction* of flow. A small PDA causes no symptoms or abnormalities on chest radiograph or ECG. A large PDA with left-to-right shunting may result in congestive heart failure and failure to thrive. Bounding pulses are palpable. A continuous murmur begins after S_1, peaks at S_2, and trails off during diastole. The chest radiograph of a large patent ductus arteriosus shows cardiomegaly, increased pulmonary vascularity, and left atrial and ventricular enlargement. The ECG shows left or biventricular hypertrophy. The PDA is best seen on ECHO using Doppler flow mapping. If pulmonary vascular resistance rises above systemic resistance (pulmonary hypertension), flow at the PDA reverses, and cyanosis is noted.

Treatment

Indomethacin decreases PGE1 levels and is often effective in closing the ductus in the premature neonate. A PDA usually closes in term infants in the first month of life. If the ductus remains patent, coil embolization or device closure in the cardiac catheterization laboratory or surgical ligation via thoracotomy or video-assisted thoracoscopic surgery may be performed.

COARCTATION OF THE AORTA

Coarctation of the aorta (Fig. 3-11) accounts for 8% of congenital heart defects and has a male-to-female predominance of 2:1. When coarctation of the aorta occurs in a girl, **Turner syndrome** must be considered. The obstruction (narrowing) is usually located in the descending aorta at the insertion site of the ductus arteriosus. The aortic valve is bicuspid in 80% of cases, and mitral valve anomalies may also be present. The coarctation results in obstruction to blood flow (between the proximal and distal aorta) and increased left ventricular afterload.

Clinical Manifestations

The degree of narrowing determines clinical severity. Infants may be asymptomatic or present with irritability, difficulty feeding, and failure to thrive. On examination, the femoral pulses are often weak and delayed or even absent, and there is upper extremity hypertension. Neonates with critical coarctation have ductal-dependent systemic blood flow and may present with circulatory collapse as the ductus closes. On cardiac examination, there is a nonspecific ejection murmur at the heart apex. The chest radiograph and ECG are normal in mild lesions. In patients with more severe obstruction, the chest radiograph may reveal an enlarged aortic knob. Right ventricular hypertrophy is seen in the neonatal ECG; left ventricular hypertrophy is more common in the older child.

Treatment

In neonates with critical coarctation of the aorta, the child's systemic blood flow is ductal dependent, and PGE1 should be started prior to surgical or catheter-based intervention. Treatment may be surgical, with end-to-end anastomosis or patch aortoplasty, or interventional, with balloon dilation angioplasty with or without stent placement. Timing and type of therapy depends on age at diagnosis, severity of illness, and related defects. Restenosis at the surgical repair site is not uncommon, especially in neonates. Persistent hypertension after intervention in the older

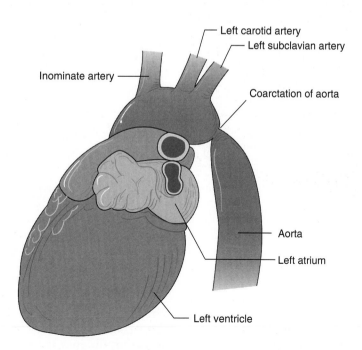

Figure 3-11 • Coarctation of the aorta.

child is not uncommon and may require β-blocker therapy.

AORTIC STENOSIS

In aortic stenosis, the valvular tissue is thickened, rigid, and domes in systole. Most commonly, the valve is bicuspid. The increased pressure generated in the left ventricle, as it attempts to direct blood flow across a stenotic valve, results in left ventricular hypertrophy and, over time, decreased compliance and ventricular performance.

Clinical Manifestations

The level of symptomatology is related to the severity of the stenosis and the level of ventricular function. Infants with minimal stenosis are asymptomatic (although with a murmur). The neonate with critical aortic stenosis has ductal-dependent systemic blood flow and may present with circulatory collapse if the ductus closes. The cardiac examination is characterized by a harsh systolic ejection murmur heard at the right upper sternal border that is preceded by an ejection click. In severe aortic stenosis, a thrill may be palpable. The more pronounced the stenosis, the louder the murmur. However, if ventricular function is highly compromised, only a soft murmur may be appreciated. The chest radiograph shows cardiomegaly. Pulmonary edema may be noted in cases with ventricular dysfunction. Left ventricular hypertrophy is seen on the ECG. In some cases a strain pattern of ST depression and inverted T waves consistent with ischemia may be noted.

Treatment

In neonates with critical aortic stenosis, the child's systemic blood flow is ductal dependent, and PGE1 should be started prior to surgical of catheter-based intervention. If intervention is required, relief of the aortic valve gradient may be accomplished by balloon valvuloplasty. Balloon valvuloplasty may result in progressive aortic regurgitation that may require aortic valve replacement with a mechanical, homograft, or autograft valve (Ross procedure).

PULMONIC STENOSIS

Pulmonic valve stenosis accounts for 5% to 8% of CHDs. The valve is domed with only a small central opening, and there is poststenotic dilatation of the main pulmonary artery. Right ventricular hypertrophy occurs over time as the ventricle attempts to maintain cardiac output. In *critical pulmonic stenosis*, a decrease in the compliance of the right ventricle increases right atrial pressure and may open the foramen ovale, producing a small right-to-left shunt.

Clinical Manifestations

Most patients are asymptomatic. Severe to critical pulmonary stenosis may cause dyspnea on exertion and angina. Right-sided congestive heart failure is rare, except in infants with critical pulmonic stenosis who may have ductal-dependent pulmonary blood flow. Characteristically, the ejection click of pulmonic stenosis varies with inspiration, and a harsh systolic ejection murmur is heard at the left upper sternal border. In severe stenosis, a thrill and right ventricular heave are palpable. On chest radiograph, heart size and pulmonary vascularity are normal, but the pulmonary artery segment is enlarged. The degree of right ventricular hypertrophy and right-axis deviation present on ECG correlates with the degree of stenosis.

Treatment

In neonates with critical pulmonary stenosis, the child's pulmonary blood flow is ductal dependent, and PGE1 should be started prior to surgical or catheter-based intervention. Definitive treatment is accomplished by balloon dilation valvuloplasty of the stenotic valve. Indications for pulmonary valvotomy include a right ventricular pressure that was three-quarters systemic or greater, or symptoms of right-sided congestive heart failure.

Table 3-5 lists the classic findings of the ten most common congenital heart lesions.

ACQUIRED STRUCTURAL HEART DISEASE

RHEUMATIC HEART DISEASE

Acute rheumatic fever causes carditis in 50% to 80% of patients. Rheumatic heart disease results from single or multiple episodes of acute rheumatic fever. **Mitral regurgitation** is the most common lesion. Aortic insufficiency may also occur, with or without mitral regurgitation. Late-stage disease may progress to mitral and/or aortic stenosis. Patients with severe

■ TABLE 3-5 Findings for the Ten Most Common Congenital Heart Lesions

Lesion	Presentation	Physical Examination	ECG	Radiograph
Atrial septal defect	Murmur	Fixed split S_2	Mild RVH	± CE, ↑ PBF
Ventricular septal defect	Murmur, CHF	Holosystolic murmur	LVH, RVH	± CE, ↑ PBF
Patent ductus	Murmur, ± CHF	Continuous murmur	LVH, ± RVH	± CE, ↑ PBF
AV canal defect	Murmur, ± CHF	Holosystolic murmur	"Superior" axis	± CE, ↑ PBF
Pulmonic stenosis	Murmur, ± cyanosis	Click, SEM	RVH	± CE, NL, or ↓ PBF
Tetralogy of Fallot	Murmur, cyanosis	SEM	RVH	± CE, ↓ PBF
Aortic stenosis	Murmur, ± CHF	Click, SEM	LVH	± CE, NL, PBF
Coarctation of aorta	Hypertension	↓ Femoral pulses	LVH	± CE, NL, PBF
Transposition of the great arteries	Cyanosis	Marked cyanosis	RVH	± CE, NL, or ↑ PBF
Single ventricle	(Variable)	(Variable)	(Variable)	(Variable)

CE, cardiac enlargement; CHF, congestive heart failure; LVH, left ventricular hypertrophy; NL, normal; PBF, pulmonary blood flow; RVH, right ventricular hypertrophy; SEM, systolic ejection murmur.

valvular involvement manifest signs and symptoms of chronic congestive heart failure. Chapter 12 discusses acute rheumatic fever.

KAWASAKI'S DISEASE

Cardiac effects may include pericarditis, myocarditis, and transient rhythm disturbances. However, it is the development of **coronary artery aneurysms**, with their potential for occlusion or rupture, that makes the disease life-threatening. Coronary artery aneurysms develop during the subacute phase (11th to 25th day) in approximately 25% of cases but regress in most patients. Early therapy with intravenous immunoglobulin decreases the incidence of coronary artery aneurysms to less than 10%. High-dose aspirin therapy given during the acute inflammatory period lessens the likelihood of aneurysm development. Low-dose aspirin is continued for 6 to 8 weeks (or indefinitely if the aneurysms do not resolve). An ECHO is used to assess ventricular function and detect coronary artery aneurysms. Chapter 11 offers a thorough discussion of Kawasaki's disease.

ENDOCARDITIS

Pathogenesis

Bacterial endocarditis is a microbial infection of the endocardium. Although it may occur on normal valves, bacterial endocarditis is much more likely to occur where there is turbulent flow on congenitally abnormal valves, valves damaged by rheumatic fever, acquired valvular lesions (mitral valve prolapse), and prosthetic replacement valves. Factors that may precipitate bacterial endocarditis include dental manipulation or infection, instrumentation of the gastrointestinal or genitourinary tract, intravenous drug abuse, an indwelling central venous catheter, and/or prior cardiac surgery.

In children, α-hemolytic streptococci (*Streptococcus viridans*) and *Staphylococcus aureus* are the most common etiologic agents. *S. viridans* accounts for approximately 67% of cases, whereas *S. aureus* is present in an estimated 20% of cases. When the infection is a complication of cardiac surgery, *Staphylococcus epidermidis* and fungi should be considered. Gram-negative organisms cause approximately 5% of cases of endocarditis in children and are more likely in neonates, immunocompromised patients, and intravenous drug abusers.

Clinical Manifestations

Fever is the most common finding in children with bacterial endocarditis. Often, a new or changing murmur is auscultated. Children with endocarditis usually display nonspecific symptoms, including chest pain, dyspnea, arthralgia, myalgia, headache, and malaise. Embolic phenomena such as hematuria and transient ischemic attack (strokes) may be present. Other embolic phenomena (Roth spots, splinter hemorrhages, petechiae, Osler nodes, and Janeway lesions) are relatively rare in children with bacterial endocarditis.

Diagnostic Evaluation

Typical laboratory findings include elevated white blood count, erythrocyte sedimentation rate (ESR), and C-reactive protein (CRP). Anemia is common. Hematuria (with red blood casts) may be seen on urinalysis. Multiple blood cultures increase the probability of discovering the pathogen. An ECHO is used to define vegetations and/or thrombi in the heart.

Treatment

Medical management consists of 6 weeks of intravenous antibiotics directed against the isolated pathogen. Surgery is indicated for endocarditis when medical treatment is unsuccessful, refractory congestive heart failure exists, serious embolic complications intervene, myocardial abscesses develop, or there is refractory prosthetic valve disease.

Antibiotic prophylaxis is necessary for high-risk patients. Antibiotic regimens to prevent endocarditis during dental, respiratory, gastrointestinal, or genitourinary procedures include oral amoxicillin or parenteral ampicillin and gentamicin prior to the procedure.

🔑 3-2 KEY POINTS

1. Patients with congenitally abnormal valves, valves damaged by rheumatic fever, acquired valvular lesions (mitral valve prolapse), or prosthetic replacement valves are at increased risk for endocarditis.
2. α-Hemolytic streptococci (*Streptococcus viridans*) and *Staphylococcus aureus* are the most common etiologic agents in endocarditis.
3. Patients at risk for the development of endocarditis require antibiotic prophylaxis prior to procedures that may result in bacteremia.

CORONARY ARTERY DISEASE

Coronary artery disease is rare in childhood. The atherosclerotic process appears to begin early in life. Evidence indicates that progression of atherosclerotic lesions is influenced by genetic factors (familial hypercholesterolemia) and lifestyle (cigarette smoking; high-cholesterol diet, high saturated-fat diet). Certain diseases place children at an increased risk for hypercholesterolemia (e.g., some storage and metabolic diseases, renal failure, diabetes, hepatitis, systemic lupus erythematosus). Because many lifetime habits are formed during childhood, the opportunity exists for prevention of coronary artery disease.

FUNCTIONAL HEART DISEASE

MYOCARDITIS

Most cases of myocarditis in the developed world result from viral infection of the myocardium, predominantly **enteroviruses** (coxsackie B virus and echovirus). It is unclear whether the myocardial damage results from direct viral invasion or an autoimmune antibody response.

Clinical Manifestations

If myocardial damage is mild, patients are asymptomatic; the diagnosis may be made by finding ST- and T-wave changes on an ECG done for an unrelated reason. Severe myocardial damage presents with fulminant congestive heart failure and arrhythmia. Common symptoms include fever, dyspnea, fatigue, and chest pain (usually caused by a secondary pericarditis). Tachycardia, evidence of congestive heart failure, and S_3 ventricular gallop may be appreciated on examination. The ECG often reveals ST-segment depression, T-wave inversion, and low voltage. Arrhythmias and conduction defects may also be present. Heart size on chest radiograph varies from mild to markedly enlarged. The ECHO reveals ventricles that are dilatated and/or poorly functioning. Pericardial effusion is common. Viral etiology should be investigated by viral culture and polymerase chain reaction (PCR) from the throat, stool, blood, and pericardial fluid, if present. In select cases, endomyocardial biopsy is indicated to confirm diagnosis.

Treatment

Therapy for patients with viral myocarditis is supportive to maintain perfusion and oxygen delivery. Ventricular arrhythmias, conduction abnormalities, and congestive heart failure are treated as indicated. Intravenous immunoglobulin and/or steroids are given to minimize further damage to the myocardium. The prognosis for patients with myocarditis is directly related to the extent of myocardial damage.

DILATED CARDIOMYOPATHY

Dilated or congestive cardiomyopathy is characterized by myocardial dysfunction and ventricular dilatation. In idiopathic cases (most common), the cause is theorized to be a recent undiagnosed episode of myocarditis. Dilated cardiomyopathy can also be caused by neuromuscular disease (Duchenne muscular dystrophy) or drug toxicity (anthracyclines).

Clinical Manifestations

Signs and symptoms are related to the resultant congestive heart failure and pulmonary edema. Symptoms include dyspnea, orthopnea, and paroxysmal nocturnal dyspnea. The cardiac examination reveals an S_3 gallop rhythm and often a murmur consistent with mitral regurgitation. As right heart failure worsens, dependent edema, a right ventricular heave, and pulsus alternans (beat-to-beat variability in pulse magnitude) may be noted. The heart is enlarged on chest radiograph, often accompanied by pulmonary edema. The ECG is notable for broadening of the QRS complexes and nonspecific ST- and T-wave ischemic changes. Ventricular function is evaluated by ECHO.

Treatment

Initial treatment includes fluid restriction and diuretics (to reduce preload), inotropic agents and vasodilators (to improve myocardial contractility and decrease afterload), and anticoagulants (to prevent thrombus formation). Antiarrhythmic medications are reserved for treatment of potentially fatal ventricular arrhythmias. If medical therapy fails, heart transplantation may be necessary.

HYPERTROPHIC OBSTRUCTIVE CARDIOMYOPATHY

Also known as idiopathic hypertrophic subaortic stenosis, hypertrophic cardiomyopathy is a disorder in which the ventricular septum is significantly thickened, resulting in left ventricular outflow tract obstruction. In the thickened stiff left ventricle, diastolic function is compromised and systolic function is preserved. Abnormal motion of the mitral valve results in mitral insufficiency. Inheritance is dominant with incomplete penetrance.

Clinical Manifestations

Most cases are asymptomatic and discovered as a result of evaluation of a heart murmur. When present (generally in adolescence), symptoms include dyspnea on exertion, chest pain, and syncope. A systolic ejection murmur at the left lower sternal border and/or apex may be accompanied by the soft, holosystolic murmur of mitral regurgitation and an S_3 gallop. There may be a bisferious (double-peaked) pulse, left ventricular heave, and thrill. The chest radiograph shows normal vascularity and mild left ventricular enlargement. ECG illustrates left-axis deviation, left ventricular hypertrophy, and possible ST- and T-wave changes consistent with ischemia or strain. The ECHO is diagnostic.

Unfortunately, hypertrophic cardiomyopathy may also present as sudden death during physical activity in an otherwise healthy, asymptomatic person with undiagnosed disease.

Treatment

Therapy is centered on preventing fatal ventricular arrhythmias and decreasing the stiffness of the left ventricle with negative inotropic medications (calcium channel blockers, β-adrenergic blocking agents). The avoidance of competitive sports is essential because sudden death during exertion is a significant risk (4% to 6% of affected patients a year).

🔑 3-3 KEY POINTS

1. Most cases of myocarditis in North America result from viral infection of the myocardium.
2. Dilated or congestive cardiomyopathy is characterized by myocardial dysfunction and ventricular dilatation; it is usually idiopathic.
3. Therapy for dilated cardiomyopathy includes fluid restriction and diuretics, inotropic agents and vasodilators, and anticoagulants. Antiarrhythmic medications are used to control potentially fatal ventricular arrhythmias.
4. In hypertrophic cardiomyopathy, the ventricular septum is thickened, resulting in left ventricular outflow tract obstruction.
5. Hypertrophic cardiomyopathy may present as sudden death during physical exertion in an asymptomatic, otherwise healthy individual.
6. Therapy for hypertrophic cardiomyopathy focuses on preventing fatal ventricular arrhythmias and decreasing the stiffness of the left ventricle with negative inotropic medications.

ARRHYTHMIAS

Arrhythmias in children are much less common than in adults but can be just as life-threatening. Arrhythmias result from disorders of impulse formation, impulse conduction, or both, and they are generally classified as follows.

Bradyarrhythmias
- Sinus node dysfunction
- Conduction block

Tachyarrhythmias
- Narrow QRS
- Wide QRS

Premature Beats
- Atrial
- Ventricular

Arrhythmias may result from congenital, functional, or acquired structural heart disease; electrolyte disturbances (potassium, calcium, and magnesium); drug toxicity; poisoning; or an acquired systemic disorder. Table 3-6 lists the etiologies predisposing children to arrhythmias.

BRADYARRHYTHMIAS

Bradyarrhythmias result from either depressed automaticity at the sinus node (sinus node dysfunction) or conduction block at the atrioventricular node or bundle of His (AV block). Bradyarrhythmias that may result from sinus node dysfunction include sinus bradycardia, junctional bradycardia, ectopic atrial bradycardia, and sinus pauses. Bradyarrhythmias that may result from AV block include first-degree heart block, second-degree heart block, and third-degree (complete) heart block.

Differential Diagnosis

Figure 3-12 shows the rhythm strips of various bradycardias. **Sinus bradycardia** is caused by a decreased rate of impulse generation at the sinus node. It may be associated with increased vagal tone, hypoxia, central nervous system disorders with increased intracranial pressure, hypothyroidism, hyperkalemia, hypothermia, drug intoxication (digoxin, β-blockers, calcium channel blockers), and prior atrial surgery. It is also a normal finding in healthy athletic teenagers. The ECG reveals a normal P wave with normal AV conduction at rates less than 100 beats per minute (bpm) in the

TABLE 3-6 Factors Predisposing to *Arrhythmias*

Congenital heart disease

Supraventricular arrhythmias:

Ebstein anomaly (may also present with WPW syndrome), atrial septal defects, atrial surgery, L-transportation of the great arteries, after Fontan operation

Ventricular arrhythmias:

Aortic valve disease, pulmonary valve disease, after Tetralogy of Fallot repair, anomalous left coronary artery, RV dysplasia

Heart block (varying degrees):

After open-heart surgery (Ebstein anomaly, L-transportation of the great arteries, systemic lupus erythematosus, L-transportation of the great arteries)

Isolated conduction system disorders

WPW syndrome

Prolonged QT-interval syndromes

Associated with systemic illness

Infectious myocarditis

Kawasaki's disease

Idiopathic dilatated or hypertrophic cardiomyopathy

Friedrich ataxia (atrial tachycardia or fibrillation)

Muscular dystrophies (Duchenne, periodic paralysis)

Glycogen storage diseases (Pompe disease)

Collagen vascular diseases (rheumatic carditis, systemic lupus erythematosus, periarteritis nodosa, dermatomyositis)

Endocrine disorders (hyperthyroidism, adrenal dysfunction)

Metabolic and electrolyte disturbances (hypomagnesemia, hyperkalemia, hypocalcemia, hypoxia)

Lyme's disease

Drug toxicity

Chemotherapeutic agents

Tricyclic antidepressants

Cocaine

Anti arrythmia drugs (Digitalis, β-adrenergic blockers, calcium blockers)

Asthma medications (sympathomimetics)

Blunt chest trauma (myocardial contusion)

Increased intracranial pressure

WPW, Wolff-Parkinson-White; RV, right ventricle.

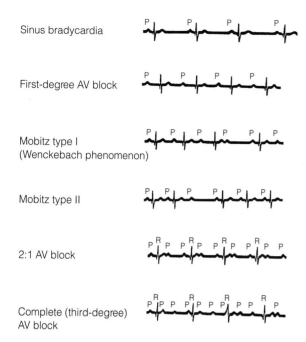

Sinus bradycardia

First-degree AV block

Mobitz type I
(Wenckebach phenomenon)

Mobitz type II

2:1 AV block

Complete (third-degree)
AV block

Figure 3-12 • Bradyarrhythmias.

neonate and 60 bpm in the older child. When sinus bradycardia becomes too slow, sinus pauses or escape rhythms (ectopic atrial bradycardia or ectopic atrial rhythm, junctional bradycardia or junctional rhythm, or a slow idioventricular ventricular rhythm) may occur. Patients with sinus bradycardia can increase their heart rate appropriately when stimulated.

First-degree heart block usually results from slowing of atrioventricular conduction at the level of the AV node. It is associated with increased vagal tone, medication administration (digoxin and β-blocker), infectious etiologies (viral myocarditis, Lyme's disease), hypothermia, electrolyte abnormalities (hypo/hyperkalemia, hypo/hypercalcemia, and hypomagnesemia), CHD (ASD, atrioventricular canal defect, Ebstein anomaly, TAPVC, and l-transposition of the great arteries or "corrected transposition"), rheumatic fever, and cardiomyopathy. First-degree AV block is characterized on ECG by PR interval prolongation for age and rate. Otherwise, the rhythm is regular, originates in the sinus node, and has a normal QRS morphology.

Second-degree heart block refers to episodic interruption of AV nodal conduction ("dropped beats"). Some P waves are followed by QRS complexes; others are not.

- **Mobitz type I (Wenckebach)** denotes progressive prolongation of the PR interval over several beats until a QRS is dropped. This cycle repeats itself

often, although the number of beats in a cycle may not be constant. The QRS configuration is normal. Etiologies for this rhythm are the same as those for first-degree heart block.

- **Mobitz type II** is caused by abrupt failure of atrioventricular conduction below the AV node in the bundle of His-Purkinje fiber system. It is a more serious bradycardia than first-degree heart block or Wenckebach because it can progress to complete heart block. On ECG, there is sudden AV conduction failure with a dropped QRS after a normal P wave. No preceding PR interval prolongation is seen in normal conducted impulses.
- **Fixed-ratio AV block** is an arrhythmia in which the QRS complex follows only after every second (third or fourth) P wave, causing 2:1 (3:1 or 4:1) AV block. There is a normal PR interval in conducted beats. There is usually a normal or slightly prolonged QRS. Fixed-ratio block results from either AV node or His bundle injury, and intracardiac recordings are required to distinguish the site of injury. Patients may progress to complete heart block.

Third-degree heart block exists when no atrial impulses are conducted to the ventricles. The atrial rhythm and rate are normal for the patient's age, and the ventricular rate is slowed markedly (40 to 55 bpm). If an escape rhythm arises from the AV node (*junctional rhythm*), the QRS interval is of normal duration, but if an escape rhythm arises from the distal His bundle or Purkinje fibers, the QRS interval is prolonged (*idioventricular rhythm*). Congenital complete AV block can be an isolated abnormality or can be associated with l-transposition of the great arteries, atrioventricular canal defect, or maternal lupus erythematosus. Other causes include open-heart surgery (especially after large ventricular septal defect closure), cardiomyopathy, or Lyme's disease. Newborns with congenital complete heart block may present with hydrops fetalis.

Treatment

No intervention is necessary for sinus bradycardia if cardiac output is maintained. Figure 3-13 shows a management algorithm for sinus bradycardia.

No treatment is necessary for first- or second-degree heart block (Mobitz type I). Mobitz type II, fixed-ratio AV block, and third-degree heart block all require pacemaker placement. In Mobitz type II and fixed-ratio AV block, prophylactic pacemaker insertion is essential to protect the patient should he or she progress to complete heart block with inadequate cardiac output away from medical care.

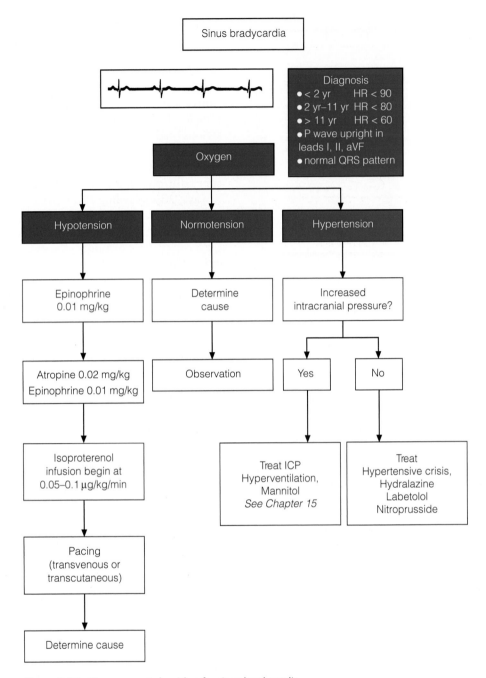

Figure 3-13 • Management algorithm for sinus bradycardia.

If the child with complete heart block is hemodynamically unstable, transcutaneous or transvenous pacing can be performed acutely, and permanent transvenous or epicardial pacemaker placement can be performed later. Third-degree heart block is managed with either ventricular demand pacing or AV sequential pacing. Figure 3-14 is a management algorithm for AV block.

TACHYARRHYTHMIAS

Tachyarrhythmias arise from abnormal impulse formation caused by enhanced automaticity or a reentrant circuit. Narrow-complex tachycardias have a QRS morphology identical to that of normal sinus rhythm. Most SVTs are narrow-complex in appearance. Narrow-complex tachycardias may be caused

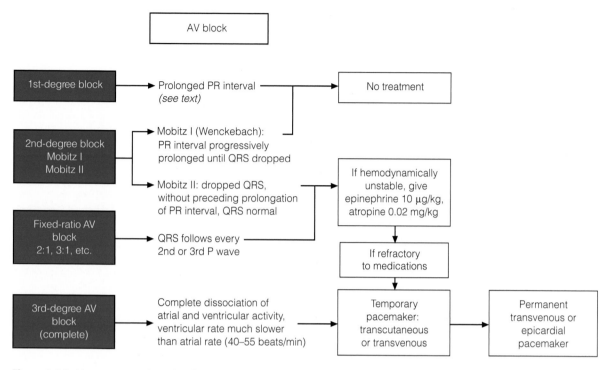

Figure 3-14 • Management algorithm for AV block.

by increased automaticity (e.g., sinus tachycardia, ectopic atrial tachycardia, junctional ectopic tachycardia, atrial fibrillation) or a reentrant circuit. Reentrant circuits include either orthodromic reentrant tachycardia (ORT) or antidromic reentrant tachycardia (ART). In ORT, the SVT propagates down the AV node and up the bypass tract. Because the ventricles are depolarized in the normal fashion, down the AV node, the *QRS complex is narrow*. In ART, the SVT propagates down the bypass tract and up the AV node. Because the ventricles are depolarized down the bypass tract and the ventricles depolarize at different times, the *QRS complex is widened*. Narrow-complex AV reciprocating tachycardias include AV node reentrant tachycardia; WPW syndrome orthodromic tachycardia (accessory pathway not concealed on ECG—short PR interval with delta wave); orthodromic atrioventricular reciprocating tachycardia (accessory pathway concealed on ECG—normal PR interval and no delta wave); sinoatrial reentrant tachycardia; and atrial flutter. Narrow-complex tachycardias are relatively well tolerated acutely. Patients with WPW syndrome have antegrade impulse propagation through both the AV node and

the accessory pathway. Characteristic findings on ECG include a short PR interval and delta wave (Fig. 3-15).

Conversely, wide-complex tachycardias, defined as tachycardias with a QRS more than 0.12 seconds, are a medical emergency. Wide-complex tachycardias include ventricular tachycardia, ventricular fibrillation, WPW syndrome antidromic reentrant tachycardia, and orthodromic SVT with aberrancy.

Differential Diagnosis

Figure 3-16 shows the rhythm strips of the various tachyarrhythmias.
The causes of tachyarrhythmia are as follows.

Narrow-Complex Tachycardias
- *Sinus tachycardia:* Fever, stress, dehydration, and anemia.
- *ORT (most common nonsinus tachycardia SVT):* Most cases result from a concealed bypass tract AV node reentrant tachycardia, WPW syndrome, Ebstein anomaly (associated with WPW syndrome), L-transposition of the great arteries.

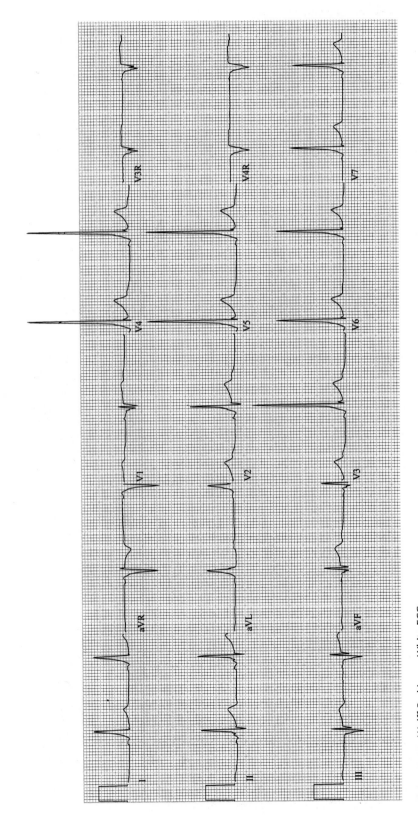

Figure 3-15 • Wolff-Parkinson-White ECG.

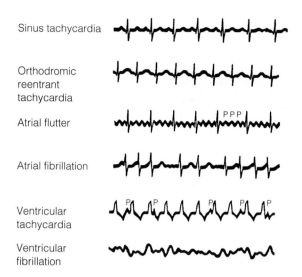

Figure 3-16 • Tachydysrhythmia.

- *Atrial flutter*: Atrial surgery (D-TGA status post Mustard/Senning procedure, ASD status post repair Hemi-Fontan, Fontan), myocarditis, structural heart disease with dilatated atria (Ebstein anomaly, tricuspid atresia, rheumatic heart disease of the mitral valve), severe tricuspid regurgitation.
- *Atrial fibrillation*: Most often seen with left atrial enlargement (rheumatic heart disease of the mitral valve, VSD, systemic to pulmonary artery palliative shunt placement); other causes that result in right atrial or biatrial enlargement include Ebstein anomaly, WPW syndrome, and myocarditis.

Wide-Complex Tachycardia

- *Ventricular tachycardia*: Congenital or acquired heart disease resulting in ventricular dilatation or hypertrophy or ventricular suture line, drug ingestion, or WPW syndrome with ART.
- *Ventricular fibrillation*: Terminal rhythm that develops after hypoxia, ischemia, or high-voltage electrical injury; predisposing factors include WPW syndrome and long QT syndrome.

Treatment

Narrow-Complex Tachycardia

Treatment of sinus tachycardia involves correcting the underlying cause of the tachycardia. Figure 3-17 outlines a management algorithm for supraventricular tachycardia. Treatment for stable narrow-complex tachycardia progresses from vagal maneuvers to pharmacotherapy to cardioversion. Vagal maneuvers (ice to face and carotid massage) enhance vagal tone to slow conduction in the AV node and often result in termination of the arrhythmia.

If vagal maneuvers are ineffective, adenosine may be given to block the AV node and break the reentrant SVT. The reentrant SVT, whose circuit involves the AV node (AV node reentrant tachycardia, WPW syndrome–type ORT, concealed bypass tract–type ORT), is likely to break with the administration of adenosine. Adenosine is ineffective on a narrow-complex tachycardia that results from increased automaticity or a reentrant mechanism that does not involve the AV node (sinus tachycardia, ectopic atrial tachycardia, junctional ectopic tachycardia, atrial flutter, or sinoatrial reentrant tachycardia). If adenosine returns the child to normal sinus rhythm and WPW is not suspected (no delta wave seen after conversion of tachycardia), the child may be started on digoxin to reduce the risk of future events. If adenosine therapy reveals WPW syndrome (short PR interval and delta wave noted after conversion of tachycardia), a β-blocker should be used. The use of digoxin in patients with WPW may slow the conduction across the AV node, leading to preferential depolarization down the accessory pathway in an antidromic fashion. This antidromic conduction may result in ventricular fibrillation if atrial fibrillation or some other fast atrial arrhythmia is present.

Treatment for hemodynamically stable atrial flutter may include digoxin, β-blockers, procainamide, amiodarone, sotalol, or a quinidine/digoxin combination. When attempting pharmacologic conversion of the atrial flutter, the patient should be loaded with digoxin prior to procainamide administration. Procainamide has vagolytic activity that could inadvertently increase the ventricular rate and cause acute hemodynamic deterioration.

If atrial fibrillation has been present for more than a few days, anticoagulation is needed before converting the rhythm to decrease the risk of embolization of possible intra-atrial clots. An alternative to anticoagulation is transesophageal echocardiography to assess for clots. If no clots are seen, cardioversion may proceed, although with a slightly increased risk of thromboembolism relative to anticoagulation. Quinidine, procainamide, or amiodarone can be effective in pharmacologic conversion of atrial fibrillation, and quinidine and procainamide are good long-term maintenance drugs. Synchronized cardioversion converts most cases to sinus rhythm.

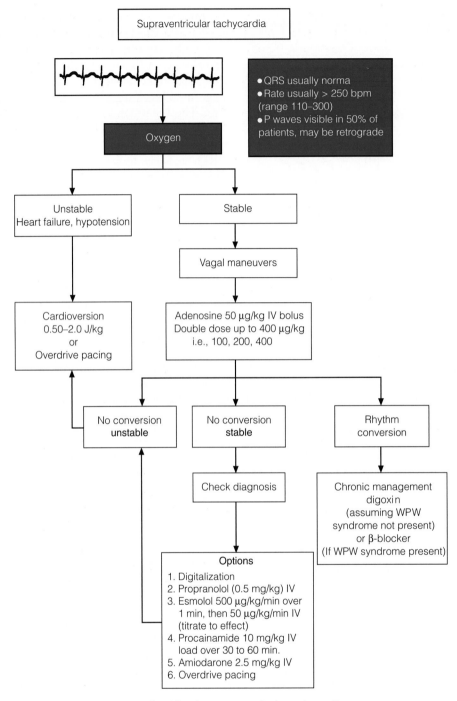

Figure 3-17 • Management algorithm for supraventricular tachycardia.

When unstable narrow-complex tachycardia is present and the patient has congestive heart failure or hypotension, cardioversion or transesophageal overdrive pacing is indicated. Synchronized cardioversion is required to avoid the inadvertent development of ventricular fibrillation.

Most chronic cases of SVT with the exception of atrial fibrillation are amenable to radiofrequency ablation.

Wide-Complex Tachycardia

Wide-complex ventricular tachycardia caused by WPW syndrome should be treated with antidromic conduction or orthodromic SVT with aberrancy as if the patient has ventricular tachycardia. Hypotensive or unresponsive patients should be treated immediately with cardiopulmonary resuscitation and synchronized cardioversion. After cardioversion, sinus rhythm can be maintained with intravenous lidocaine or amiodarone. Normotensive patients with acute-onset ventricular tachycardia can be treated with

intravenous lidocaine or amiodarone in an attempt to break the arrhythmia without cardioversion.

Children with ventricular fibrillation should receive CPR and must be defibrillated with nonsynchronized cardioversion. Giving epinephrine may turn fine fibrillation into coarse fibrillation and allow successful defibrillation. Figures 3-18 and 3-19 outline the management algorithms for ventricular

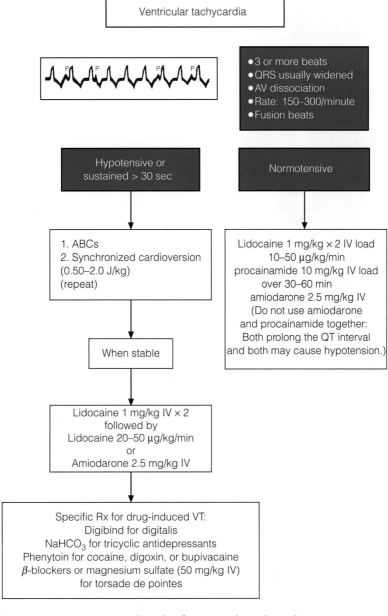

Figure 3-18 • Management algorithm for ventricular tachycardia.

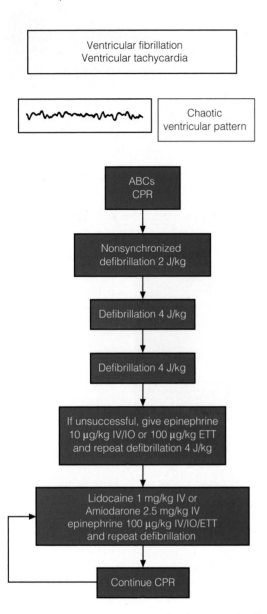

Figure 3-19 • Management algorithm for ventricular fibrillation.

tachycardia and ventricular fibrillation/pulseless ventricular tachycardia, respectively.

Many chronic cases of ventricular tachycardia are amenable to radiofrequency ablation.

3-4 KEY POINTS

1. Bradyarrhythmias with widened QRS complexes are likely to be escape rhythms from the His bundle or Purkinje system (idioventricular rhythm) and are at high risk for progression to complete heart block.
2. Symptomatic sinus bradycardia, second-degree heart block (Mobitz type II and fixed-ratio AV block), and third-degree heart block all need pacing.
3. Narrow-complex tachycardias tend to be well tolerated acutely, whereas wide-complex tachycardias are considered a medical emergency.
4. Wide-complex tachycardia caused by supraventricular tachycardia (SVT)—Wolfe-Parkinson-White (WPW) syndrome with antidromic reentrant tachycardia (ART) or SVT with aberrancy—should be treated as though the patient has ventricular tachycardia.
5. When treating SVT, rule out WPW syndrome because the treatment for WPW-associated SVT is different from that for non-WPW SVT.

Additional Suggested Reading

Andrews R, Tulloh R, Sharland G, et al. Outcome of staged reconstructive surgery for hypoplastic left heart syndrome following antenatal diagnosis. *Arch Dis Child*. 2001;85:474–477.

Batra AS, Lewis AB. Acute myocarditis. *Curr Opin Pediatr*. 2001;13:234–239.

Hoyer A, Silberbach M. Infective endocarditis. *Pediatr Rev*. 2005;26:394–400.

McDaniel NL. Ventricular and atrial septal defects. *Pediatr Rev*. 2001;22:265–270.

Gutgesell HP, Barton DM, Elgin KN. Coarctation of the aorta in the neonate: associated conditions, management, and early outcome. *Am J Cardiol*. 2001; 88:457–459

Tingelstad J. Consultation with the specialist: cardiac dysrhythmias. *Pediatr Rev*. 2001;22:91–94.

Development

DEVELOPMENTAL MILESTONES

Intellectual and physical development in infants and children each occur in an orderly and sequential manner. Table 4-1 lists the normal progression of developmental milestones. The information is subdivided into gross motor, visual motor (or fine motor–adaptive), language, and social milestones.

The two developmental screens most commonly used by pediatricians are the **Denver II** developmental screening test and the Clinical Adaptive Test/Clinical Linguistic and Auditory Milestone Scale **(CAT/CLAMS)**. The Denver II evaluates children from 0 to 6 years of age and divides streams of development into gross motor, fine motor—adaptive, language, and personal-social. The CAT rates problem-solving and visual motor ability, and the CLAMS assesses language development from birth to 36 months of age.

Sometimes the developmental process does not progress appropriately. **Developmental delay** refers to a performance significantly below average in a given skill area. A **developmental quotient** (DQ) below 70 constitutes developmental delay. The DQ reflects the child's rate of development: DQ = (developmental age ÷ chronological age) × 100. **Developmental dissociation** refers to a substantial difference in the rate of development between two skill areas. An example of a developmental discrepancy between gross motor and language development is a child with isolated mental retardation whose gross motor development is normal. *Language is the best indicator of future intellectual achievement.* Language development is divided into two streams, receptive and expressive, each assigned a separate DQ.

Premature infants require age-adjusted parameters for assessment of their developmental achievement. Until 2 years of age, a child's chronological age should take into account the gestational age at birth. For example, at his or her 9-month checkup, a former premature infant born at 28 weeks' gestation should be able to perform skills appropriate for a child 6 months of age.

Sexual development is covered in Chapter 21.

DEVELOPMENTAL DELAY

MENTAL RETARDATION

Mental retardation, as defined in the *Diagnostic and Statistical Manual of Mental Disorders, Fourth Edition (DSM-IV)*, involves (a) IQ (intellectual quotient) of 70 or less; (b) onset before 18 years of age, and (c) functional impairment in adaptive functioning (in at least two of these areas: communication, self-care, home living, social/interpersonal skills, use of community resources, self-direction, academic skills, work, leisure, health, and safety).

An IQ of 50 to 55 to 70 denotes **mild** retardation, 35 to 40 to 50 to 55 denotes **moderate** retardation, 20 to 25 to 35 to 40 denotes **severe** retardation, and below 20 to 25 denotes **profound** retardation. (Note: An alternate method of classifying mental retardation based on levels of support needed has proved less useful clinically.) The great majority of affected patients (85%) are classified in the mild range. Mild retardation is more likely to be caused by environmental factors, whereas most cases of severe retardation are biologic (genetic, neurologic, metabolic) in origin. The most commonly used IQ tests in the pediatric population are the **Wechsler** scales (preschool and school age) and the **Stanford-Binet** (school age). Mental retardation may come to the attention of the pediatrician when the child exhibits developmental

■ TABLE 4-1 Commonly Quizzed Developmental Milestones

Age	Gross Motor	Fine (Visual) Motor	Language	Social
1 mo	Raises head slightly from prone	Follows with eyes to midline only; tight grasp	Alerts/startles to sound	Fixes on face
2 mo			Smiles responsively	Recognizes parent
3 mo	Holds head up	Hands open at rest	Coos	Reaches for familiar objects or people
4–5 mo	Rolls front to back, back to front; sits well supported	Grasps with both hands together	Orients to voice	Enjoys observing environment
6 mo	Sits well unsupported	Transfers hand to hand; reaches with either hand	Babbles	Recognizes strangers
9 mo	Crawls, cruises, pulls to stand	Uses pincer grasp; finger-feeds	Begins to use "dada/mama"; understands "no"	Plays pat-a-cake
12 mo	Walks alone	Throws, releases objects	1–8 words other than "dada/mama"; follows one-step commands	Imitates; comes when called; cooperates with dressing
15 mo	Walks backward; creeps upstairs	Builds two-block tower; scribbles		
18 mo	Runs	Feeds self (messily) with utensils	Points to body parts when asked	Plays around (not with) other children
24 mo	Walks well up and down stairs; squats and recovers	Removes clothing; builds five-block tower	Understands two-step commands; stranger understands half of speech; two-word combinations	Parallel play
3 yr	Pedals tricycle; throws ball overhand	Draws a circle	Three-word sentences; uses plurals, pronouns, past tense; knows first and last names; stranger understands three fourths of speech	Group play; shares
4 yr	Alternates feet going down stairs; skips	Catches ball; dresses alone	100% of speech intelligible	Imaginative play
5 yr		Ties shoes	Prints first name	Plays cooperative games; understands "rules" and abides by them

delay in one or more areas. Occasionally, dysmorphisms are present that suggest a syndrome (Down's syndrome, fragile X syndrome). Laboratory testing may be beneficial when a genetic cause is suggested and the parents desire more children. Co-morbid conditions (cerebral palsy, behavioral disorders, and seizures) are common and may be specific to the syndrome. Treatment is interdisciplinary, supportive, and symptom specific, with the goals of maximizing function and quality of life.

SPEECH AND LANGUAGE DELAY

Our ability to speak impacts our ability to communicate with others and develop social relationships. Speech delay or difficulty is the most common developmental concern raised by parents. As many as 15% of preschoolers have some sort of language delay at one time or another. Persistent speech delay that significantly impacts a child's ability to communicate becomes a speech disorder. In many cases, no underlying biologic abnormality (genetic syndrome, neuromuscular disease) exists to explain the disorder.

Language disorders result in the inability to understand or acquire the vocabulary, grammatical rules, or conversation patterns of the language. **Speech disorders** involve difficulty producing the speech sounds and the rhythm of speech. **Phonetic disorders** are problems with the articulation of the language. Speech and phonetic disorders are expressive disorders, whereas language disorders may affect both expressive and receptive language skills.

Disfluency describes interruption in the flow of speech. Developmental disfluency occurs in many preschoolers, resolves by 4 years of age, and is not pathologic. True disfluency **(stuttering)** is characterized by signs of tension and struggle when speaking, repetition or complete speech blockage, and significant compromise in the ability to communicate.

Parental concern is a good predictor of the need for further workup. Because many young children are uncomfortable exhibiting their speech for strangers, the history should concentrate on discerning the quantity and quality of the child's speech. *Any child with suspected language delay should receive a full audiologic (hearing) assessment.* (Note: The most common cause of mild-to-moderate hearing loss in a young child is chronic otitis media with effusions.) This should be followed by referral to a speech pathologist for further workup and treatment (if indicated). Early and intensive therapy can result in significant improvement in communication skills over time.

4-1 KEY POINTS

1. Developmental quotient (DQ) is calculated as follows: DQ = (developmental age ÷ chronological age) × 100.
2. Language is the best indicator of future intellectual achievement.
3. Until 2 years of age, a child's chronological age should be adjusted for gestational age at birth.
4. The Wechsler preschool scale is used to assess intelligence quotient (IQ) in preschoolers.
5. Disfluency may be developmental in children 3 and 4 years of age. Disfluency, accompanied by tension, struggle, and/or total word blockage *or* that severely limits communication should be considered true disfluency (stuttering) necessitating referral to a speech therapist.
6. Any child with a suspected speech or language disorder should be referred for a full hearing evaluation.

VARIATIONS IN DEVELOPMENTAL PATTERNS

ATTENTION DEFICIT HYPERACTIVITY DISORDER

Attention deficit hyperactivity disorder (ADHD) is a syndrome composed of **inattention, hyperactivity,** and **impulsivity** to the extent that the behavior is maladaptive and inconsistent with the developmental stage of the child. ADHD may be found in 5% of girls and 10% of boys in elementary school. School performance and peer relationships in particular suffer; these patients are at risk for the development of low self-esteem. Up to 70% of those affected with ADHD as a child have persistent symptoms into adulthood.

DIFFERENTIAL DIAGNOSIS

Attention deficit disorder (ADD) may occur without the element of hyperactivity. Inattentiveness is the primary symptom. These children are typically diagnosed later than their hyperactive peers, even throughout middle and high school years.

Clinical Manifestations

For a diagnosis of ADHD to be made, a child must meet the criteria outlined in the *DSM-IV* (Table 4-2). The diagnosis of ADHD requires the persistent presence of

■ **TABLE 4-2** Diagnostic Criteria for Attention Deficit Hyperactivity Disorder

Symptoms of inattention

    Failing to give attention to detail

    Difficulty completing tasks

    Difficulty organizing activities

    Avoids activities that require sustained mental effort

    Easily distracted by external forces

    Forgetful in daily activities

Symptoms of hyperactivity

    Fidgets and squirms

    Unable to remain in position

    Feelings of restlessness

    Unable to enjoy activities quietly

    Talks excessively

Symptoms of impulsivity

    Difficulty waiting turn

    Interrupts others

NOTE: These symptoms should be present in two or more settings and result in impaired functioning. In addition, the symptoms must be present prior to the patient reaching 7 years of age.
Adapted from American Psychiatric Association. Diagnostic and statistical manual of mental disorders. 4th ed. Washington, DC: American Psychiatric Association, 1994.

inattention, hyperactivity, and impulsiveness in multiple environments (e.g., in school and at home). The symptoms must be present for at least 6 months and are usually present by 7 years of age. However, the signs of ADHD may be minimized in settings that are able to provide immediate reinforcement, are new to the child, or are highly supervised. With this in mind, a child may not display any signs of ADHD when in the pediatrician's office.

Assessment

To assess a child with possible ADHD, a physician must rely on information obtained from parents and teachers. Various rating scales (depending on the patient's age) are available for teacher and parent use. The Conner's Parent and Teacher Rating Scales are the most commonly used for school-age children. A complete physical examination should be performed, but normally the sensory, physical, and neurologic examinations are normal.

Management

The treatment goal is to provide symptom reduction throughout the entire day. The treatment program for ADHD requires a multidisciplinary approach. Emotional supports should be made available for the patient and parents. A behavior management program must be developed to assist both the parents and teachers with discipline. The patient's academic needs should be met; up to 25% of children with ADHD also have a learning disability. Co-morbid conditions are common and may include aggression problems, oppositional defiant disorder, conduct problems, and mood disorders.

Pharmacologic treatments have been proven to be superior to behavior modification alone. Psycho-stimulants, including **methylphenidate, dextroamphetamine**, and **mixed amphetamine salts** (Adderall), have a long history of use. All are designated as controlled substances. These drugs work by increasing the availability of dopamine and norepinephrine in the central nervous system (CNS). Side effects include insomnia and anorexia; sometimes tics and dyskinesias may develop. However, recent Food and Drug Administration (FDA) approval for **atomoxetine** in the treatment of childhood ADHD has led to an increase in the use of this non-stimulant medication. Atomoxetine (Strattera) is a highly specific norepinephrine reuptake inhibitor with a low incidence of side effects and low abuse potential. Pharmacologic treatment should never be given in isolation, and at least once a year the patient deserves a trial off medications.

PERVASIVE DEVELOPMENTAL DISORDER

Pervasive developmental disorder (PDD) represents a spectrum of chronic nonprogressive developmental disabilities involving impairments in social interaction, communication, and behavior. Table 4-3 lists the *DSM-IV* criteria. Autism is a form of PDD, as is Asperger's syndrome. PDD is seen in 2 to 6 children per 1,000 children and is four times more common in boys. Most children present between 18 months and 3 years of age, but symptoms can be present from infancy (impaired attachment). No single underlying cause has been identified. *Long-term epidemiologic studies have not shown an association between the measles-mumps-rubella (MMR) vaccine or thimerosal* (a preservative formerly present in some vaccines) *and the development of autism.*

TABLE 4-3 Diagnostic Criteria for Pervasive Developmental Disorder

Impairments in social interactions

Lack of nonverbal behaviors

Lack of peer relationships

Lack of showing interest

Lack of emotional reciprocity

Impairments in communication

Developmental language delay

Unable to sustain a conversation with others

Use of repetitive language

Lack of social play

Presence of stereotypic behaviors

Inflexible adherence to rituals

Stereotypic motor mannerisms

Preoccupation with objects

Adapted from American Psychiatric Association. Diagnostic and statistical manual of mental disorders. 4th ed. Washington, DC: American Psychiatric Association, 1994.

Clinical Manifestations

Children with **autism** have significant language and communication abnormalities and problems with social interactions. They use very limited eye contact, do not exhibit reciprocal communication, and do not engage in pretend play. These children usually display stereotypic and/or repetitive behavior patterns and may have an attachment to or fascination with unusual objects. Children with **PDD-NOS** ("not otherwise specified") have less severe disruptions in social relationships, communication, and behavior; PDD-NOS has also been referred to in the literature as "subthreshold autism."

Asperger's syndrome is characterized by difficulty forming relationships and/or relating to others and development of intense interest in very specific topics (dinosaurs, ancient Egyptian mummies). Although people with Asperger do not have an obvious language

disorder, they do not pick up on nonverbal cues, and they do not understand abstract forms of language such as metaphors and sarcasm. Children with Asperger usually want to form friendships, but their inability to pick up on subtle social cues makes this difficult.

Management

No pharmacologic treatment is available for PDD. Some children will benefit from medication designed to target specific symptoms such as anxiety, hyperactivity, and perseverative behaviors. Treatment involves behavioral therapy, improving communication, and providing parental support. (Note: At the present time, dietary manipulation, supplements, secretin infusion, and medication [antibiotics, intravenous immunoglobulin, chelation] are being studied but have not been proven effective.) What is clear is that early recognition and intervention lead to better clinical outcomes. The best prognostic indicator of future success is the extent of language development present during the preschool years.

4-2 KEY POINTS

1. The elements of attention deficit hyperactivity disorder (ADHD) are inattentiveness, hyperactivity, and impulsivity. Attention deficit disorder (ADD) has inattention as the primary symptom.
2. Atomoxetine is a highly specific norepinephrine reuptake inhibitor approved for use in childhood ADHD. It is not a stimulant, has few side effects, and has low abuse potential.
3. Pervasive developmental disorder (PDD) represents a spectrum of chronic nonprogressive developmental disabilities involving impairments in social interaction, communication, and behavior. Autism, PDD-NOS (not otherwise specified), and Asperger's syndrome are forms of PDD.
4. Neither the measles-mumps-rubella (MMR) vaccine nor thimerosal is associated with the development of autism.

Additional Suggested Reading

Agin MC. The "late talker"—when silence isn't golden. *Contemp Pediatr.* 2004;21:22–32.

American Academy of Pediatrics. Clinical practice guideline: diagnosis and evaluation of the child with attention-deficit/hyperactivity disorder. *Pediatrics.* 2000;105:1158–1170.

Feldman HM. Evaluation and management of speech disorders in preschool children. *Pediatr Rev.* 2005;26:131–141.

Madsen KM, Hviid A, Vestergaard M. A population-based study of measles, mumps, and rubella vaccination and autism. *N Engl J Med.* 2002;347:1477–1482.

Madsen KM, Lauritsen MB, Pederson CB, et al. Thimerosal and the occurrence of autism: negative ecological evidence from Danish population-based data. *Pediatrics.* 2003;112(3):604–606.

Michelson D, Faries D, Wernicke J, et al. Atomoxetine in the treatment of children and adolescents with attention-deficit/hyperactivity disorder: a randomized, placebo-controlled, dose-response study. *Pediatrics.* 2001;108:1–9.

Nash PL, Coury DL. Screening tools assist with diagnosis of autistic spectrum disorders. *Pediatr Ann.* 2003;32:664–671.

Simms MD, Schum RL. Preschool children who have atypical patterns of development. *Pediatr Rev.* 2000;21:147–158.

5 Dermatology

VIRAL EXANTHEMS

CLINICAL MANIFESTATIONS

Certain viral exanthems are characteristic for particular viral illnesses. Although **measles** is uncommon in developed countries where vaccines are used, it continues to be a major health problem worldwide. The incubation period is 8 to 12 days after initial exposure to the paramyxovirus; there are no signs or symptoms during this stage. A prodrome follows, consisting of malaise, high fever, and the classic triad of cough, coryza, and conjunctivitis. Within 2 to 3 days of the onset of symptoms, characteristic Koplik spots (small irregular red spots with central gray or bluish white specks) appear on the buccal mucosa. Approximately 5 days after the onset of symptoms, an erythematous maculopapular rash erupts on the head and spreads caudally, lasting 4 to 5 days. Diagnosis is made by the distinctive history and characteristic clinical findings; however, it may be confirmed by serologic testing. Severe complications include acute encephalitis (which may result in brain damage) and subacute sclerosing panencephalitis.

Rubella is generally innocuous when acquired postnatally, but when a fetus is infected during gestation the results can be devastating. For details on congenital rubella, see Chapter 13. Rubella is caused by rubella virus, an RNA togavirus. Clinical manifestations in postnatally acquired rubella are absent in many cases. There is no prodrome during the incubation period of 14 to 21 days. When symptoms do occur, rubella is characterized by an erythematous, maculopapular, discrete rash, with generalized lymphadenopathy and slight fever. The rash rarely lasts longer than 5 days. Fever may accompany the onset of rash. Transient polyarthralgia and polyarthritis are common in adolescents. Encephalitis and thrombocytopenia are rare complications. Postnatally acquired rubella is confirmed by serologic testing. The diagnosis of rubella is often difficult because the symptoms are mild and may be confused with those of enteroviral infection, roseola, toxoplasmosis, infectious mononucleosis, mild measles, and scarlet fever.

Roseola infantum is a common acute disease of infants and young children caused by human herpesvirus 6 (HHV-6). The illness begins with an abrupt fever characterized by temperatures of 103°F to 106°F (39.4° to 41.0°C) that persist for 1 to 5 days. During the fever, the child generally appears well and has no physical findings to explain the fever. On the third or fourth day of illness, a maculopapular rash appears on the trunk and spreads peripherally. The rash typically appears as the fever resolves. Initially, leukocytosis up to 20,000 per μL with a left shift may exist, but by the second day of illness, leukopenia and neutropenia may be noted. Complications are uncommon, although febrile seizures may occur because of the rapid increase in temperature during the onset of infection.

Erythema infectiosum (Fifth disease) is a mild, self-limited, systemic illness caused by the DNA-containing parvovirus B19. It primarily occurs in epidemics. Usually there is no prodrome, and fever may be absent or low grade. The rash progresses through three stages. It begins as a marked erythema of the cheeks, which gives a "**slapped cheek**" appearance. A lacy or reticulate, erythematous, pruritic rash then starts on the arms and spreads to the trunk and legs. The third stage is characterized by fluctuations in the severity of the rash and usually lasts 2 to 3 weeks. Fluctuations occur with temperature changes and exposure to sunlight. Complications include arthritis, hemolytic anemia, and encephalopathy. Parvovirus B19 infection during pregnancy is associated with fetal hydrops and death of the fetus. In some patients with parvovirus B19 infection, a petechial eruption may develop in a gloves-and-stocking distribution.

Hand-foot-and-mouth disease is a common acute disease of young children during the spring and summer caused by coxsackie A viruses. There is usually a prodrome of fever, anorexia, and oral pain, followed by crops of ulcers on the tongue and oral mucosa and a vesicular rash on the hands, feet, and occasionally the buttocks. The individual vesicles often have a "football" shape with surrounding erythema. Diagnosis is made by the history and the constellation of symptoms.

Varicella (chickenpox) is a highly contagious disease caused by primary infection with varicella-zoster virus. It is usually a mild, self-limited disease in normal children. Its severity can range from a few lesions and a low-grade fever to hundreds of lesions and a temperature up to 105°F (40.6°C). Fatal disseminated disease may occur in immunocompromised children or in neonates whose mothers develop the infection within 1 week of delivery. After an incubation period of 10 to 21 days, there is a prodrome consisting of mild fever, malaise, anorexia, and occasionally a scarlatiniform or morbilliform rash. The characteristic pruritic rash occurs the following day, appearing first on the trunk and then spreading peripherally. The rash begins as red papules and develops rapidly into clear vesicles that are approximately 1 to 2 mm in diameter. The vesicles then become cloudy, break, and form scabs. The lesions occur in widely scattered "crops," so several stages of lesions are usually present at the same time. Vesicles often occur on mucous membranes. Patients are infectious from 24 hours before the appearance of the rash until all the lesions are crusted, which usually occurs 1 week after the onset of the rash.

Chickenpox is a clinical diagnosis. In unclear cases, a Tzanck test, looking for multinucleated giant cells, can be performed on a vesicle, or a pharyngeal swab or swab of vesicular fluid can be sent for viral culture. Most centers now perform direct fluorescent antibody (DFA) testing, which can rapidly identify the presence of infected cells. Other confirmatory techniques include viral culture for varicella (which may take a week to obtain results) and polymerase chain reaction (PCR) testing. Progressive varicella with meningoencephalitis, hepatitis, and pneumonitis may occur in immunocompromised children and is associated with a 20% mortality rate. Immunization with varicella vaccine has reduced the frequency of this infection in the United States.

Herpes zoster (shingles) represents a reactivation of varicella-zoster virus infection and occurs predominantly in adults who previously have had varicella and have circulating antibodies. After chickenpox, varicella-zoster virus retreats to the dorsal root ganglion; as a result, it follows a dermatomal distribution when reactivated. Although herpes zoster occurs in children, it is uncommon in those younger than 10 years. An attack of zoster begins with pain along the affected sensory nerve and is accompanied by fever and malaise. A vesicular eruption then appears in crops confined to the dermatomal distribution and clears in 7 to 14 days. The rash may last as long as 4 weeks, however, with pain persisting for weeks or months.

Other complications from zoster include encephalopathy, aseptic meningitis, Guillain-Barré's syndrome, pneumonitis, thrombocytopenic purpura, cellulitis, and arthritis. Figure 5-1 shows typical herpes zoster eruptions.

TREATMENT

In uncomplicated cases, treatment is mainly supportive. Fever is treated with acetaminophen or ibuprofen and fluids. (Note: Ibuprofen is contraindicated when varicella is suspected because of the increased risk of streptococcal cellulitis.) Aspirin should be avoided because aspirin therapy for fever in the setting of a viral infection is associated with Reye's syndrome. The itching associated with Fifth disease, varicella, and herpes zoster may be treated with an oral antihistamine medication. During chickenpox, daily bathing in lukewarm water reduces the risk of secondary bacterial infection. Herpes zoster can be quite painful, and narcotics are sometimes needed. Immunocompromised children who are exposed to someone with varicella-zoster virus infection are given varicella-zoster immune globulin within 96 hours of the exposure and observed closely. Acyclovir is effective in the treatment

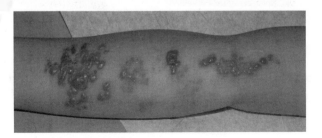

Figure 5-1 • Herpes zoster.
Image courtesy of Albert C. Yan, MD.

of both varicella and zoster; its use is indicated in immunocompromised patients. Systemic administration of antivirals, such as acyclovir, may be considered for use in patients older than 12 years, children with chronic disease, and those who have received systemic steroids for any reason. Administration of the varicella vaccine within 72 hours of exposure may prevent or lessen disease. Immunizations are available for the prevention of measles, rubella, and varicella (see Chapter 12).

5-1 KEY POINTS

1. Viral exanthems are generally benign and treated symptomatically.
2. The exanthems are differentiated by history and rash appearance.
3. Children with chickenpox are contagious from 24 hours before the onset of rash until all lesions have crusted over.

BACTERIAL RASHES

Bacterial rashes of the skin are common, and in most cases they are the result of group A β-hemolytic streptococcal or *Staphylococcus aureus* infection.

↳ NORMAL SKIN FLORA

CLINICAL MANIFESTATIONS

Bullous impetigo, which is caused by a toxin-producing strain of *S. aureus*, begins as red macules that progress to bullous (fluid-filled) eruptions on an erythematous base. These lesions range from a few millimeters to a few centimeters in diameter. After the bullae rupture, a clear, thin, varnishlike coating forms over the denuded area. *S. aureus* can be cultured from the vesicular fluid. Bullous impetigo lesions can be mistaken for cigarette burns, raising the suspicion of abuse.

Nonbullous impetigo, which is caused by both group A β-hemolytic streptococci and *S. aureus*, begins as papules that progress to vesicles and then to painless pustules measuring approximately 5 mm in diameter with a thin erythematous rim. The pustules rupture, revealing a honey-colored thin exudate that then forms a crust over a shallow ulcerated base. Local lymphadenopathy is common with streptococcal impetigo. Fever is uncommon. The causative organism can usually be isolated from the lesions.

Staphylococcal scalded skin syndrome, which is caused by exfoliative toxin-producing isolates of

S. aureus, is most common in infancy and rarely occurs beyond 5 years of age. Onset is abrupt, with diffuse erythema, marked skin tenderness, and fever. Within 12 to 24 hours of onset, superficial flaccid bullae develop and then rupture almost immediately, leaving a beefy red, weeping surface. Although widespread areas may be affected, accentuation is seen on periorificial areas of the face, as well as areas around the neck, axillae, and inguinal creases. Exfoliation is caused by a toxin and may affect most of the body, and there is usually a positive **Nikolsky sign** (separation of the epidermis on light rubbing). The initial focus of staphylococcal infection may be minor or not apparent. Unruptured bullae contain sterile fluid.

Folliculitis is an infection of the shaft of the hair follicle. Superficial folliculitis is common and easily treated. Deep forms of this infection include furuncles (boils) and carbuncles. **Furuncles** begin as superficial folliculitis and are most frequently found in areas of hair-bearing skin that are subject to friction and maceration, especially the scalp, buttocks, and axillae. **Carbuncles** are an accumulation of furuncles.

Cellulitis is a localized, acute inflammation of the skin characterized by erythema, pain, and warmth. Cellulitis in children is most often caused by group A β-hemolytic streptococcal or *S. aureus* infection. These bacteria are normal flora of the skin, and a break in the integument allows entry into the dermis and epidermis. The location of the infection is important because in rare cases the cellulitis may arise from an underlying osteomyelitis, septic arthritis, sinusitis, or deep wound infection. Before the use of *Haemophilus influenzae* type b (Hib) vaccine, *H. influenzae* type b was a significant pathogen, resulting in many cases of cellulitis by hematogenous spread. *H. influenzae* type b cellulitis is now rarely seen. Currently, *Streptococcus pneumoniae* is the most common cause of hematogenously spread cellulitis. Hematogenously spread *S. pneumoniae* often affects the face and periorbital area. Cellulitis of the face, depending on whether it results from trauma or hematogenous spread, can result from all the pathogens mentioned: group A β-hemolytic streptococci, *S. aureus*, *S. pneumoniae*, or *H. influenzae* type b.

TREATMENT

Limited nonbullous impetigo can be treated topically with mupirocin ointment. Bullous impetigo and nonbullous impetigo, if the lesions are numerous, are treated with a first-generation cephalosporin such as cephalexin, an oral drug that is effective against both staphylococci and group A streptococci. In settings where methicillin-resistant *S. aureus* is suspected, agents such as clindamycin or trimethoprim-sulfamethoxazole may be more appropriate. The caretaker can remove any honey-colored crusts with twice-daily cool compresses.

Mild to moderate cases of staphylococcal scalded skin are treated with an oral antistaphylococcal medication. Children with severe cases should be treated as though they had a second-degree burn, with meticulous fluid management and intravenous oxacillin or clindamycin.

Superficial folliculitis responds to aggressive hygiene and topical mupirocin, whereas folliculitis of the male beard is unusually recalcitrant and needs an oral antistaphylococcal drug. Simple furunculosis is treated with moist heat. Larger and deeper furuncles may need to be incised and drained. After drainage, they need only topical mupirocin treatment.

Children with mild cellulitis can be treated with an oral antibiotic, such as cephalexin or amoxicillin-clavulanic acid. Those with severe infection who have lymphangitic streaking or lymphadenopathy may be hospitalized and given a parenteral antibiotic. Facial or periorbital cellulitis (see Chapter 18) usually is treated with intravenous ampicillin-sulbactam or cefuroxime and admission to the hospital for observation. When orbital or periorbital cellulitis is present or a peripheral skin cellulitis results in lymphadenopathy or lymphangitic streaking, a blood culture should be sent to determine whether bacteremia is present.

manifests as an annular lesion with peripheral scaling, giving it the appearance of a ring (hence the name *ringworm*). Scraping of the edge of a lesion and examining the scrapings with potassium hydroxide under microscopy will reveal septated, branching hyphae. On the scalp, **tinea capitis** manifests as patches of scaling and hair loss, sometimes associated with itching and lymphadenopathy. **Tinea pedis** classically presents as scaling in a "moccasin" distribution, frequently also involving the interdigital spaces of the toes. **Tinea cruris** presents with erythema, scaling, and maceration in inguinal creases. Most superficial skin infections can be treated with topical antifungals. However, systemic antifungal agents are necessary to eradicate fungal infections of the nails or hair. Table 5-1 presents tinea infections and their treatments. Figure 5-2A and 5-2B show tinea corporis and capitis, respectively.

Tinea (pityriasis) versicolor, another type of yeast infection caused by *Malassezia furfur*, is characterized by superficial tan or hypopigmented oval scaly lesions on the neck, upper part of the back, chest, and proximal arms in a Christmas tree distribution. Dark-skinned individuals tend to have hypopigmented lesions during the summer when uninfected skin darkens from sunlight exposure. However, individual patients may demonstrate both dark- and light-colored lesions at the same time (hence the name *versicolor*). Treatment is with selenium sulfide shampoo or other antifungal

---

🔑 5-2 KEY POINTS

1. *S. aureus* and group A β-hemolytic streptococci cause most bacterial skin infections.
2. Because of the Hib vaccine, *Streptococcus pneumoniae* has replaced *Haemophilus influenzae* as the most common pathogen in hematogenously spread cellulitis.
3. The child with peripheral cellulitis with lymphadenopathy or lymphangitic streaking and the child with orbital or periorbital cellulitis should have a blood culture sent to determine whether bacteremia is present.

SUPERFICIAL FUNGAL RASHES

Essentially, three fungal organisms cause superficial tinea infections: *Trichophyton*, *Microsporum*, and *Epidermophyton*. On the skin, **tinea corporis** frequently

---

■ TABLE 5-1 Common Tinea Infections and Their Treatments

Infection	Treatment
Tinea capitis (scalp)	Oral griseofulvin, 4–6 wk
	Selenium sulfide shampoo to decrease infectivity; does not eradicate infection
Tinea corporis (body) "ringworm"	Topical antifungals (e.g., clotrimazole) for at least 4 wk; oral griseofulvin if refractory
Tinea cruris (genitocrural) "jock itch"	Same as tinea corporis
Tinea pedis (foot) "athlete's foot"	Same as tinea corporis, plus proper foot hygiene

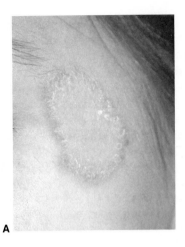 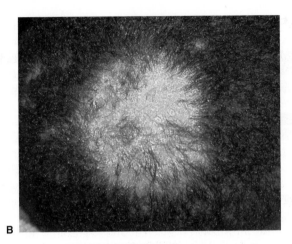

A **B**

Figure 5-2 • A: Tinea corporis. **B:** Tinea capitis.
Images courtesy of Albert C. Yan, MD.

agent. Figure 5-3 shows characteristic hypopigmented oval scaly lesions noted within tinea versicolor.

Diaper rash may result from atopic dermatitis, primary irritant dermatitis, or primary or secondary *Candida albicans* infection. Eighty percent of diaper rashes lasting more than 4 days are colonized with *Candida*. Fiery red papular lesions with peripheral scales in the skin folds and satellite lesions are typical for candidal diaper rash. Barrier creams along with topical **nystatin** are the first-line treatments of choice.

Figure 5-3 • Tinea versicolor.
Image courtesy of Albert C. Yan, MD.

ACNE

PATHOGENESIS

Acne vulgaris is caused by enlargement of sebaceous glands, increased sebum production, proliferation of *Propionibacterium acnes*, and secondary inflammatory changes. There is a predilection for face, chest, and back. Lesions progress from comedones (whiteheads), to open comedones (blackheads), to pustules, to papules, to nodules (cysts), and finally to atrophic and hypertrophic scars or keloids. Androgens are the stimulus for sebaceous gland development and secretion. At puberty, hormonal stimuli lead to increased growth and development of sebaceous follicles. Female patients with severe acne often have high levels of circulating androgens. Figure 5-4 illustrates typical acne lesions.

EPIDEMIOLOGY

Acne is a very common, self-limited, multifactorial disorder of the sebaceous follicles noted during the teenage years. Lesions may begin as early as 8 to 10 years of age. Prevalence increases steadily throughout adolescence and then decreases in adulthood. Although girls often develop acne at a younger age than boys, severe disease affects boys ten times more frequently because of higher androgen levels. In fact, 15% of all teenage boys have severe acne.

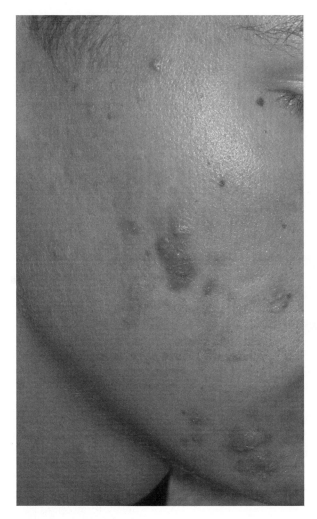

Figure 5-4 • Acne vulgaris.
Image courtesy of Albert C. Yan, MD.

RISK FACTORS

Risk factors include male gender, puberty, oily complexion, Cushing syndrome, or any other process that results in increased androgens.

CLINICAL MANIFESTATIONS

History

It is important to determine when the acne started and whether there is a family history of acne. A full menstrual history should be taken to determine a possible correlation between the onset of menses and the patient's acne exacerbations. It is also important to discuss the patient's skin care, including how the patient's acne has been treated in the past. Many drugs cause acne. Corticosteroids, androgens, danazol, iodides, and bromides often exacerbate acne. Other possible stimuli include isoniazid, lithium, halothane, vitamin B_{12}, and hyperalimentation. These drugs are not directly comedogenic but "prime" the follicular epithelium to the comedogenic effects of sebum.

Physical Examination

Distribution, morphology, and severity of lesions should be recorded. It is important to differentiate common acne from **nodulocystic** acne because the latter invariably results in hypertrophic or pitted scarring.

DIFFERENTIAL DIAGNOSIS

The differential diagnosis for acneiform rashes includes acne vulgaris, drug-induced acne, Cushing syndrome, or other pathologies that increase endogenous steroid secretion and perioral dermatitis. Rosacea, an acneiform eruption of the central face and neck, is sometimes confused with acne, but it is primarily seen in adults.

TREATMENT

Treatment should be individualized depending on the patient's gender and the severity, type, and distribution of lesions.

Benzoyl peroxide works by decreasing the colonization of *P. acnes* and decreasing the development of microcomedomes by lessening the concentration of surface free fatty acids. Topical **retinoids** (e.g., tretinoin, adapalene, tazarotene) have strong anticomedogenic activity; however, side effects may limit use and include dryness, burning, and, most important, photosensitivity by reducing the thickness of the stratum corneum layer. The use of sunscreen with a sun protective factor (SPF) of at least 15 is necessary. Topical and systemic **antibiotics** are used to prevent and decrease colonization of *P. acnes*. Topical antibiotics are also available in combination with benzoyl peroxide. The systemic antibiotics used include tetracycline, doxycycline, minocycline, and erythromycin. In some cases, oral contraceptives with low levels of androgens may also be helpful by suppressing androgen production.

To maximize the therapeutic benefits, combination therapy is usually prescribed. *Mild* acne with few comedones is treated with benzoyl peroxide and topical antibiotics. Mild acne generally responds to therapy without scarring.

The presence of many comedones with some papules and pustules is characteristic of *moderate* acne. Therapy includes benzoyl peroxide, topical retinoids, and topical or oral antibiotics. Response to treatment is variable, and scarring is a possibility with this grade of acne.

Severe acne is characterized by inflammatory papules, pustules, cysts, abscesses, and scarring. Treatment consists of topical therapy and sebaceous gland–suppressive agents, including estrogens, steroids, and oral **retinoic acid** (Accutane). Because of its teratogenicity, a negative pregnancy test must be obtained within 2 weeks of initiating retinoic acid therapy, and contraception must be used from 1 month before to 1 month after therapy. Controversial associations of isotretinoin and mood alterations have also been reported. Isotretinoin therapy usually lasts 4 to 6 months.

🔑 5-3 KEY POINTS

1. Nodulocystic acne is associated with scarring.
2. Acne is best treated with combination therapy.
3. Therapies include topical agents (benzoyl peroxide, retinoids, and antibiotics) and oral medications (antibiotics, oral contraceptives, and retinoic acid).

PSORIASIS

PATHOGENESIS

The pathogenesis of **psoriasis** is unknown. A multifactorial inheritance pattern has been proposed. Children with HLA type C6 are clearly more likely to develop the disease. Histologically, there is hyperproliferation of the epidermis, and epidermal turnover time is noted to be distinctly accelerated in those affected. The rash usually appears at sites of physical, thermal, or mechanical trauma. This is known as the **Köbner phenomenon**, a diagnostic feature of the disease.

EPIDEMIOLOGY

Psoriasis is considered by some to be an adult disease, but 10% of cases begin before 10 years of age, and 35% before 20 years of age. Fifty percent of children with psoriasis have a positive family history for the disease. If psoriasis is present during adolescence, it is likely a lifelong disease.

RISK FACTORS

HLA inheritance is part of the mode of transmission; therefore, a positive family history is a significant risk factor.

CLINICAL MANIFESTATIONS

History and Physical Examination

The nonpruritic rash consists of erythematous papules that coalesce to form plaques with sharply demarcated borders and a silvery or yellow-white scale. The scales tend to build up into layers, and their removal may result in pinpoint bleeding **(Auspitz sign)**. The rash is usually symmetric, with plaques appearing over the knees, elbows, scalp, and genital area. The scalp frequently has a thick adherent scale with alopecia at sites of involvement. The nails often demonstrate punctate stippling or pitting, detachment of the nail plate (onycholysis), and accumulation of subungual debris. Examination of the palms and soles reveals scaling and fissuring. Psoriatic arthritis may also be present in a subset of patients. Figure 5-5 demonstrates the scaly plaques noted in psoriasis.

DIFFERENTIAL DIAGNOSIS

The differential diagnosis for a psoriatic rash in children includes uncommon disorders such as Reiter's syndrome, pityriasis rubra pilaris, and lichen planus. **Reiter's syndrome**, in contrast to simple psoriasis, is a psoriaticlike rash that involves the mucous membranes. In some severe cases in which the rash is also accompanied by arthritis, the lesions of the mucous membrane are the main differentiating point between psoriasis and Reiter's syndrome. Occasionally, atopic dermatitis may be confused with psoriasis; however, eczema is pruritic and concentrated in flexural creases, whereas psoriasis is not usually pruritic and favors extensor surfaces. Scalp lesions may be confused with seborrheic dermatitis or tinea capitis.

DIAGNOSTIC EVALUATION

The diagnosis is a clinical one. Skin biopsy is seldom necessary but may show a hyperplastic epidermis,

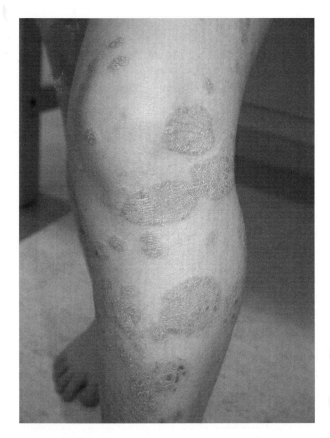

Figure 5-5 • Psoriasis.
Image courtesy of Albert C. Yan, MD.

ALLERGIC RASHES

Atopic dermatitis, urticaria, and angioedema are discussed in Chapter 11.

ERYTHEMA MULTIFORME

Erythema multiforme is an acute, self-limited, hypersensitivity reaction that is uncommon in children. Common etiologic agents include viral infection (herpesvirus, adenovirus, and Epstein-Barr virus), *Mycoplasma pneumoniae* infection, drug ingestion (especially sulfa drugs), immunizations, and food reactions.

Clinical Manifestations

In erythema multiforme, a symmetric distribution of lesions evolves through multiple morphologic stages: erythematous macules, papules, plaques, vesicles, and target lesions. The lesions change over days, not hours. Erythema multiforme tends to occur over the dorsum of the hands and feet, palms and soles, and extensor surfaces of extremities, but it may spread to the trunk. Burning and itching are common. Systemic manifestations include fever, malaise, and myalgias. The most common cause of recurrent erythema multiforme in children is herpes simplex virus.

Stevens-Johnson's syndrome is the most severe form of erythema multiforme. There is a prodrome for 1 to 14 days of fever, malaise, myalgias, arthralgias, arthritis, headache, emesis, and diarrhea. This is followed by the sudden onset of high fever, erythema multiforme skin lesions, and inflammatory bullae of two or more mucous membranes (oral mucosa, lips, bulbar conjunctiva, and anogenital area). In the most severe cases, involvement of most of the gastrointestinal, respiratory,

thinning of the papillary dermis, and dermal vessels approaching close to the surface of the skin (which explains the Auspitz sign).

TREATMENT

Psoriasis is characterized by remissions and exacerbations. The most important aspect of treating psoriasis is to educate the patient and family that the disease is a chronic and recurrent one that cannot be cured but can be controlled with conscientious therapy. No matter the location or severity of the rash, the goal of psoriasis therapy is to keep the skin well hydrated. Tar preparations may be added to the daily bath or used as an ointment. For more severe cases, natural sunlight or ultraviolet B (UVB) light is used in conjunction with the tar lubricant. For small areas of involvement, fluorinated steroids may be successful; the least potent but effective dose should be used because adrenal suppression can occur.

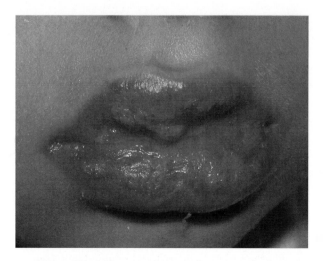

Figure 5-6 • Stevens-Johnson's syndrome.
Image courtesy of Albert C. Yan, MD.

or genitourinary tracts may be seen. Untreated, this syndrome has a mortality rate of approximately 10%. The most common causes of Stevens-Johnson's syndrome include drugs and mycoplasma infections. Figure 5-6 denotes the typical inflammatory bullae of the oral mucosa noted in Stevens-Johnson's syndrome.

Toxic epidermal necrolysis (TEN) is the most severe form of cutaneous hypersensitivity, considered by some to be a variant of Stevens-Johnson's syndrome. Although its occurrence in children is rare, it is associated with a 30% mortality rate. The pathogenesis appears to be related to upregulated expression of Fas ligand, a mediator of apoptosis. Most cases are secondary to medications, especially sulfa drugs, anticonvulsants, and nonsteroidal anti-inflammatory agents. Onset is acute, with high fever, a burning sensation of the skin and mucous membranes, and/or oral and conjunctival erythema and erosions. The presentation of the skin resembles that of staphylococcal scalded skin, with widespread erythema, tenderness, blister formation, and detachment of the epidermis causing denudation (positive Nikolsky sign). Mucous membrane involvement is severe, and the nails may be shed. Systemic complications include elevated liver enzymes, renal failure, and fluid and electrolyte imbalance. Sepsis and shock are frequent causes of death.

Treatment

For uncomplicated erythema multiforme, symptomatic treatment and reassurance are all that is necessary. Oral antihistamines, moist compresses, and oatmeal baths are helpful. The lesions resolve over a 1- to 3-week period, with some hyperpigmentation. The use of corticosteroids is controversial.

Treatment of the patient with Stevens-Johnson's syndrome includes hospitalization with barrier isolation, fluid and electrolyte support, treatment of common secondary infections of the skin, moist compresses on bullae, and colloidal baths. For oral mucosal lesions, mouthwashes with viscous lidocaine, diphenhydramine, and Maalox (aluminum hydroxide, magnesium hydroxide) are comforting. Because corneal ulceration, keratitis, uveitis, and panophthalmitis are possible, an ophthalmology consultation is recommended.

Children with toxic epidermal necrolysis are treated as though they had a full-body second-degree burn. Fluid therapy and reverse barrier isolation are critical to survival; many patients are treated in an intensive care or burn center unit. Intravenous immunoglobulin has been used with some success in several series of patients with TEN, presumably because of its effects of binding or modulating the effect of Fas ligand.

5-5 KEY POINTS

Stevens-Johnson's syndrome is erythema multiforme with oral mucosal bullae, whereas toxic epidermal necrolysis (TEN) is similar to staphylococcal scalded skin in that both result in sloughing of the epidermal layer.

HYPERPIGMENTED LESIONS

With the incidence of melanoma increasing, it is very important to identify suspicious lesions and understand risk factors. Children with fair skin, excessive sun exposure, and multiple nevi are at increased risk for skin cancer.

CONGENITAL NEVI

Congenital nevi are classified based on their size. Large or giant nevi are greater than 20 cm, small nevi are less than 2 cm, and intermediate nevi are between 2 and 20 cm. Research has shown an ill-defined but increased risk of melanoma in patients with congenital nevi. Congenital nevi must be followed annually for changes and may require complete excision. Giant nevi have an increased risk of melanoma (between 5% and 15%).

There is also an association with neurocutaneous melanosis, so patients with lesions over the head and spine, or with multiple associated satellite nevi, require an MRI to evaluate for central nervous system (CNS) involvement.

COMMON ACQUIRED NEVI

Many children go on to develop nevi, reaching a maximum number in early adulthood. Patients with more than 15 common acquired moles have an increased risk for melanoma in the future. Moles need to be assessed by using the ABCDs. Moles with **asymmetry**, irregular **borders**, variations in **color**, and **diameter** larger than 6 mm have atypical features and may require excision.

A **Spitz nevus** is a smooth pink to brown dome-shaped papule. These nevi are benign but may need to be removed if they grow rapidly. A **halo nevus** is a mole with a depigmented ring around it. These lesions are generally benign in children but may be associated with the presence of vitiligo or melanoma at another site.

PREVENTION

A large amount of childhood sun exposure and frequent sunburns are associated with increased risk for the development of moles and skin cancer. Sun protection with a sunblock having an SPF of 15 or more against UVB and ultraviolet A (UVA) light is recommended.

🔑 5-6 KEY POINTS

1. Moles need to be assessed for asymmetry, irregular borders, color, and size.
2. Sunblock against ultraviolet B and A (UVB and UVA) light is recommended to decrease the risk of melanoma.

Additional Suggested Reading

Hansen RC. Atopic dermatitis: taming "the itch that rashes." *Contemp Pediatr*. 2003;7:79–97:

Krowchuk DP. Managing adolescent acne: a guide for pediatricians. *Pediatr Rev*. 2005,26:250–261.

Leaute-Labreze C, Lamireau T Chawki D, et al. Diagnosis, classification, and management of erythema multiforme and Stevens-Johnson's syndrome. *Arch Dis Child*. 2000;25:965–972.

6 Endocrinology

DIABETES MELLITUS

DIABETES MELLITUS (TYPE 1)

Pathogenesis

Diabetes mellitus is a chronic metabolic disorder characterized by hyperglycemia and abnormal energy metabolism caused by absent or diminished insulin secretion. **Diabetes mellitus type 1** (type 1 DM) results from lack of insulin production in the β cells of the pancreas. Although the precise etiology of type 1 DM is unknown, genetic, autoimmune, and environmental factors have all been implicated.

After 90% of β-cell function has been destroyed, loss of insulin secretion becomes clinically significant. With the loss of insulin, the major anabolic hormone, a catabolic state develops, which decreases peripheral glucose utilization and increases hepatic glucose production by gluconeogenesis and glycogenolysis. The lack of insulin prevents glucose from entering the cell, and hyperglycemia results. The production of ketoacids is brought about by an increase in the catabolic mediators glucagon, epinephrine, growth hormone (GH), and cortisol. These messengers trigger lipolysis, fatty acid release, and ketoacid synthesis. When the blood glucose concentration exceeds 180 mg per dL, the resultant glycosuria causes an osmotic diuresis with increased urine output (polyuria). If insulin deficiency is severe, ketones are produced in significant quantities, the blood's native buffering capacity is overwhelmed, and **diabetic ketoacidosis** (DKA) results.

DKA is characterized by hyperglycemia, metabolic acidosis (ketoacidosis), dehydration, and lethargy. It is a medical emergency that, in severe cases, may progress to coma and death. The most common cause of DKA in the known diabetic is inadequate insulin dosing. The condition can also be triggered by insulin resistance, which is exacerbated by an intercurrent illness or extreme physiologic stress. Frequently, new-onset diabetics present in DKA. The most severe complication of DKA management is cerebral edema.

In addition to DKA, the other major complication seen in type 1 DM is hypoglycemia from insulin overdose, decreased caloric intake, or increased exercise without a concomitant increase in calories.

Epidemiology and Risk Factors

Type 1 DM is the most common endocrine disease in childhood, occurring in 1 in 500 children and adolescents. The main risk factor for type 1 DM is a positive family history. The presence of DR3 and DR4 major histocompatibility antigens increases the lifetime risk for an individual developing type 1 DM, as does having a first-degree relative with type 1 DM. There is a 50% concordance among identical twins. The presence of anti–islet cell antibodies in 85% of individuals with recent-onset DM and the increased appearance of other autoimmune diseases in children with type 1 DM make the case for an autoimmune etiology. The environmental role in disease pathogenesis remains unclear. No particular virus has been determined to be directly responsible.

Clinical Manifestations

History and Physical Examination

A history of new-onset weight loss, polydipsia, polyphagia, and polyuria is consistent with type 1 diabetes mellitus. The physical examination is generally normal in type 1 diabetes mellitus unless DKA is present.

When DKA is suspected in a child with known type 1 DM, important historic information includes the usual insulin dose, the last insulin dose, the child's diet over the previous day, and whether the child has been ill and emotionally or physically stressed. The child with DKA appears acutely ill and suffers from moderate to profound dehydration. Symptoms include polyuria, polydipsia, fatigue, headache, nausea, emesis, and abdominal pain. The child's mental status may vary from confused to comatose. On physical examination, tachycardia and hyperpnea (Kussmaul respirations) are generally noted. There may be a fruity odor to the breath because of the ketosis. Intravascular volume depletion may be so marked that hypotension may be detected. Although cerebral edema is rare, it often is fatal. Changing mental status, unequal pupils, decorticate or decerebrate posturing, and/or seizures indicate cerebral edema. Early identification and aggressive management of increased intracranial pressure are pivotal to improve outcome.

Symptoms of hypoglycemia are caused by catecholamine release (trembling, diaphoresis, flushing, and tachycardia) and to cerebral glucopenia (sleepiness, confusion, mood changes, seizures, and coma).

Differential Diagnosis

Secondary diabetes may occur when there is insulin antagonism from excess glucocorticoids (Cushing syndrome or iatrogenic), hyperthyroidism, pheochromocytoma, GH excess, or with medications such as thiazide diuretics.

Diagnostic Evaluation

Glucosuria, ketonuria and a random plasma glucose level greater than 200 mg per dL are consistent with a diagnosis of diabetes mellitus. If early diabetes is suspected, a 2-hour postprandial blood glucose concentration is the first value to become abnormal. A fasting blood glucose concentration greater than 126 mg per dL and a 2-hour postprandial blood glucose concentration greater than 200 mg per dL are suggestive of diabetes. Islet cell antibodies in the serum may be found in the new-onset insulin-dependent diabetic; poorly controlled diabetics have high levels of glycosylated hemoglobin.

In children with suspected DKA, the serum glucose concentration is grossly elevated, and the venous pH and serum P_{CO_2} are low. Metabolic acidosis from ketosis results in diminished pH, and the response to metabolic acidosis is a compensatory respiratory alkalosis and a drop in serum P_{CO_2}. Because of the osmotic diuresis, blood urea nitrogen is elevated, and there is loss of phosphate, calcium, and potassium. Although there is a total body loss of potassium, serum potassium may be low, normal, or even high depending on the level of acidosis. When acidosis is present, protons move from the extracellular space to the intracellular space and potassium moves from the intracellular space to the extracellular space to maintain electroneutrality. Until the catabolic state is reversed with insulin, the urine is positive for ketones; until the serum concentration of glucose falls below 180 mg per dL, the urine is positive for glucose.

Treatment

The immediate goals of treatment of new-onset diabetes mellitus and DKA are to reverse the catabolic state through exogenous insulin therapy and to restore fluid and electrolyte balance.

The child with type 1 DM is treated through insulin replacement, diet, exercise, psychological support, and regular medical follow-up. Patient education has a vital role. Current therapy requires frequent blood glucose monitoring and carbohydrate counting. The patient learns how to tailor insulin dosing based on the glucose level and the current meal. The newly diagnosed diabetic requires 0.5 to 1.0 U per kg of insulin per day. Most diabetics take insulin two to three times a day. It is customary to give two thirds of the total daily dose before breakfast and one third before dinner and bedtime, and the human insulin is divided between short-acting Humalog insulin and intermediate-acting neutral protamine Hagedorn (NPH) insulin. An insulin pump has now become available that delivers a basal amount of insulin throughout the day, with bolus doses of short-acting insulin given at mealtimes. At times of medical, surgical, or emotional stress, additional insulin may be needed. Glycosylated hemoglobin levels should be monitored every 3 months to assess average glycemic control.

If hypoglycemia occurs, a child may ingest a carbohydrate snack to increase the serum glucose concentration. If the child is vomiting, Monogel instant glucose or cake icing may be applied to the buccal mucosa to provide glucose. If the child is stuporous or having a seizure, intravenous glucose or intramuscular glucagon may be given.

DKA is a medical emergency. Initial fluid resuscitation is accomplished by giving a normal saline or lactated Ringer solution, 10 mL per kg intravenous bolus. While the fluid bolus is running in, the total fluid deficit is calculated based on the amount of dehydration.

The fluid deficit should be replaced over a 48-hour period. The level of hyperglycemia is assessed, and an insulin drip is started at 0.1 U/kg/hour. The goal is to decrease the serum glucose 50 to 100 mg/dL/ hour. A glucose level that falls too quickly could precipitate cerebral edema. When serum glucose approaches 250 to 300 mg per dL, dextrose should be added to normal saline and the electrolyte solution to avoid hypoglycemia. Hyperglycemia, acidosis and ketone production correct with insulin therapy. Until there is adequate insulin, the body will continue to produce ketoacids. Frequent monitoring of blood glucose level, electrolytes, and acid–base status is crucial.

Prognosis

The Diabetes Control and Complications Trial demonstrated that intensive management and tight glycemic control reduce the risk of diabetes complications by 50% to 75%. Complications from diabetes include microvascular disease of the eye (retinopathy), kidney (nephropathy), and nerves (neuropathy). Microvascular's disease is generally not seen until the child has been insulin dependent for a minimum of 10 years. Accelerated large vessel atherosclerotic disease can lead to myocardial infarction or stroke. Diabetic children should have annual urine collections to screen for microalbuminuria, annual ophthalmologic examinations, and annual screening for hyperlipidemia.

DIABETES MELLITUS TYPE 2

Pathogenesis

Diabetes mellitus type 2 (type 2 DM) is a polygenic condition that results from relative insulin resistance. This insulin resistance initially causes a compensatory increase in insulin secretion; however, with time there is a progressive decline in the glucose-stimulated insulin secretion.

Epidemiology

Type 2 DM accounts for 2% to 3% of all diabetes in children. However, the incidence is increasing because of the high prevalence of obesity. Most cases occur during early adolescence around the onset of puberty. Prevalence is highest in Native Americans, African Americans, and Hispanics. Genetic susceptibility is important; however, environmental factors, including obesity, physical inactivity, and diet, play a major role.

History and Physical Examination

Many patients are asymptomatic at presentation. Others may have symptoms similar to those of type 1 diabetics. There is usually a positive family history. On physical examination, obesity is noted, with a body mass index (BMI) usually greater than 30 kg per m^2. Often associated with type 2 DM is acanthosis nigricans, a skin condition involving hyperpigmentation and thickening of the skin folds, found primarily on the back of the neck and flexor areas.

Treatment

Currently, the mainstay of treatment is insulin therapy. Metformin is the only oral hypoglycemic agents used for treatment in children older than 10 years with type 2 DM; other oral hypoglycemic use is primarily anecdotal. More research is needed in this area. In addition to medical therapy, lifestyle changes in diet and exercise are particularly important.

6-1 KEY POINTS

1. Diabetes mellitus (DM) is a chronic metabolic disorder characterized by hyperglycemia and abnormal energy metabolism caused by absent or diminished insulin secretion or action at the cellular level.
2. Type 1 DM results from a lack of insulin production in the β cells of the pancreas.
3. A history of new-onset weight loss, polydipsia, polyphagia, and polyuria is consistent with type 1 DM.
4. Long-term complications from type 1 DM include microvascular disease (retinopathy, nephropathy, and neuropathy) and accelerated large vessel atherosclerotic disease.
5. The percentage of type 2 DM cases in children is rising.

DIABETES INSIPIDUS

In central **diabetes insipidus,** there is loss of antidiuretic hormone secretion from the posterior pituitary gland and an inability to concentrate the urine. Diabetes insipidus can occur after head trauma or with a brain tumor or central nervous system (CNS) infection. Surgical interruption of the pituitary stalk during craniopharyngioma removal often results in diabetes insipidus. Only rarely is diabetes insipidus an isolated idiopathic disorder.

CLINICAL MANIFESTATIONS

The child with diabetes insipidus has abrupt-onset polydipsia and polyuria. If the cause of the diabetes insipidus is a brain tumor impinging on the pituitary gland, focal neurologic signs and visual abnormalities may be noted.

The increased urine output may reach 5 to 10 L per day, with a urine specific gravity and urine osmolality that are quite low. Over time, serum sodium and serum osmolality increase as hemoconcentration occurs from free water loss. In unclear cases, the water deprivation test is used to document diabetes insipidus. Demonstration of antidiuretic hormone (ADH) secretion is critical in differentiating ADH-deficient (central) diabetes insipidus from nephrogenic diabetes insipidus, a rare X-linked recessive disease in which the collecting ducts do not respond to ADH.

TREATMENT

Desmopressin acetate (DDAVP), an ADH analogue, is given intranasally, subcutaneously, or orally to stimulate the kidneys to retain water and reverse the polyuria, polydipsia, and hypernatremia.

🔑 6-2 KEY POINTS

1. In central diabetes insipidus, there is loss of antidiuretic hormone (ADH) secretion and an inability to concentrate the urine.
2. Diabetes insipidus can occur after head trauma or with a brain tumor or central nervous system (CNS) infection.

SHORT STATURE

Short stature is a common concern of parents. Normal causes include familial (genetic) short stature and constitutional delay. Eighty percent of cases of short stature are attributable to these two causes. Pathologic causes may result in either disproportionate or proportionate short stature. Etiologies that result in proportionate short stature are much more prevalent than those of disproportionate short stature.

Disorders that result in disproportionate short stature affect the long bones predominantly and include rickets, which is caused by activated vitamin D deficiency, and achondroplasia, an autosomal dominant disorder.

Diseases that cause proportionate short stature may result from either a prenatal or postnatal insult to the growth process. Prenatal etiologies include intrauterine growth retardation, placental dysfunction, intrauterine infections, teratogens, and chromosomal abnormalities. The most common chromosomal abnormalities that result in short stature are trisomy 21 and Turner syndrome. Postnatal causes include malnutrition, chronic systemic diseases, psychosocial deprivation, drugs, and endocrine disorders. Common endocrine defects that result in short stature include hypothyroidism, GH deficiency, glucocorticoid excess, and precocious puberty. Of note, with precocious puberty there is initial accelerated growth but with compromise of final adult height and thus subsequent short stature compared to genetic potential.

DIFFERENTIAL DIAGNOSIS

Children with familial short stature establish growth curves at or below the fifth percentile by 2 years of age. They are otherwise completely healthy, with a normal physical examination. These children have a normal bone age, and puberty occurs at the expected time. Short stature is usually found in at least one parent, but height inheritance is complex, and the diminutive ancestor may be more distant.

Children with constitutional delay grow and develop at or below the fifth percentile at normal growth velocities. This results in a curve parallel to the fifth percentile. Puberty is significantly delayed, which results in a delay in the bone age. Because these children fail to enter puberty at the usual age, their short stature and sexual immaturity are accentuated when their peers enter puberty. Family members are usually of average height, but there is often a history of short stature in childhood and delayed puberty. The parents of children with constitutional delay should be counseled that their child's growth is a normal variant and the child will likely mature to the height expected for their family.

GH deficiency accounts for approximately 5% of cases of short stature referred to endocrinologists. Children with classic GH deficiency grow at a diminished growth velocity (less than 5 cm per year) and have delayed skeletal maturation. A history of birth asphyxia or neonatal hypoglycemia or physical findings of microphallus, cleft palate, or other midline defects are suggestive of idiopathic GH deficiency. GH deficiency secondary to hypothalamic or pituitary tumor usually is associated with other neurologic or visual impairments. In an older child with more recent onset of subnormal growth, the index of suspicion for tumor should be high.

Primary hypothyroidism causes marked growth failure because of a diminished growth velocity and skeletal maturation. Thyroxine (T_4), triiodothyronine resin uptake (T_3RU), thyroid-stimulating hormone (TSH), and thyroid antibodies should be measured, even in the absence of symptoms, to rule out any degree of hypothyroidism when evaluating short stature. Primary hypothyroidism is treated with levothyroxine (Synthroid).

Cushing disease is a rare cause of short stature. Hypercortisolism, from either exogenous steroid therapy or endogenous oversecretion, may have a profound growth-suppression effect. Usually, other stigmata of Cushing syndrome are present if growth suppression has occurred.

Chronic systemic diseases can result in short stature from lack of caloric absorption or increased metabolic demands. Cyanotic heart disease, cystic fibrosis, poorly controlled DM, chronic renal failure, human immunodeficiency (HIV) infection, and severe rheumatoid arthritis are disorders that increase metabolic demands and diminish growth. Alternatively, inflammatory bowel disease, celiac sprue, and cystic fibrosis can reduce caloric absorption and produce short stature.

Some children who live in emotionally or physically abusive or neglectful environments develop functional GH deficiency. Children with **psychosocial deprivation** may have bizarre behaviors that include food hoarding, pica, and encopresis, as well as immature speech, disturbed sleep-wake cycles, and an increased pain tolerance. Clinically, they resemble children with GH deficiency, with marked retardation of bone age and pubertal delay. If GH testing is done while the child remains in the hostile environment, there is a blunted GH response; when the child is removed from the deprived environment, GH testing reverts to normal and catch-up growth is noted.

One of the manifestations of **Turner syndrome** (discussed in detail in Chapter 9) is short stature. The clinical manifestations of Turner syndrome can sometimes be subtle. Given that the incidence of Turner syndrome is 1 in 2,500 females, gonadotropins and karyotype testing are indicated in the female adolescent with short stature and delayed puberty. Elevated gonadotropins, indicating primary ovarian failure, and a 45,XO karyotype is diagnostic.

Chronic administration of certain **medications** may result in poor growth. Such drugs include steroids, dextroamphetamine (Dexedrine), and methylphenidate (Ritalin).

CLINICAL MANIFESTATIONS

History

Important historical information includes the child's prenatal and birth history, the pattern of growth, the presence of chronic disease, long-term medication use, the achievement of developmental milestones, and the growth and pubertal patterns of the patient's parents and siblings. Obtaining and evaluating the child's growth charts are vitally important. A thorough feeding history, including what, how, and by whom the child is fed, is also required.

Physical Examination

The majority of physical examinations done on children with short stature are normal. It is critical to plot the child's height and weight on the appropriate growth curve for age. In addition to height, arm span and upper-to-lower-body segment ratio are measured to check for pathologic disproportionate causes of short stature. In young children, the head circumference should also be evaluated to check for failure to thrive. In children with failure to thrive, weight and height are diminished and the head circumference is often spared. When examining the child with short stature, the physician may find dysmorphic features in a pattern suggestive of a particular syndrome. The integument should be examined for cyanosis indicating potential congenital heart disease, abnormal pigmentation noted in Cushing syndrome, the stigmata of hypothyroidism, and bruises and poor hygiene indicative of psychosocial deprivation. The thyroid is palpated to determine its size, its consistency, and the presence of thyroid nodules. The lungs and heart are examined to identify chronic cardiopulmonary disease. Abdominal tenderness or bloating may indicate inflammatory bowel disease or celiac sprue. Tanner staging for both boys and girls must be documented to help differentiate among familial short stature, constitutional delay, and precocious puberty. A thorough neurologic and funduscopic examination may reveal underlying CNS disease resulting in GH deficiency.

DIAGNOSTIC EVALUATION

Because most cases of short stature result from either familial short stature or constitutional delay, diagnostic studies are generally not necessary unless abnormalities are found on examination. A bone age (anteroposterior radiograph of the left wrist) assessment helps delineate familial short stature from constitutional delay. An advanced bone age likely indicates precocious puberty; a normal bone age, familial short stature; and a delayed bone age, constitutional delay.

Thyroid function tests must be done to rule out hypothyroidism. Urinalysis and renal function tests are needed to rule out chronic renal disease. A complete blood count with differential and an erythrocyte sedimentation rate may reveal evidence of chronic systemic infection. The child's nutritional status can be examined through the serum albumin and total protein counts. A screen for insulinlike growth factor-1 (IGF-1) and insulinlike growth factor binding protein-3 (IGF-BP3) may be ordered to look for GH deficiency. If a chromosomal anomaly is considered, obtaining a karyotype may be helpful. An MRI of the head may identify a hypothalamic or pituitary process that is resulting in decreased GH secretion from the pituitary.

TREATMENT

The child with familial short stature has few therapeutic options. For most children with constitutional delay, reassurance that the child's short stature is a normal variant suffices. In some select patients with no signs of puberty by 14 years of age, a 4- to 6-month treatment with the appropriate sex hormone may help to modestly increase stature and pubertal development for psychological support until true pubertal development begins.

Children with GH deficiency are managed with biosynthetic human GH by subcutaneous injection every day or by a depot form of growth hormone that is given one to two times per month. Accelerated growth velocity on GH treatment results in catch-up growth in most children. An MRI of the brain should be ordered prior to initiating GH therapy. GH therapy is needed into adulthood because of its effects on bone mass and lipid metabolism. If puberty is delayed beyond 14 years of age, the addition of sex steroids may be considered, both to augment the growth response to GH and to stimulate secondary sexual development.

Primary hypothyroidism is treated with levothyroxine (Synthroid). After several weeks of therapy, the growth velocity generally returns to normal. Unlike GH therapy, levothyroxine therapy does not promote catch-up growth.

To manage the short stature associated with Cushing disease, the physician must identify and treat the etiology. Girls with short stature caused by Turner syndrome may receive GH to increase their final adult height. Short stature caused by psychosocial deprivation is treated by removing the child from the environment. Short stature caused by medications is reversed by discontinuing the offending medication.

🔑 6-3 KEY POINTS

1. Eighty percent of cases of short stature result from normal growth and development and are caused by either familial (genetic) short stature or constitutional delay.
2. Pathologic causes may result in either disproportionate or proportionate short stature; proportionate short stature is more prevalent than disproportionate short stature.
3. The most common pathologic etiologies of proportionate short stature include growth hormone (GH) deficiency, primary hypothyroidism, Cushing disease, chronic systemic diseases, psychosocial deprivation, Turner syndrome, and medications.

THYROID DYSFUNCTION

HYPERTHYROIDISM

Most cases of hyperthyroidism in children are caused by **Graves' disease**. Other causes include a hyperfunctioning "hot" thyroid nodule or acute suppurative thyroiditis. Graves' disease, an autoimmune disorder, is caused by circulating thyroid-stimulating immunoglobulins binding to thyrotropin receptors on thyroid cells, which results in diffuse hyperplasia and increased levels of free T_4. Neonatal Graves' disease follows transplacental passage of maternal thyroid-stimulating immunoglobulins.

Clinical Manifestations

Symptoms include a voracious appetite (without weight gain or with weight loss), heat intolerance, emotional lability, restlessness, excessive sweating, frequent loose stools, and poor sleep. Exophthalmos is uncommon in children. Older children may complain of palpitations. There is often a change in behavior and school performance. On physical examination, the child may be flushed, fidgety, and warm, with proptosis, a hyperactive precordium, resting tachycardia, and a widened pulse pressure. The thyroid gland is generally enlarged, smooth, firm (but not hard), and nontender, with a bruit on auscultation of the gland. Often a fine tremor is noted, and proximal muscle weakness is present. Acute-onset tachycardia, hyperthermia, diaphoresis, fever, nausea, and vomiting indicate thyroid storm (malignant hyperthyroidism), which can be life-threatening but is rare in children.

Infants with neonatal Graves' disease tend to stare, are jittery and hyperactive, and have an increased appetite and poor weight gain. Tachycardia is usually present, and thyromegaly may be palpable.

In hyperthyroidism, T_4 levels are elevated, T_3RU is elevated, and TSH is suppressed.

Treatment

Neonatal Graves' disease generally resolves over the first several months of life. In the infant hemodynamically compromised by hyperthyroidism, parenteral fluids, digoxin, and propranolol may be necessary.

Propylthiouracil (PTU), methimazole, or radioiodine may be used to treat Graves' disease and must be titrated carefully because too high a dose can result in hypothyroidism. Fifty percent of children with Graves' disease have a spontaneous remission and may be taken off antithyroid medication after 12 to 24 months of treatment. Those children who do not have remission of their disease continue on the antithyroid drug; levothyroxine is added to prevent hypothyroidism.

HYPOTHYROIDISM

Congenital hypothyroidism is discussed in Chapter 13. The most common cause of juvenile or acquired hypothyroidism is **Hashimoto thyroiditis**, which is a chronic lymphocytic thyroiditis that results in autoimmune destruction of the thyroid gland. Other causes of hypothyroidism include panhypopituitarism, ectopic thyroid dysgenesis, administration of antithyroid medications, and surgical or radioactive iodine ablation for treatment of hyperthyroidism. The incidence of hypothyroidism in girls is four times greater than in boys. There is often a family history of Graves' disease or Hashimoto thyroiditis. Most children present at adolescence; it is unusual to develop thyroiditis before 5 years of age.

Clinical Manifestations

Symptoms include cold intolerance, diminished appetite, lethargy, and constipation. Physical findings include slow linear growth, delayed puberty, immature body proportions, coarse puffy facies, dry thin hair, dry skin, and deep tendon reflexes with a delayed relaxation time.

Thyroid function tests reveal a depressed total T_4 serum concentration and a depressed T_3RU level. If primary hypothyroidism is present, an elevated serum TSH concentration is noted. If secondary hypothyroidism is present, the TSH level may be depressed, normal, or mildly elevated. The detection of thyroid autoantibodies indicates an autoimmune basis for disease, whereas palpation of a thyroid nodule should prompt evaluation with a thyroid scan.

Treatment

Thyroid replacement with synthetic levothyroxine is provided and adjusted to maintain normal serum-free T_4 levels, normal TSH levels, and normal growth and development. Thyroid function tests should be monitored frequently.

🔑 6-4 KEY POINTS

1. Most cases of hyperthyroidism in children are caused by Graves' disease, which is an autoimmune-induced thyroid hyperplasia.
2. Neonatal Graves' disease results from transplacental passage of maternal thyroid-stimulating immunoglobulins.
3. In primary hyperthyroidism, T_4 levels are elevated, T_3RU is elevated, and TSH is suppressed.
4. Medical therapy for Graves' disease consists of propylthiouracil administration.
5. The most common cause of juvenile or acquired hypothyroidism is Hashimoto thyroiditis, which is a chronic lymphocytic thyroiditis that results in autoimmune destruction of the thyroid gland.
6. Thyroid function tests in hypothyroidism reveal a decreased T_4 serum concentration, decreased T_3RU, and elevated serum TSH concentration.
7. Hypothyroidism is treated with synthetic levothyroxine.

ADRENAL DYSFUNCTION

CONGENITAL ADRENAL HYPERPLASIA

The clinical characteristics of congenital adrenal hyperplasia depend on which enzyme in the pathway of steroidogenesis is deficient. Figure 6-1 is a schematic of steroidogenesis in the adrenal cortex.

21-Hydroxylase deficiency accounts for 90% of the cases of congenital adrenal hyperplasia. The disease is inherited as an autosomal recessive trait and tends to occur as either classic salt-wasting 21-hydroxylase deficiency or as virilizing 21-hydroxylase deficiency. 21-Hydroxylase is needed to produce aldosterone and cortisol. 21-Hydroxylase deficiency results in a buildup of the precursors of aldosterone and cortisol. Specifically, 17-hydroxyprogesterone increases, which is then metabolized to dehydroepiandrosterone and androstenedione. Both forms of 21-hydroxylase deficiency result in decreased cortisol and aldosterone secretion, increased adrenocorticotropin hormone (ACTH), and increased 17-hydroxyprogesterone and 17-hydroxypregnenolone.

11-Hydroxylase deficiency accounts for 5% of the cases of congenital adrenal hyperplasia and is also inherited as an autosomal recessive trait. Similar to 21-hydroxylase deficiency, 11-hydroxylase deficiency impairs the production of aldosterone and cortisol. 11-Hydroxylase converts 11-deoxycortisol to cortisol and deoxycorticosterone to corticosterone in the aldosterone pathway. With reduction or absence of 11-hydroxylase, cortisol and aldosterone precursors build up and are shunted to androgen synthesis.

Clinical Manifestations

In congenital 21-hydroxylase deficiency, female infants are born with ambiguous genitalia. Clitoromegaly and labioscrotal fusion may result in erroneous male sex assignment. There is normal ovarian development, and internal genital structures are female. Male infants born with the defect have no genital abnormalities. Symptoms of emesis, salt wasting, dehydration, and shock develop in the first 2 to 4 weeks of life. Hyponatremia and hyperkalemia result from lack of aldosterone, and hypoglycemia results from decreased levels of cortisol. Worsening hyponatremic dehydration culminates in

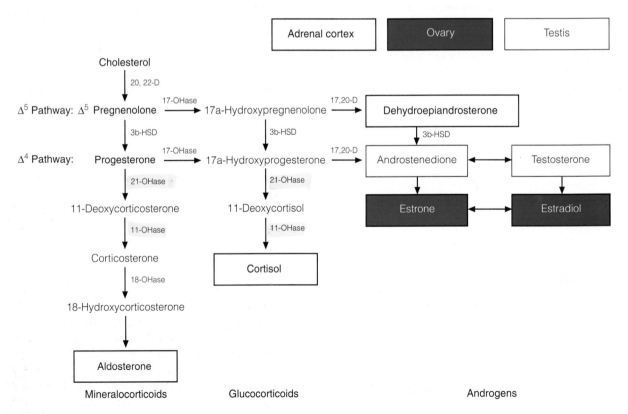

Figure 6-1 • A schematic of steroidogenesis in the adrenal cortex.

shock and acidosis in severe cases. The diagnosis of 21-hydroxylase deficiency is made by documenting elevated serum levels of 17-hydroxyprogesterone.

In 11-hydroxylase deficiency, there is overproduction of deoxycorticosterone, which has mineralocorticoid activity and results in hypernatremia, hypokalemia, and hypertension. Diagnosis is based on the measurement of increased levels of 11-deoxycortisol and deoxycorticosterone in the serum or their metabolites in the urine. Serum androstenedione and testosterone are also elevated, and renin and aldosterone levels are depressed.

Treatment

Therapy for 21-hydroxylase deficiency includes cortisol and mineralocorticoid therapy. Cortisol therapy reduces ACTH secretion and overproduction of androgens, and mineralocorticoid administration is adjusted to normalize serum renin levels. Surgical correction of female genital abnormalities is accomplished early. The linear growth and sexual development of children with 21-hydroxylase deficiency must be monitored closely. Undertreatment, as indicated by elevated 17-hydroxyprogesterone, androstenedione, and renin levels and by accelerated advancement of skeletal maturity, leads to excessive growth, premature sexual hair growth, and virilization of the child. Ultimately, undertreatment may lead to premature epiphyseal fusion and adult short stature. Overtreatment with cortisol suppresses growth and may cause symptoms of hypercortisolism.

🔑 6-5 KEY POINTS

1. 21-Hydroxylase deficiency accounts for 90% of the cases of congenital adrenal hyperplasia.
2. In congenital 21-hydroxylase deficiency, female infants are born with ambiguous genitalia, whereas male infants born with the defect have no genital abnormalities.
3. In salt-wasting 21-hydroxylase deficiency, symptoms of emesis, salt wasting, dehydration, and shock develop in the first 2 to 4 weeks of life.
4. The diagnosis of congenital adrenal hyperplasia is made by documenting elevated levels of 17-hydroxyprogesterone in the serum.
5. Therapy for 21-hydroxylase deficiency includes cortisol and mineralocorticoid therapy.

PRECOCIOUS PUBERTY

True **precocious puberty** is defined as secondary sex characteristics presenting in girls before 7.5 years of age and in boys before 9 years of age and may be either gonadotropin-dependent or gonadotropin-independent. True central (gonadotropin-dependent) precocious puberty is more common in girls than in boys. Precocious puberty in girls is usually idiopathic, whereas in boys there is a greater incidence of CNS pathology. Tumors causing gonadotropin-dependent precocious puberty (GDPP) include gliomas, embryonic germ cell tumors, and hamartomas. Other causes of GDPP include hydrocephalus, head injury, and CNS infection or congenital malformation.

Gonadotropin-independent precocious puberty (GIPP) is extremely rare and is seen in McCune-Albright's syndrome (polyostotic fibrous dysplasia of bone), familial precocious puberty in boys (familial testitoxicosis), Leydig cell tumors, and ectopic human chorionic gonadotropin (HCG) production by neoplasms such as hepatic and pineal tumors.

Precocious thelarche refers to isolated early breast development. The usual age of onset is 12 to 24 months. Premature thelarche is likely caused by small transient bursts of estrogen from the prepubertal ovary or from increased sensitivity to low levels of estrogen in the prepubertal female. **Premature adrenarche** refers to the early appearance of sexual hair before 8 years of age in girls and 9 years of age in boys. This benign condition is caused by early maturation of adrenal androgen secretion.

Clinical Manifestations

In precocious thelarche, gonadotropin and serum estrogen levels are in the prepubertal range, and linear growth acceleration and advancing skeletal maturation are not present. This nonprogressive, benign condition is distinguished from true precocious puberty by the normal growth rate and bone age noted with premature thelarche.

In premature adrenarche, the levels of adrenal androgens are normal for pubertal stage but elevated for chronologic age. The child's bone age is usually slightly advanced. Children with premature adrenarche must be evaluated for other causes of increased androgen production, such as congenital adrenal hyperplasia, polycystic ovarian syndrome, or adrenal tumor. In children with evidence of significant androgen effect (advanced bone age, growth acceleration, and acne), measurement of adrenal steroids and androgens before and after ACTH administration is used to identify those with congenital adrenal hyperplasia.

The clinical manifestations of GDPP include premature development of secondary sexual characteristics and an accompanying growth spurt. If the GDPP is secondary to pathology of the CNS, focal neurologic signs are often present. Diagnosis is based on advanced bone age and pubertal levels of gonadotropins and estrogen or testosterone. A pubertal pattern of elevated gonadotropins after infusion of gonadotropin-releasing hormone (GnRH) is indicative of GDPP. In GIPP, gonadotropins are low, and GnRH has no effect on gonadotropin levels.

Treatment

Premature thelarche is a benign condition that does not require any treatment. Premature adrenarche that is not caused by congenital adrenal hyperplasia, tumor, or polycystic ovarian syndrome is also a benign condition. GDPP is treated with injections of long-acting preparations of GnRH (leuprolide). GnRH analogues suppress gonadotropin release and thereby decrease secondary sex characteristics, slow skeletal growth, and prevent the fusion of long bone epiphyseal plates. GIPP is managed by treating the underlying disease process.

PUBERTAL DELAY

Pubertal delay is characterized by a delay in the onset of puberty or in the rate of progression through normal sexual development. In females, this refers to the absence of secondary sex characteristics at 13 years of age or the absence of menarche 5 years from the onset of sexual development. In males, pubertal delay denotes the absence of secondary sex characteristics at 14 years of age or the failure to complete genital growth 5 years from the onset of puberty. Constitutional delay is the cause for 90% to 95% of cases. In these children the bone age is delayed, growth is slow, and puberty simply appears late. There is usually a positive family history.

Differential Diagnosis

Systemic disease can delay puberty in both sexes. Pubertal delay may be caused by primary gonadal failure or hypergonadotropic hypogonadism. Examples of this include Turner syndrome or autoimmune ovarian failure (in girls) and Klinefelter's syndrome (in boys). Hypogonadotropic hypogonadism is caused by hypothalamic/pituitary axis dysfunction. Examples include Kallmann's syndrome, isolated gonadotropic

deficiency, hypothalamic and pituitary tumors, hypopituitarism, and anorexia nervosa. Other endocrine disorders including hypothyroidism may also delay or advance puberty.

Clinical Manifestations

The history and physical examination should include an examination of growth trends, the timing of puberty in other family members, and an assessment of the patient's current Tanner staging. Laboratory evaluation is helpful, including a bone age, testosterone and estradiol levels, gonadotropins, follicle-stimulating hormone (FSH) and luteinizing hormone (LH), prolactin, and thyroid function testing. Screening to look for systemic disease is also indicated.

Treatment

In the case of constitutional delay, a short course of sex steroids may be needed to initiate pubertal development. Psychosocial support is also important. If permanent hypogonadism is determined to be the etiology, sex steroid replacement is initiated at the normal time of puberty and continued for a lifetime.

⚲ 6-6 KEY POINTS

1. True precocious puberty is defined as secondary sex characteristics presenting in girls before 7.5 years of age and in boys before 9 years of age and may be either gonadotropin-dependent or independent.

2. True central (gonadotropin-dependent) precocious puberty is more common in girls than in boys. Precocious puberty in girls is usually idiopathic, whereas precocious puberty in boys is often caused by tumors of the central nervous system (CNS).

3. The clinical manifestations of gonadotropin-dependent precocious puberty (GDPP) include premature development of secondary sexual characteristics and an accompanying growth spurt.

4. GDPP is treated with injections of long-acting preparations of gonadotropin-releasing hormone (GnRH).

5. The most common cause of pubertal delay is constitutional delay.

CUSHING SYNDROME

Cushing syndrome is a constellation of symptoms and signs that result from high cortisol levels. It is caused by either endogenous overproduction of cortisol or excessive exogenous treatment with pharmacologic doses of cortisol. Endogenous causes include Cushing disease and adrenal tumors. Cushing disease, also known as bilateral adrenal hyperplasia, is the most common etiology of Cushing syndrome in children older than 7 years. In most instances, it is caused by a microadenoma of the pituitary gland resulting in ACTH oversecretion. Rarely, in the young child or infant, a malignant carcinoma of the adrenal gland is seen. Most adrenal tumors that cause Cushing syndrome are adenomas. Ectopic ACTH secretion may occur with some tumors; however, this is exceedingly rare in children.

Clinical Manifestations

The classic signs and symptoms of Cushing syndrome include slow growth with pubertal arrest, "moon" facies, buffalo hump, truncal obesity, abdominal striae, acne, hyperpigmentation, hypertension, fatigue, muscle weakness, and emotional and mental changes. Most adrenal tumors are virilizing.

Initial laboratory studies include documentation of an elevated serum cortisol level and an increased 24-hour urine free cortisol test. If hypercortisolism is demonstrated, the dexamethasone suppression test is performed to document the presence of Cushing syndrome. Dexamethasone is given in the late evening, and a cortisol level is measured the next morning. Failure of the dexamethasone to suppress the morning cortisol level is consistent with Cushing syndrome. A prolonged dexamethasone suppression test is used to differentiate Cushing disease from an adrenal tumor. When evaluating a child with Cushing syndrome, obtaining MRI scans of the pituitary and CT scans of the adrenal glands is helpful to determine if additional pathology exists.

Treatment

Adrenal tumors require surgical removal. Similarly, bilateral adrenal hyperplasia is treated with surgical excision of the pituitary adenoma. Transsphenoidal microsurgery is the most effective method of microadenoma removal. Perioperative stress dosing of glucocorticoids is needed to avoid adrenal insufficiency. Postoperatively, the patient may develop mineralocorticoid deficiency in addition to the glucocorticoid deficiency.

6-7 KEY POINTS

1. Cushing syndrome is a constellation of symptoms and signs that result from high cortisol levels and is caused by either endogenous overproduction of cortisol or excessive exogenous treatment with pharmacologic doses of cortisol. Cushing disease is the most common noniatrogenic cause of Cushing syndrome.
2. The classic signs and symptoms of Cushing syndrome include "moon" facies, buffalo hump, truncal obesity, abdominal striae, acne, decreased growth velocity, hypertension, and muscle weakness.

ADDISON DISEASE

Addison disease, or primary adrenal insufficiency, may be congenital or acquired and results in decreased cortisol secretion. Depending on the disease process, there may be a concomitant decrease in aldosterone release. In the newborn, primary adrenal insufficiency may be caused by adrenal hypoplasia, ACTH unresponsiveness, adrenal hemorrhage, or ischemic infarction with sepsis (Waterhouse-Friderichsen's syndrome). In older children and adolescents, autoimmune adrenal insufficiency is most common. It may occur alone or in association with another autoimmune endocrinopathy such as thyroiditis or type 1 DM. Tuberculosis, hemorrhage, fungal infection, neoplastic infiltration, and HIV infection may also cause destruction of the adrenal gland. Adrenoleukodystrophy is an X-linked recessive disorder of long-chain fatty acid metabolism that results in adrenal insufficiency and progressive neurologic dysfunction.

In contrast to primary adrenal insufficiency, **secondary adrenal insufficiency** is caused by ACTH deficiency. The most common cause of ACTH deficiency is chronic steroid therapy that results in suppression of pituitary ACTH. Pituitary tumors and craniopharyngioma also result in depressed pituitary ACTH secretion from either destruction of the pituitary gland or pituitary compression.

Clinical Manifestations

Symptoms from primary adrenal insufficiency include weakness, nausea, vomiting, weight loss, headache, emotional lability, and salt craving. Physical findings include postural hypotension and increased pigmentation over joints and on scar tissue, lips, nipples, and the buccal mucosa. The postural hypotension and salt craving are caused by lack of aldosterone, whereas the increased pigmentation because of increased ACTH secretion. Melanocyte-stimulating hormone is a by-product of the ACTH biosynthetic pathway. Adrenal crisis is characterized by fever, vomiting, dehydration, and shock. It may be precipitated by intercurrent illness, trauma, or surgery.

Electrolyte abnormalities include hyponatremia, hyperkalemia, hypoglycemia, and mild metabolic acidosis from dehydration. An elevated baseline ACTH with a concurrent low cortisol level is consistent with primary adrenal insufficiency. The serum cortisol level by definition is low and is unresponsive to injection of ACTH (corticotropin stimulation test). If the corticotropin stimulation test is abnormal, a prolonged ACTH stimulation test is necessary to rule out secondary adrenal insufficiency.

Treatment

Adrenal crisis, also known as Addisonian crisis, is a life-threatening condition that should be treated without delay. Correction of electrolyte abnormalities and dehydration is required immediately with 5% dextrose in normal saline and stress dose intravenous glucocorticoids.

Long-term management consists of maintenance doses of oral glucocorticoids and mineralocorticoids. The glucocorticoid dose is increased during times of acute metabolic stress to avoid adrenal insufficiency.

6-8 KEY POINTS

1. Primary adrenal insufficiency may be congenital or acquired and results in decreased cortisol and aldosterone secretion, whereas secondary adrenal insufficiency is caused by adrenocorticotropin hormone (ACTH) deficiency.
2. Symptoms of primary adrenal insufficiency include weakness, nausea, vomiting, weight loss, salt craving, postural hypotension, and increased pigmentation.
3. An adrenal crisis is characterized by fever, vomiting, dehydration, and shock. It may be precipitated by intercurrent illness, trauma, or surgery.
4. Electrolyte abnormalities found in adrenal crisis include hyponatremia, hyperkalemia, hypoglycemia, and metabolic acidosis from dehydration.

Additional Suggested Reading

Chianese J, Adam HM. Short stature. *Pediatr Rev.* 2005;26:36–37.

Diabetes Control and Complications Trial Research Group. The effect of intensive treatment of diabetes on the development and progression of long-term complications in insulin-dependent diabetes mellitus. *N Engl J Med.* 1993;329:977–986.

Foley TP. Hypothyroidism. *Pediatr Rev.* 2004;25: 94–100.

Levine LS. Congenital adrenal hyperplasia. *Pediatr Rev.* 2000;21:159–171.

Nesmith JD. Type 2 diabetes mellitus in children and adolescents. *Pediatr Rev.* 2001;22:147–152.

Ratner Kaufman F. Type 1 diabetes mellitus. *Pediatr Rev.* 2003;24:291–300.

Root AW. Precocious puberty. *Pediatr Rev.* 2000;21:10–19.

Saborio P, Tipton GA, Chan JCH. Diabetes insipidus. *Pediatr Rev.* 2000;21:122–129.

7 Fluid, Electrolyte, and pH Management

A human is born with 90% of his or her body weight as water. Body composition changes dramatically over the first year of life as muscle mass increases. By 1 year of age, a child's total body water approaches the adult level of 60% body weight. **Electrolyte homeostasis, fluid distribution**, and **pH balance** are critical to the maintenance of normal physiology. The younger the patient, the more intolerant he or she is to challenges to these systems.

MAINTENANCE FLUIDS

The amount of fluid needed to maintain normal body function is directly related to caloric expenditure, which in turn is related to a child's weight. The **Holliday-Segar method** is useful for calculating daily maintenance fluids: 100 mL/kg/day for the first 10 kg, plus 50 mL/kg/day for the next 10 kg, plus 25 mL/kg/day for each additional kg thereafter. For practical purposes, it is often more useful to calculate an hourly rate using 4 mL/kg/hr (first 10 kg body weight), 2 mL/kg/hr (second 10 kg body weight), and 1 mL/kg/hr (each additional kilogram).

Here is an example of calculating maintenance fluid requirements for a 22-kg child:

Daily rate: (100 mL/kg/day × 10 kg)
  + (50 mL/kg/day × 10 kg) + (25 mL/kg/day × 2 kg)
  = 1,550 mL per day
Hourly rate: 1,550 mL per day ÷ 24 hours per day
  = 65 mL per hour
Short-cut method: (4 mL per hour × 10 kg)
  + (2 mL per hour × 10 kg) + (1 mL per hour × 2 kg)
  = 62 mL per hour

For each 100 mL of maintenance fluids, a child needs 3 mEq of sodium and 2 mEq of potassium, as well as a carbohydrate source (dextrose). In general, one-fourth normal saline with 5% dextrose (10% in infants) and 20 mEq per L KCl meets maintenance glucose and electrolyte needs. One-half normal saline with KCl is often used in adolescents and adults.

DEHYDRATION

Dehydration in the pediatric patient is usually secondary to **vomiting** and/or **diarrhea**. Infants and toddlers are particularly susceptible because of the limited ability of the immature kidney to conserve water and electrolytes and because of the child's dependence on caretakers to meet his or her needs. When addressing dehydration, it is important to consider **maintenance fluid** needs as well as **replacement** of the initial deficit and **ongoing losses**.

CLINICAL MANIFESTATIONS

History

A careful history clarifies the differential and provides information concerning the acuity, source, and quantity of fluid lost, all of which influence treatment. Recent **weight loss** and **decreased urine output** are important benchmarks of the degree of deficiency. The color, consistency, frequency, and volume of stool and/or emesis may influence initial diagnostic and therapeutic measures.

Many chronic medical illnesses may present acutely with dehydration, including diabetes, metabolic disorders, cystic fibrosis, and congenital adrenal hyperplasia. Polyuria in the presence of physical signs of dehydration may indicate diabetes mellitus, diabetes insipidus, or renal tubular acidosis. Children who are neglected or refuse to drink because of severe oropharyngeal pain may also develop significant dehydration.

Physical Examination

No single physical examination or laboratory finding accurately assesses a patient's degree of dehydration (Table 7-1). A child's primary mechanism of compensating for decreased plasma volume is **tachycardia; hypotension** is a very late and ominous finding.

DIAGNOSTIC EVALUATION

Serum electrolyte levels help guide the choice of fluid composition and rate of replacement. Dehydration may be isotonic, hypotonic (hyponatremic), or hypertonic (hypernatremic), depending on the nature of the fluid lost and the replacement fluids provided by the caretaker.

Isotonic dehydration is the most common form and suggests that either compensation has occurred or that water losses roughly parallel sodium losses. **Hypotonic (hyponatremic) dehydration** is defined by a serum sodium less than 130 mEq per L. Children who lose electrolytes in their stool and are supplemented with free water or very dilute juices may present in this manner. **Hypertonic (hypernatremic) dehydration** (Na ≥ 150 mEq per L) is uncommon in children but implies an excessive loss of free water compared with electrolyte loss (e.g., diabetes insipidus). Of note, patients with hyponatremic dehydration tend to appear more dehydrated, whereas those with hypernatremic dehydration may not appear as clinically compromised because intravascular volume is preserved.

Usually, the serum bicarbonate concentration is decreased secondary to metabolic acidosis. However, protracted vomiting may result in alkalosis and a high bicarbonate level as a result of acid loss from gastric secretions (see "Metabolic Alkalosis" later).

TABLE 7-1 Clinical Estimation of Degree of Dehydration[a]			
	Mild	**Moderate**	**Severe**
Weight loss	<5%	5%–10%	>10%
Vital signs			
Heart rate	Increased	Increased	Greatly increased
Respiratory rate	Normal	Normal	Increased
Blood pressure	Normal	Normal (orthostasis)	Decreased
Skin			
Capillary refill	<2 sec	2–3 sec	>3 sec
Mucous membranes	Normal/dry	Dry	Dry
Anterior fontanelle	Normal	Depressed	Depressed
Eyes			
Tearing	Normal/absent	Absent	Absent
Appearance	Normal	Sunken	Sunken
Mental status	Normal	Altered	Depressed
Laboratory values			
Urine osmolarity	600 mOsm/L	800 mOsm/L	Maximal
Urine specific gravity	1.020	1.025	Maximal
Blood urea nitrogen	<20	Elevated	High
Blood pH	Normal	Mildly acidotic	Moderate/profound acidosis
Stage of shock	Not in shock	Compensated shock	Uncompensated shock

[a]Infants exhibit greater weight loss per degree of dehydration (5% mild, 10% moderate, 15% severe), whereas adolescents exhibit less weight loss per degree of dehydration (3% mild, 5%–6% moderate, 7–9% severe).

With significant dehydration, perfusion of the kidneys may be impaired. This will be reflected in elevations of the serum blood urea nitrogen (BUN) and creatinine (Cr) levels as glomerular filtration rate falls. A BUN-to Cr ratio greater than 20 is consistent with prerenal failure.

TREATMENT

Oral rehydration therapy (ORT) is the preferred treatment for mild to moderate dehydration. The World Health Organization recommends that solutions contain 90 mEq per L sodium, 20 mEq per L potassium, and 20g per L glucose. Commercial preparations that approximate these concentrations are available. Free water may precipitate hyponatremia and is contraindicated. ORT is particularly labor intensive, requiring small volumes of fluid given very frequently. Administered correctly, it is extremely effective.

Severe dehydration leads to life-threatening **hypovolemic shock**. Children in hypovolemic shock should receive 20 mL per kg intravenous boluses of isotonic fluid (normal saline or Ringer lactate) until their condition stabilizes (see Chapter 1). Both fluids are isotonic, resulting in improved intravascular volume without fluid shifts. Clinical estimation of degree of dehydration and serum electrolyte studies tailor subsequent management.

Most **deficits** are replaced over 24 hours, with half given in the first 8 hours and the rest over the next 16 hours. One notable exception is the child with hypernatremic dehydration, in whom the deficit should be replaced over 48 to 72 hours to prevent excessive fluid shifts and brain edema. **Ongoing losses** (usually in stool) are replaced milliliter for milliliter with intravenous fluid comparable in electrolyte content with that being lost.

For example, an 18-kg infant with a normal serum sodium judged to be 10% dehydrated has lost an estimated 2,000 mL of fluid (1,000 mL = 1 kg). Half the deficit is replaced over the first 8 hours, with the balance given over the next 16 hours. Maintenance therapy must also be included. The child received a 20 mL per kg bolus initially.

1. 2,000 mL ÷ 2 = 1,000 mL (half the total deficit); 360 mL (20 mL per kg) has already been replaced. Therefore, 640 mL is given over the first 8 hours at 80 mL per hour. This should be added to the 56 mL per hour the child requires to meet maintenance needs. Rate = 80 mL per hour + 56 mL per hour = 136 mL per hour.

2. The second half (1,000 mL) is replaced over the next 16 hours (63 mL per hour) along with the maintenance rate (56 mL per hour). Rate = 63 mL per hour + 56 mL per hour = 119 mL per hour.

The composition of the **replacement fluid** varies depending on the initial laboratory values. Replacement (and maintenance) fluid should be **potassium free** until the patient urinates. Sodium bicarbonate therapy may be indicated if the pH and serum bicarbonate levels remain dangerously low after the initial boluses. In general, ongoing gastrointestinal losses are replaced with one-half normal saline. Urine electrolyte and osmolality studies should be obtained if ongoing losses result from an abnormal renal process.

Patients with profound hyperglycemia or electrolyte disturbances because of an ongoing underlying pathologic process (e.g., diabetic ketoacidosis) may require more specialized management discussed elsewhere in this chapter.

7-1 KEY POINTS

1. Maintenance fluids may be calculated by the Holliday-Segar method or using the hourly rate method.
2. Children are more susceptible to severe dehydration than adults.
3. The history and physical examination are the best determinants of the degree of dehydration. Tachycardia is an early sign. Hypotension occurs very late in children, and its absence does not rule out significant dehydration requiring intervention.
4. Oral rehydration therapy can be highly effective but is very labor intensive.
5. If intravenous fluids are required, initial 20 mL per kg boluses of normal saline or Ringer lactate should be given until the patient's condition stabilizes.
6. When calculating fluid needs, remember to replace previous losses, keep up with ongoing output, and provide maintenance therapy.
7. Potassium should not be added to replacement or maintenance fluids until urine output is assured.

HYPONATREMIA

Hyponatremia (serum sodium level less than 130 mEq per L) may occur in the face of decreased, normal, or increased total body sodium content. In children, the most common setting is dehydration. Other causes include syndrome of inappropriate secretion of antidiuretic hormone (SIADH), water intoxication, renal or congestive heart failure, and adrenal insufficiency.

CLINICAL MANIFESTATIONS

History and Physical Examination

The severity of clinical manifestations depends on both the **level of sodium** in the extracellular space and the **rate of change** from normal. Falling levels that occur over several days are better tolerated than rapid losses. Anorexia and nausea are early, nonspecific complaints. Neurologic findings include confusion, lethargy, and decreased deep tendon reflexes. **Seizures** and **respiratory arrest** are late, life-threatening complications.

DIAGNOSTIC EVALUATION

The laboratory workup of hyponatremia includes serum electrolytes, glucose, blood urea nitrogen and creatinine, serum osmolality, liver function tests, protein, and lipid levels. These laboratory values reveal the severity of the deficit and may suggest an underlying cause. The measured serum sodium needs to be "corrected" in the setting of hyperglycemia. For every 100 mg per dL rise in glucose (above "normal" 100 mg per dL), add 1.6 mEq Na^+ to the *measured* value to get the *true* value. Urine sodium (U_{Na}) and specific gravity (USG) also assist in diagnosis.

TREATMENT

Dehydration is treated with fluid resuscitation as discussed previously. Hyponatremia related to other causes requires fluid restriction and treatment of the underlying disorder. The cautious use of 3% hypertonic saline is limited to life-threatening situations (i.e., intractable seizures). Serum sodium correction should not exceed 1 to 2 mEq per L because of the risk of central pontine myelinolysis.

HYPERNATREMIA

Hypernatremia is uncommon in children in the absence of dehydration (discussed earlier). Signs and symptoms include muscle weakness, irritability, and lethargy. Seizures and coma are the major complications. Hypernatremic dehydration is treated with infusion of isotonic saline. Serum sodium correction

should not exceed 1 to 2 mEq per L because of the risk of cerebral edema.

HYPERKALEMIA

Normal serum potassium values range from 3.5 to 5.7 mEq per L; a measurement of 5.8 mEq/L or greater is considered **hyperkalemia**. In children, the most common cause of an abnormally high potassium level is artifactual because of the hemolysis of red cells during sample collection. Transcellular shifts in hydrogen ions increase serum potassium without changing total body content; for every unit reduction in arterial pH, plasma potassium increases 0.2 to 0.4 mEq per L. Disorders and medications that interfere with renal excretion of the electrolyte precipitate true hyperkalemia.

DIFFERENTIAL DIAGNOSIS

Common causes of hyperkalemia include the following:

- Acidosis
- Severe dehydration
- Potassium-sparing diuretics (spironolactone)
- Excessive parenteral infusion
- Renal failure

Other less common but important conditions to consider include the following:

- Adrenal corticoid deficiency (i.e., Addison's disease)
- Renal tubular acidosis
- Massive crush injury with rhabdomyolysis
- β-Blocker or digitalis ingestions
- Excessive supplementation

CLINICAL MANIFESTATIONS

Paresthesias and weakness are the earliest symptoms; flaccid paralysis and tetany occur late. Cardiac involvement correlates with specific progressive **ECG changes**;

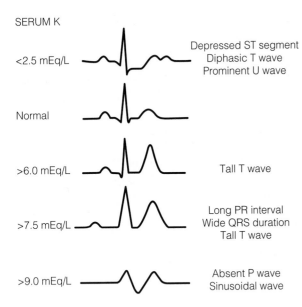

SERUM K

<2.5 mEq/L — Depressed ST segment / Diphasic T wave / Prominent U wave

Normal

>6.0 mEq/L — Tall T wave

>7.5 mEq/L — Long PR interval / Wide QRS duration / Tall T wave

>9.0 mEq/L — Absent P wave / Sinusoidal wave

Figure 7-1 • ECG findings of hyperkalemia (Lead II).

T-wave elevation ("peaking") is followed by loss of P waves, widening QRS complexes, and ST segment depression (Fig. 7-1). Ventricular fibrillation and cardiac arrest occur at serum levels greater than 9 mEq per L.

TREATMENT

Calcium gluconate protects the heart by stabilizing the cardiac cell membrane. Infusion of sodium bicarbonate or insulin (and glucose) drives potassium into the cells. Cation exchange resins (e.g., Kayexalate) and hemodialysis are the only measures that actually remove potassium from the body.

7-3 KEY POINTS

1. Progressive electrocardiogram (ECG) changes associated with hyperkalemia include peaked T waves, loss of P waves, and widening of the QRS complex.
2. Treatment options include calcium gluconate, sodium bicarbonate or insulin/glucose, cation exchange resins, and hemodialysis.

HYPOKALEMIA

Hypokalemia in the pediatric population is usually encountered in cases of alkalosis secondary to vomiting, administration of loop diuretics (furosemide), or diabetic ketoacidosis. Signs and symptoms include weakness, tetany, constipation, polyuria, and polydipsia. Muscle breakdown leading to myoglobinuria may compromise renal function. ECG changes (prolonged Q-T interval, T wave flattening) are noted at levels less than or equal to 2.5 mEq per L; cardiac arrhythmias (ventricular tachycardia/fibrillation) can occur and are more likely if the patient is being treated with digoxin. Blood pressure changes and urine electrolyte content assist in diagnosis (Fig. 7-2). Treatment consists of correcting pH (when increased) and replenishing potassium stores orally or intravenously.

METABOLIC ACIDOSIS

The extracellular fluid pH (the negative logarithm of the hydrogen ion concentration) is kept in a very narrow range (normal: 7.4), largely as a result of the **bicarbonate buffer system**. Hydrogen ions (H^+) combine with HCO_3^- to form H_2CO_3, which is transformed into water and CO_2. The kidneys control excretion of HCO_3^- (bicarbonate), whereas CO_2 is expired by the lungs. The addition of excessive H^-, the loss of HCO_3^-, or abnormal renal or pulmonary function can all affect this buffering system and lead to acid–base disturbances.

Metabolic acidosis (pH ≤ 7.35) results from the loss of HCO_3^- or the addition of H^+ in the extracellular fluid. It is the most common acid–base disorder encountered in the pediatric population. Causes include increased acid intake or production, decreased renal excretion, or increased renal or gastrointestinal bicarbonate loss. $PaCO_2$ begins to drop almost immediately because of increased ventilation; the compensation is complete within 24 hours. In the presence of a metabolic acidosis, the expected $PaCO_2 = 1.5 \times HCO_3^- + 8$ (±2). If the measured $PaCO_2$ is higher than expected, there is a primary respiratory acidosis. If it is lower than expected, there is primary respiratory alkalosis (see "Respiratory Acidosis and Alkalosis").

CLINICAL MANIFESTATIONS

Hyperpnea is the most consistent clinical finding in metabolic acidosis. Severe acidemia affects multiple organ systems: cardiac contractility is impaired, cardiac output is reduced, and the heart becomes vulnerable to arrhythmias. Protein breakdown is accelerated, and mental status changes occur. Other signs and symptoms are specific to the underlying disorder. Important laboratory studies include serum electrolytes, blood urea nitrogen, creatinine, glucose, venous or arterial blood

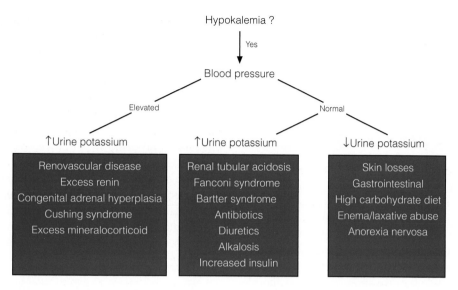

Figure 7-2 • Evaluation of hypokalemia.

gas, and urine dipstick for pH and glucose. These studies help quantify the acidosis and may suggest the underlying condition. The difference between the sums of the measured cations ($Na^+ + K^+$) and anions ($Cl^- + HCO_3^-$), termed the **anion gap**, is normally 12 ± 4; Table 7-2 lists conditions associated with changes in the anion gap.

TREATMENT

The intravenous administration of sodium bicarbonate should be reserved for cases in which the serum pH is less than 7.0 and the cause is unknown or slow to reverse (i.e., most normal anion gap acidosis). Boluses are reserved for extreme situations; in general, the

■ **TABLE 7-2** Changes in the Anion Gap		
Increased Anion Gap[a]	**Normal Anion Gap**	**Decreased Anion Gap**
Hypokalemia	Diarrhea	Hyperkalemia
Hypocalcemia	Renal tubular acidosis	Hypercalcemia
Hypomagnesemia	Hyperalimentation	Hypermagnesemia
Hyperphosphatemia	Hypoaldosteronism	Hypoalbuminemia
Lactic acidosis	Lithium ingestion	
Diabetic ketoacidosis		
Renal failure/uremia		
Salicylate ingestion		
Ethylene glycol, ethanol, methanol ingestion		

[a]The mnemonic MUDPILES is helpful for recalling several clinical conditions that result in metabolic acidosis with a high anion gap: **m**ethanol ingestion; **u**remia; **d**iabetic ketoacidosis; **p**araldehyde ingestion; **i**soniazid ingestion, iron ingestion, and inborn errors of metabolism; **l**actic acidosis; **e**thanol ingestion; and **s**alicylate ingestion.

infusion should be slow and relatively isotonic. Patients receiving alkali therapy require frequent pH, sodium, potassium, calcium, and mental status monitoring. Complications include alkalosis (overcorrection), hypokalemia, hypernatremia/hyperosmolarity, and hypocalcemia.

METABOLIC ALKALOSIS

Metabolic alkalosis (pH $\geq$ 7.45) is much less common than acidosis in children. "Contraction" alkalosis results from the loss of fluid high in H^+ or Cl^- as may occur with protracted gastric vomiting (pyloric stenosis, bulimia) or chronic thiazide or loop diuretic administration. Patients with cystic fibrosis may develop metabolic alkalosis because of excessive electrolyte losses in the sweat. Other causes include laxative abuse and other chloride-wasting diarrheas. Volume expansion and chloride replacement correct the alkalosis unless it results from disorders of mineralocorticoid excess (e.g., renal artery stenosis, adrenal disorders, steroid use); potassium supplements are also necessary in these cases.

The goal is diagnosis and resolution of the underlying disorder. Complications of severe alkalosis include reduction in coronary blood flow and arrhythmias, hypoventilation, seizures, and decreased potassium, magnesium, and phosphate levels.

RESPIRATORY ACIDOSIS AND ALKALOSIS

Normal $PaCO_2$ levels range from 39 to 41 mm Hg. Any process that causes respiratory insufficiency (CNS depression, chest wall muscle weakness, pulmonary or cardiopulmonary diseases) results in a primary elevation in the $PaCO_2$, termed *respiratory acidosis*. This is followed by renal bicarbonate reabsorption and a compensatory rise in the serum bicarbonate measurement (secondary metabolic alkalosis). Conversely, respiratory alkalosis results from a primary reduction in the $PaCO_2$. The kidney responds by increasing the urine bicarbonate concentration (secondary metabolic acidosis). Causes of respiratory alkalosis include lung disease, mechanical ventilation, or any process (metabolic or neurologic) that results in a sustained increase in the respiratory rate.

Of note, both respiratory acidosis and alkalosis may occur as compensation for other primary metabolic pH disturbances.

🔑 7-4 KEY POINTS

1. Metabolic acidosis is a relatively common disorder in pediatric patients.
2. The equation $PaCO_2 = 1.5 \times HCO_3^- + 8 \ (\pm 2)$ can help distinguish between primary and secondary metabolic acidosis.
3. An increased respiratory rate is the most consistent physical finding in metabolic acidosis.
4. Measurement of the anion gap may aid in diagnosis.
5. $NaHCO_3$ (sodium bicarbonate) should be used only when acidosis is severe or difficult to correct.
6. Contraction alkalosis may result from protracted vomiting from pyloric stenosis or with diuretic therapy.

Additional Suggested Reading

Moritz ML, Ayus JC. Disorders of water metabolism in children: hyponatremia and hypernatremia. *Pediatr Rev.* 2002;23:371–380.

Roberts KB. Fluid and electrolytes: parenteral fluid therapy. *Pediatr Rev.* 2001;22:380–387.

Schwaderer AL, Schwartz GJ. Acidosis and alkalosis. *Pediatr Rev.* 2004;25:350–357.

Gastroenterology

ABDOMINAL PAIN

Abdominal pain is one of the most common symptoms the pediatrician sees, and it has a complex differential diagnosis. Abdominal pain may be acute or chronic/recurrent (at least three episodes within 3 months), and it may represent a surgical or medical condition. Chronic/recurrent abdominal pain occurs in approximately 10% of children 5 to 15 years of age, and less than 10% of these cases result from an organic cause.

DIFFERENTIAL DIAGNOSIS

Infectious conditions (including bacterial and viral gastroenteritis) are the most common cause of abdominal pain. Mesenteric lymphadenitis may cause persistent pain following an infection. Group A streptococcal infections, urinary tract infections, and lower lobe pneumonias may also present with abdominal pain. Pelvic inflammatory disease (PID) is an important consideration in adolescent females. Viral hepatitis, infectious mononucleosis, and herpes zoster are more uncommon infections that may need to be considered.

Noninfectious medical diseases are less common and include both primary gastrointestinal (GI) and genitourinary pathology and systemic diseases. Cholecystitis, pancreatitis, gastritis, and peptic ulcer disease are uncommon in children but warrant consideration. Abdominal pain is a primary feature in Henoch-Schönlein purpura (HSP), but also may be seen in other vasculitides, including Kawasaki disease, polyarteritis nodosa, and lupus erythematosus. If the pain is recurrent, the differential diagnosis must be expanded. Constipation and functional abdominal pain are frequent complaints evaluated by a pediatrician. Lactase deficiency results in recurrent pain with exposure to dairy food. Sickle cell disease, ulcerative colitis, and Crohn disease are chronic conditions in which pain is a major symptom. More rare causes include abdominal migraines, seizures, Hirschsprung disease, and malignancy, including leukemia as well as solid tumors.

Appendicitis is the most common surgical cause of abdominal pain. Intussusception is an important pediatric disease that presents with intermittent but severe pain and striking lethargy. Incarcerated hernia, volvulus, bowel obstruction, and testicular torsion represent surgical emergencies. Trauma can lead to significant intra-abdominal injury and pain.

Urologic obstruction at any level is an important consideration. Ureteropelvic junction obstruction, hydronephrosis, and renal stones can cause significant pain.

Gynecologic causes are an important part of the differential diagnosis in adolescent girls. Pregnancy should always be considered, especially if symptoms are consistent with an ectopic pregnancy. Dysmenorrhea, ovarian cysts, mittelschmerz, PID, cervicitis, endometriosis, and ovarian or adnexal torsion are all potential problems in this population.

Psychiatric causes of abdominal pain are uncommon in children. True malingering is unusual, as are conversion disorders. However, many children do experience abdominal pain in the setting of stress, especially in the context of school, and mild intermittent pain also can be seen in children with depression.

CLINICAL MANIFESTATIONS

History

The history should localize the pain and determine its quality and temporal characteristics and its exacerbating and alleviating factors. With "inflammatory" pain, the child tends to lie still, whereas with "colicky" pain, the child cannot remain still. Colicky pain usually results from obstruction, whereas inflammatory pain is caused by an infected or perforated organ or viscus. It is important to ascertain whether the child has any drug or food allergies or has had previous abdominal surgeries. With a history of previous laparotomy, small bowel obstruction becomes more likely. Pain may be accompanied by anorexia, nausea, emesis, diarrhea, or constipation. If the pain wakes the child at night, an organic cause is more likely. Bilious emesis indicates obstruction (or less commonly, ileus), whereas bloody emesis points to an upper GI bleeding source (esophagitis, gastritis, or duodenitis). Bloody or mucinous diarrhea suggests bacterial enterocolitis.

Stooling characteristics are important because constipation is a common etiology of chronic abdominal pain. Dysuria and abdominal pain are indicative of a urinary tract infection, whereas sore throat and abdominal pain implicate pharyngitis. There may be a history of trauma. Obtaining a good sexual history in the adolescent is critical. If there is a history of vaginal discharge and fever, PID should be considered. Inquiring about ill contacts can give helpful clues to the diagnosis because viral gastroenteritis is quite contagious and very common. A family history of lactose intolerance, Crohn disease, ulcerative colitis, or irritable bowel syndrome increases the likelihood of these diagnoses because they are genetically based. Changes in the child's environment (home, friends, school) or behavior (poor school performance, increasingly argumentative) may suggest that the abdominal pain is not the result of organic disease.

Physical Examination

The goal of the abdominal examination is to ascertain whether the child has an abdominal process that requires surgical intervention. Watching the child walk, climb onto the examination table, and interact with both parents and staff before formally examining the child's abdomen helps one to gain an appreciation for the degree of incapacitation or emotional overlay that may be present. The abdomen should be inspected, auscultated, and palpated. Peritoneal signs include rebound tenderness, guarding, psoas or obturator signs, and rigidity of the abdominal wall. Unless the diagnosis is thought to be uncomplicated viral gastroenteritis, a rectal examination should be performed to detect tenderness or hard stool and to obtain stool for guaiac testing. If the patient is an adolescent female, a pelvic examination should be performed.

Cervical motion tenderness is consistent with PID. In the setting of chronic abdominal pain, the growth curve should be examined for any alterations in weight gain or linear growth, which may be a sign of a chronic condition such as inflammatory bowel disease (IBD).

DIAGNOSTIC EVALUATION

The diagnostic test strategy is dictated by the history and findings on the physical examination. If the cause of the pain is thought to be a surgical one, a surgical consultation should be obtained because surgical causes are the most likely to require immediate intervention.

A complete blood count with manual differential, serum electrolytes and chemistries, amylase, lipase, stool guaiac examination, urinalysis, and radiographic studies should be performed if there has been abdominal trauma or an acute surgical condition is suspected. Blood should also be typed for possible transfusion. A barium swallow with upper GI examination, a pH probe, or an endoscopic examination may be used to evaluate for reflux. When uncomplicated viral gastroenteritis is the most likely cause, no studies need be performed, but if bacterial enterocolitis is being considered, stool should be obtained for culture. Group A streptococcal pharyngitis and PID require appropriate cultures. In some severe cases of constipation, abdominal radiographs may be indicated. To diagnose a urinary tract infection, a urinalysis and urine culture should be performed.

TREATMENT

Treatment is directed at the underlying cause of the pain. Surgical problems are treated accordingly. Group A streptococcal pharyngitis, urinary tract infections, and PID require appropriate antibiotics. Individuals with lactase deficiency will improve with a lactose-free diet or exogenous lactase replacement. Patients with reflux esophagitis benefit from small frequent meals (rather than infrequent large ones), sitting upright for 30 minutes after a meal or sleeping at a 45-degree angle after eating, avoidance of late evening meals, a prokinetic agent, and an H_2 blocker and/or proton pump antagonist. Children with abdominal pain exacerbated by stress require patience, reassurance, and in rare cases professional psychiatric assistance. Constipation can be treated with prune juice, mineral oil, MiraLax, or lactulose. In some cases, disimpaction, cathartics, or enemas may be required.

APPENDICITIS

Appendicitis is the most common indication for abdominal surgery in childhood. Appendicitis results from bacterial invasion of the appendix, which is more likely when the lumen is obstructed by a fecalith, parasite, or lymph node. Appendicitis occurs most frequently in children between 10 and 15 years of age. Less than 10% of patients are younger than 5 years.

Clinical Manifestations

Classically, fever, emesis, anorexia, and diffuse periumbilical pain develop. Subsequently, pain and abdominal tenderness localize to the right lower quadrant as the parietal peritoneum becomes inflamed. Guarding, rebound tenderness, and obturator and psoas signs are commonly found. The appendix tends to perforate approximately 36 hours after pain begins. The incidence of perforation and diffuse peritonitis is higher in children younger than 2 years when diagnosis may be delayed. Atypical presentations are common in childhood, especially with retrocecal appendicitis, which may present with periumbilical pain and diarrhea. Retrocecal appendicitis usually does not induce right lower quadrant pain until after perforation. Bacterial enterocolitis caused by *Campylobacter* and *Yersinia* may mimic appendicitis because both can result in right lower quadrant abdominal pain and tenderness. Diagnosis of appendicitis is established clinically by history and by physical examination, which should include a rectal examination to detect tenderness or a mass. A moderately elevated white blood cell count with a left shift is often seen in appendicitis. A plain film of the abdomen may demonstrate a fecalith. An inflamed appendix may be noted on ultrasound, but CT scans have a higher yield.

Treatment

Laparotomy and appendectomy should be performed before perforation. When appendicitis results in perforation, the patient should be given ampicillin, gentamicin, and metronidazole (Flagyl) to treat peritonitis from intestinal flora. The mortality rate rises significantly with perforation.

INTUSSUSCEPTION

Intussusception results from telescoping of one part of the intestine into another. Intussusception causes impaired venous return, bowel edema and ischemia, necrosis, and perforation. It is one of the most common causes of intestinal obstruction in infancy. Most intussusceptions are ileocolic; the ileum invaginates into the colon at the ileocecal valve. A previous viral infection may cause hypertrophy of the Peyer patches or mesenteric nodes, which are hypothesized to act as the lead point in intussusception. A specific lead point is identified in only approximately 5% of cases but should be sought in neonates or in children older than 5 years. Recognizable lead points in intussusception include Meckel diverticulum, an intestinal polyp, lymphoma, or a foreign body. Intussusception has also been associated with HSP, but in this setting is usually ileal-ileal. It can be very difficult to distinguish HSP complicated by intussusception from the inflammatory abdominal pain seen in simple HSP.

Clinical Manifestations

Violent episodes of irritability, colicky pain, and emesis are interspersed with relatively normal periods. Rectal bleeding occurs in 80% of patients but only rarely in the form of the classic "currant jelly" stools (stools containing bright red blood and mucus). The degree of lethargy shown by the child may be striking. A tubular mass is palpable in approximately 80% of patients. A plain abdominal film may show a paucity of gas in the right lower quadrant or evidence of obstruction with air-fluid levels. A barium enema or air enema demonstrates a coiled-spring appearance to the bowel, which is diagnostic. Stool should be tested for occult blood.

Treatment

Fluid resuscitation with normal saline or lactated Ringer solution is usually necessary. Hydrostatic reduction with barium enema or pneumatic reduction with air enema is successful in 75% of cases if performed in the first 48 hours. Peritoneal signs are an absolute contraindication to this procedure. Laparotomy and direct reduction is indicated when reduction by enema is either unsuccessful or contraindicated. The immediate recurrence rate is approximately 15%. When a specific lead point is identified, the recurrence rate is higher.

8-3 KEY POINTS

1. Most intussusceptions are ileocolic, in which the ileum invaginates into the colon at the ileocecal valve.
2. Violent episodes of irritability, colicky pain, and emesis are interspersed with relatively normal periods. Rectal bleeding may occur, but only rarely in the form of the classic "currant jelly" stools.
3. Hydrostatic reduction with barium enema or pneumatic reduction with air enema is successful in 75% of cases.

EMESIS

Vomiting is one of the most common presenting symptoms in pediatrics and can be caused by both GI and non-GI pathologies. Complications of severe, persistent emesis include dehydration and hypochloremic, hypokalemic metabolic alkalosis. Forceful emesis can result in a Mallory-Weiss tear of the esophagus at the gastroesophageal junction or erosion of the gastric cardia; chronic emesis can result in distal esophagitis.

DIFFERENTIAL DIAGNOSIS

Table 8-1 lists the most common causes of vomiting in the pediatric population.

■ **TABLE 8-1** Differential Diagnosis of Vomiting in Children

Infectious	Gastrointestinal: Infant
Viral gastroenteritis (especially rotavirus and Norwalk virus)	Gastroesophageal reflux
	Cow or soy milk protein intolerance
Bacterial enterocolitis/sepsis	Bowel obstruction[a]
Hepatitis	Duodenal atresia
Food poisoning	Pyloric stenosis
Staphylococcus aureus	Malrotation with or without volvulus
Clostridium perfringens	
Salmonella	Incarcerated hernia
Pelvic inflammatory disease	Intussusception
Peritonitis	Meckel diverticulum with torsion
Pharyngitis	
Pneumonia	Hirschsprung disease
Otitis media	
Tonsillitis	*Gastrointestinal: Child*
Urinary tract infection	Appendicitis
	Eosinophilic gastroenteritis
Metabolic	
Diabetic ketoacidosis	Pancreatitis
Inborn errors of metabolism	Hepatitis
	Cholecystitis
Other	Bowel obstruction
Adrenal insufficiency	Malrotation
Renal failure	Incarcerated hernia
Hepatic failure	Intussusception
Central Nervous System	Meckel diverticulum with torsion
Increased intracranial pressure	Adhesions
Ventricular-peritoneal shunt malfunction	Superior mesenteri artery syndrome
Meningitis	Posttraumatic obstruction[b]
Encephalitis	
Labyrinthitis	*Respiratory*
Migraine	Reactive airway disease
Reye syndrome	*Oncology*
Seizure	Chemotherapeutic agents
Tumor	
Gynecologic	
Pregnancy	

(Continued)

TABLE 8-1 Differential Diagnosis of Vomiting in Children (*continued*)

Toxic ingestion
Salicylates
Theophylline
Caustic agents
Digoxin
Lead
Emotional
"Psychogenic"
Bulimia

[a]Malrotation with or without volvulus is much more likely in an infant than in a child.
[b]From duodenal hematoma, ruptured viscus, or superior mesenteric artery syndrome.

CLINICAL MANIFESTATIONS

History

In infants, the history should differentiate between true vomiting and "spitting up" (gastroesophageal reflux) and whether the emesis is acute or chronic. Frequency, appearance (bloody or bilious), amount, and timing of the emesis are important. Emesis shortly after feeding in the infant is probably gastroesophageal reflux. If the emesis is projectile and the child is 1 to 3 months of age, pyloric stenosis must be considered. Poor weight gain and emesis may indicate pyloric stenosis or a metabolic disorder. Macrolide antibiotics are known to cause emesis and diarrhea; chemotherapeutic agents and some toxic ingestions cause emesis. If the child has a ventricular-peritoneal shunt, vomiting may be a sign of shunt obstruction and increased intracranial pressure. Emesis with seizure or headache or both may indicate an intracranial process. Diarrhea, emesis, and fever are seen with gastroenteritis. Fever, abdominal pain, and emesis are typical for appendicitis, whereas bilious emesis and abdominal pain are seen with intestinal obstruction. Emesis and syncope may result from pregnancy.

Physical Examination

On physical examination, the initial assessment should focus on the child's vital signs and hydration status. Chapter 7 discusses signs and symptoms of dehydration. A bulging fontanelle or papilledema implicates increased intracranial pressure as the cause of the emesis. Emesis is common in infectious pharyngitis. The lung fields should be auscultated for crackles or an asymmetric examination to rule out pneumonia. Emesis and vaginal discharge in the female adolescent warrant a pelvic examination to evaluate for PID. The abdominal examination should focus on bowel sounds and the presence of distention, tenderness, or masses. Hypoactive bowel sounds may indicate ileus or obstruction, whereas hyperactive bowel sounds suggest gastroenteritis. Abdominal mass with emesis may indicate intussusception or malignancy. Tenderness on examination is suggestive of appendicitis, pancreatitis, cholecystitis, peritonitis, or PID.

DIAGNOSTIC EVALUATION

Specific laboratory studies depend on the suspected cause. Appropriate cultures and a complete blood count with manual differential should be sent if an infectious cause is deemed likely and the vomiting is significant. A chest radiograph will rule out pneumonia. If a surgical process within the abdomen is considered, upright and supine abdominal films should be obtained, along with a complete blood count and electrolyte and chemistry panels. Amylase and lipase should be sent to detect pancreatitis. If vomiting is prolonged or the patient is significantly dehydrated, electrolytes will help guide replacement therapy. An ammonia level, serum amino acids, and urine organic acids should be sent if metabolic disease is suspected. Urinalysis and urine culture should be obtained to rule out urinary tract infection and assess degree of dehydration.

TREATMENT

If the cause appears to be a self-limited nonsurgical infectious process (viral gastroenteritis or bacterial enterocolitis) and the patient is not significantly dehydrated, outpatient therapy is indicated. Oral rehydration therapy (ORT), discussed in Chapter 7, is recommended for dehydrated infants. For older children, fluids should be encouraged, with cautious advancement to a soft, bland diet as tolerated. Children who are severely dehydrated or unable to orally hydrate themselves effectively should be admitted to the hospital.

A surgical consultation should be obtained if indicated. If ventricular-peritoneal shunt malfunction is a possibility, the standard of care dictates that a CT of the head and a shunt series be obtained in tandem with a neurosurgical consultation.

🔑 8-4 KEY POINTS

1. Most cases of emesis are caused by gastro-esophageal reflux, acute gastroenteritis, or non-GI infectious disorders such as tonsillitis, otitis media, or urinary tract infection.
2. Most children with uncomplicated viral gastroenteritis and mild dehydration can be treated as outpatients with oral rehydration therapy (ORT).

PYLORIC STENOSIS

Pyloric stenosis is an important cause of gastric outlet obstruction and vomiting in the first 2 to 3 months of life. Peak incidence occurs at 2 to 4 weeks of life, with an incidence of 1 in 500 infants. Male infants are affected 4:1 over female infants, and pyloric stenosis occurs more frequently in infants with a family history of the condition. Current evidence suggests that erythromycin therapy may precipitate pyloric stenosis.

Clinical Manifestations

Projectile nonbilious vomiting is the cardinal feature of the disorder. Physical findings vary with the severity of the obstruction. Dehydration and poor weight gain are common when the diagnosis is delayed. Hypokalemic, hypochloremic metabolic alkalosis with dehydration is seen secondary to persistent emesis in the most severe cases. The classic finding of an olive-sized, muscular, mobile, nontender mass in the epigastric area occurs in most cases. Visible gastric peristaltic waves may be seen. Ultrasonography reveals the hypertrophic pylorus. Upper GI study may show the classic "string sign."

Treatment

Initial treatment involves nasogastric tube placement and correction of dehydration, alkalosis, and electrolyte abnormalities. Pyloromyotomy should take place as soon as the metabolic anomalies are corrected satisfactorily.

🔑 8-5 KEY POINTS

1. Pyloric stenosis is an important cause of gastric outlet obstruction and emesis in the first 2 months of life, with a peak incidence at 2 to 4 weeks of life.
2. Projectile nonbilious vomiting is the cardinal feature of this disorder.
3. Pyloromyotomy should take place as soon as the metabolic anomalies are corrected satisfactorily.

MALROTATION AND VOLVULUS

Malrotation occurs when the small intestines rotate abnormally in utero, resulting in malposition in the abdomen and abnormal posterior fixation of the mesentery. When the intestine attaches improperly to the mesentery, it is at risk for twisting on its vascular supply; the twisting phenomenon is called volvulus. The most common age of presentation is less than 1 month of age.

Clinical Manifestations

The history almost always includes bilious emesis. In older children, a history of past attacks is occasionally elicited. Physical examination may reveal abdominal distention or shock. Blood-stained emesis or stool may be noted. Abdominal radiographs typically show gas in the stomach with a paucity of air in the intestine. An upper GI series with small bowel follow-through confirms the diagnosis by illustrating the abnormal position of the ligament of Treitz and the cecum. A positive stool guaiac examination is a poor prognostic sign, indicating significant bowel ischemia.

Treatment

Operative correction of the malrotation and the volvulus should be undertaken as soon as possible because bowel ischemia, metabolic acidosis, and sepsis can progress quickly to death.

8-6 KEY POINTS

1. Malrotation occurs when the intestines rotate abnormally in utero, resulting in malposition in the abdomen and abnormal posterior fixation of the mesentery. When the intestine attaches improperly, it is at risk for volvulus.
2. An upper GI series with small bowel follow-through confirms the diagnosis by demonstrating the abnormal position of the ligament of Treitz and the cecum.

GASTROESOPHAGEAL REFLUX

Gastroesophageal reflux (GER) is the regurgitation of stomach contents into the esophagus because of an incompetent lower esophageal sphincter. A small degree of reflux is common in all infants, and it is only infants who have moderate to severe chronic reflux that tend to come to the pediatrician's attention. In this group, complications include failure to thrive, aspiration pneumonia, esophagitis, choking or apneic episodes, hematemesis, anemia, and chronic fussiness.

DIFFERENTIAL DIAGNOSIS

Incompetence of the lower esophageal sphincter may be the result of prematurity, esophageal disease, obstructive lung disease, overdistention of the stomach caused by overeating, or medication (theophylline). If the infant is having forceful emesis or projectile vomiting, reflux is not the most likely cause, and the differential diagnosis for emesis just discussed should be considered.

The differential diagnosis for GER in the adolescent may include pneumonia, costochondritis, pericarditis, pulmonary embolism, arrhythmias, ischemia because of an anomalous coronary artery, pancreatitis, cholecystitis, peptic ulcer disease, and panic attacks.

CLINICAL MANIFESTATIONS

History

It is important to determine if the infant is "spitting up" or having projectile emesis and if the emesis is bloody or bilious. One of the most common causes of GER is overfeeding, so a careful history should include what formula the infant eats, how it is mixed, how much the infant eats during each feeding, and how often the child is fed. If the emesis is independent of meals, it is probably not reflux. A history of coughing, gagging, and arching of the back with extensor posturing during feeding may result from direct aspiration, whereas the presence of these symptoms soon after feeding may suggest GER. In severe reflux, the infant may have poor weight gain.

In the older child, GER is often manifested as epigastric abdominal or chest pain. A careful history will reveal the pain's location, severity, whether it radiates, and whether it is constant or intermittent. Burning epigastric or chest pain is probably reflux in the adolescent, especially if it occurs after meals when the patient lies down.

Physical Examination

In most cases, the physical examination of the child with GER is normal. In severe cases, infants present with poor weight gain or failure to thrive.

DIAGNOSTIC EVALUATION

The diagnosis of mild reflux is made by the characteristic history. In moderate or severe reflux, the diagnosis of GER may be confirmed by pH probe placement in the esophagus or upper GI endoscopy. An abdominal ultrasound and barium swallow are useful to confirm normal anatomy and normal gastric emptying. The child with mild to moderate reflux generally has an unremarkable complete blood count and electrolyte panel. If the chest examination is abnormal in the presence of reflux, a chest radiograph should be obtained to look for aspiration pneumonia or changes caused by recurrent aspiration.

TREATMENT

Infants with GER should receive small, frequent feedings in the upright position and be maintained in the prone head-up position for at least 20 minutes after a feeding. Feeds should be thickened with cereal. If these measures fail, metoclopramide may be used to improve gastric motility and increase the rate of gastric emptying. If esophagitis is suspected, an H_2 blocker (e.g., ranitidine) or a proton pump inhibitor (e.g., omeprazole) may be useful.

In severe cases where medical management fails, a Nissen fundoplication may be necessary. In this procedure, the fundus of the stomach is wrapped around the distal esophagus to increase lower esophageal sphincter pressure.

Older children or adolescents with reflux should also have small, frequent meals, eat slowly, and maintain the upright position after meals. Meals after 7 PM should be discouraged, and the medications just mentioned may be useful.

8-7 KEY POINTS

1. Most cases of gastroesophageal reflux (GER) occur in the infant and adolescent populations and do not require medical intervention.
2. Most infants with moderate GER respond to small, frequent feedings in the upright position, thickened feeds with rice cereal, and maintenance of the prone head-up position for at least 20 minutes after feeding.
3. The most common symptoms of GER in the adolescent are burning epigastric pain and chest pain.

DIARRHEA

Diarrhea is defined as an increase in the frequency and the water content of stools. Viral gastroenteritis accounts for 70% to 80% of acute diarrhea in most developed countries. The complications of acute diarrhea include dehydration, electrolyte and acid–base disturbance, bacteremia and sepsis, and malnutrition in chronic cases. **Enteritis** refers to small bowel inflammation, whereas **colitis** refers to large bowel inflammation.

DIFFERENTIAL DIAGNOSIS

Table 8-2 lists the most common causes of diarrhea in the pediatric population of the Western world.

CLINICAL MANIFESTATIONS

History

The history should ascertain whether the diarrhea is acute or chronic/recurrent and establish the frequency,

TABLE 8-2 Differential Diagnosis of Diarrhea in Children

Acute Diarrhea	Chronic Diarrhea
Intraintestinal Infections	*Renal*
Viral gastroenteritis	Hemolytic uremic syndrome
Rotavirus	
Enterovirus	
Adenovirus	*Vasculitis*
Norwalk agent	Henoch-Schönlein purpura
Bacterial enterocolitis	
Shigella	
Salmonella	*Infectious*
Yersinia	Parasites
Campylobacter	Amoebiasis
Escherichia coli (enteroinvasive/ enteropathogenic)	Giardiasis
	Cryptosporidium
Clostridium difficile	*Gastrointestinal*
Neisseria gonorrhoeae	Cow/soy milk intolerance
Chlamydia Trachomatis	Overfeeding
	Ulcerative colitis
Extraintestinal Infections	Crohn disease
Otitis media	Hirschsprung disease
Urinary tract infection	Lactase deficiency
	Irritable bowel disease
Gastrointestinal	Encopresis
Intussusception	Excessive fructose intake
Appendicitis	Cystic fibrosi
Hyperconcentrated infant formula	Celiac sprue
Cystic fibrosis	*Allergy*
	Food allergies
Toxic Ingestion	
Iron, mercury, lead, fluoride ingestion	
Medication Induced	
Any antibiotic, chemotherapeutic agents	

appearance (bloody, mucosal, currant jelly), amount, consistency, and color of the diarrhea. Dietary indiscretions and manipulations may result in diarrhea. Small infants have diarrhea when they are fed concentrated formula. If the child has traveled out of the country, a parasitic or bacterial enterocolitis must be considered. Weight loss or lack of weight gain in association with diarrhea indicates more severe disease. Certain medications, especially antibiotics and chemotherapeutic agents, may cause diarrhea. Viral gastroenteritis is highly contagious, so sick contacts are likely. If a close contact of the child has contact with raw poultry, salmonella should be considered. Foul-smelling diarrhea that floats in the toilet is likely steatorrhea and may result from cystic fibrosis or fat malabsorption from other causes.

Physical Examination

Chapter 7 discusses signs and symptoms of dehydration, which are critical in the evaluation of a patient with diarrhea. An attempt should be made to determine the degree of dehydration to guide therapy. The abdominal examination focuses on bowel sounds and the presence of distention, tenderness, or masses. Hypoactive bowel sounds point to intestinal obstruction. Hyperactive sounds are consistent with gastroenteritis. Abdominal mass with diarrhea could indicate intussusception or malignancy.

DIAGNOSTIC EVALUATION

When evaluating a child with diarrhea, inspecting the stool is critical to evaluation and formulation of a treatment plan. If there is a history of blood and/or mucous in the stool, bacterial cultures should be obtained. Rapid tests for rotavirus and adenovirus are available. Rotavirus causes 65% of infant diarrhea during the winter months.

If a bacterial pathogen is being considered and the child is younger than 3 months, a blood culture should be performed because the incidence of secondary bacteremia from salmonella enterocolitis is high in this age group. When there is a history of long-term or multiple antibiotic use, a *Clostridium difficile* toxin assay should be sent. Children with chronic diarrhea, a history of foreign travel or recent camping, or immunocompromise need stools examined for ova and parasites. If the child appears toxic, or moderate to severe dehydration is noted, a complete blood count with manual differential, electrolyte panel, and urine analysis is indicated. Urinary tract infection is evaluated by urine dipstick, urine microscopy, and urine culture.

TREATMENT

For uncomplicated viral gastroenteritis without significant dehydration, the current recommendations are to feed through the diarrhea. The continuation of normal feedings results in less intestinal denudement, improved nutritional absorption, and a faster return to a normal stooling pattern. If the infant is also vomiting, one feed may be replaced with Rice-Lyte or Pedialyte to calm the stomach, with subsequent return to normal feeds. The parents often need to give smaller feedings more frequently to accommodate the intestinal irritation from the gastroenteritis and to minimize emesis. Infants who do not tolerate their regular formula but are not significantly dehydrated or toxic appearing may be orally rehydrated at home. See Chapter 7 for details on ORT.

For the infant 0 to 12 months old with diarrhea for more than 5 days, with suspected enterocolitis, or with exposure to salmonella, a stool culture should be obtained. A blood culture should be performed if the infant is younger than 3 months. If the stool culture is positive and the infant is afebrile and does not appear toxic, the infant can be reexamined and observed at home. If the stool culture is positive and the infant is febrile, the infant's age determines therapy:

- The infant younger than 3 months is admitted to the hospital; a blood culture is obtained, and intravenous antibiotics are started. A lumbar puncture and urinalysis should also be considered in this age group.
- The infant older than 3 months is admitted to the hospital; a blood culture should be sent, but antibiotics may be withheld pending the results of the blood culture.
- Any infant with a positive stool culture who looks toxic or has a positive blood culture is admitted for intravenous antibiotics and evaluation for pyelonephritis, meningitis, pneumonia, and osteomyelitis.

Older children with viral gastroenteritis should be encouraged to drink isotonic fluids. Any fluid with a high carbohydrate load should be diluted with water. Admission is indicated for the child who is more than 5% dehydrated and cannot orally rehydrate himself or herself effectively. See Chapter 7 for details on intravenous rehydration.

Viral gastroenteritis requires no pharmacologic therapy. Antidiarrheal medications are contraindicated because they may cause toxic megacolon. In general, antibiotics are not indicated for bacterial enterocolitis. Exceptions include colitis caused by *Salmonella typhi*,

Shigella, and *C. difficile*. Chapter 12 offers a summary of the bacterial pathogens and their treatment. Parasitic GI infections should be treated with the appropriate antimicrobial. Antibiotic-related diarrhea remits when the offending antibiotic is discontinued. Intussusception is treated by hydrostatic reduction with barium enema, air enema, and/or surgery.

🔑 8-8 KEY POINTS

1. The most common cause of diarrhea in children is viral gastroenteritis.
2. Bacteremia is more likely in infants younger than 3 months with bacterial enterocolitis.
3. Most children with uncomplicated viral gastroenteritis or bacterial enterocolitis can be rehydrated orally.
4. Antidiarrheal medications should be avoided in children with acute diarrhea.
5. Infants with diarrhea should be fed as close to their normal diet as possible. Recovery is faster because there is less sloughing of the intestinal mucosa.

CONSTIPATION

Constipation is defined as the infrequent passage of hard, dry stools. Constipated infants fail to empty the colon completely with bowel movements and over time stretch the smooth muscle of the colon, resulting in a functional ileus. In contrast to constipation, **obstipation** is the absence of bowel movements. Beyond the neonatal period, the most common cause (90% to 95%) of constipation is caused by voluntary withholding or functional constipation. Intentional withholding is often noted from the very beginning of toilet training. A family history of similar problems is often obtained. Stool retention may be caused by conflicts in toilet training but is usually caused by pain on defecation, which creates a fear of defecation and further retention. Voluntary withholding of stool increases distention of the rectum, which decreases rectal sensation, necessitating an even greater fecal mass to initiate the urge to defecate. Complications of stool retention include impaction, abdominal pain, overflow diarrhea resulting from leakage around the fecal mass, anal fissure, rectal bleeding, and urinary tract infection caused by extrinsic pressure on the urethra.

Encopresis, which is daytime or nighttime soiling by formed stools in children beyond the age of expected toilet training (4 to 5 years), is another complication of constipation. In older children, it is important to ask specifically about soiling because such information may not be expressed because of embarrassment. These children are unable to sense the need to defecate because of stretching of the internal sphincter by the retained fecal mass.

Organic causes of failure to defecate include decreased peristalsis, decreased expulsion, and anatomic malformation. Organic etiologies are delineated in the following section.

DIFFERENTIAL DIAGNOSIS

Nonorganic
- Functional constipation (intentional withholding)
- Dysfunctional toilet training

Organic
- *Dietary*: Low-fiber diet, inadequate fluid intake
- *GI*: Functional ileus, Hirschsprung disease, anal stenosis, rectal abscess or fissure, stricture following necrotizing enterocolitis (NEC), collagen vascular diseases
- *Drugs or toxins*: Lead, narcotics, phenothiazines, vincristine, anticholinergics
- *Neuromuscular*: Meningomyelocele, tethered spinal cord, infant botulism, absent abdominal muscles (prune belly syndrome)
- *Metabolic*: Cystic fibrosis, hypothyroidism, hypokalemia, hypercalcemia
- *Endocrine*: Hypothyroidism

CLINICAL MANIFESTATIONS

History and Physical Examination

Abdominal pain caused by constipation is often diffuse and constant. The pain may be accompanied by nausea, but vomiting is unusual. Stools are hard, difficult to pass, and infrequent. Particular foods can exacerbate constipation. Discussion of the psychological state of the child helps determine whether voluntary withholding is the most likely diagnosis. A medication history is essential. If a history of diarrhea or fecal spotting alternating with periods of constipation exists, a diagnosis of Hirschsprung disease or encopresis should be entertained. An organic cause of constipation (cystic fibrosis) is more likely in a patient who did not pass meconium in the first 24 hours of life.

On examination, the abdomen is diffusely uncomfortable rather than tender, and the left colon may be easily palpable and full of feces. Rectal examination usually reveals a rectal vault full of feces. Fissure or any other rectal processes can make defecation painful, so direct examination is warranted.

DIAGNOSTIC EVALUATION

If the diagnosis is unclear, a plain abdominal film can be helpful because a colon full of feces makes the diagnosis of constipation. Thyroid studies, including free T_4, TSH, and T_3RU levels, are indicated if hypothyroidism is suspected. If hypokalemia or hypocalcemia is a potential cause, an electrolyte and chemistry panel may be obtained. A rectal mucosal biopsy is required to make the diagnosis of Hirschsprung disease. A lead level assists in diagnosing plumbism as the cause of constipation. Genetic testing or a sweat test can confirm suspected cystic fibrosis.

TREATMENT

Most children with functional constipation can be treated through dietary changes. The child's fluid intake should be increased, the amount of simple carbohydrates (junk food) decreased, and the amount of fiber and bulk in the diet (leafy vegetables, cereals) increased. The child should begin daily ingestion of undiluted prune juice or apple juice. Several high-fiber juice products are also now available. Senna or Colace should be reserved for children in whom dietary measures are insufficient. The routine use of laxatives or enemas is discouraged.

The constipated child with impaction may be manually disimpacted or may receive a Fleet enema with a stool softener (mineral oil), osmotic agent (lactulose, MiraLax), or peristalsis inducer (senna). Anal fissures are treated by softening the stools, avoiding the insertion of objects in the anus (thermometer), keeping the rectum as clean as possible, and applying petroleum jelly locally with each diaper change. Hirschsprung disease should be managed in consultation with a pediatric surgeon and gastroenterologist.

In children with cystic fibrosis and those who have received vincristine, constipation can be so persistent and intractable that GoLYTELY clean-outs are needed. GoLYTELY (polyethylene glycol-electrolyte solution) is a powerful osmotic cathartic. In some severe cases, constipation because of psychological causes requires counseling or psychotherapy.

🔑 8-9 KEY POINTS

1. Constipation is defined as infrequent passage of hard, dry stools. Constipated patients fail to completely empty the colon with bowel movements and over time stretch the smooth muscle of the colon, resulting in a functional ileus.
2. Failure to defecate resulting from organic causes may be caused by decreased peristalsis, decreased expulsion, and anatomic malformation.
3. In infancy, constipation is commonly associated with anal fissure.
4. Beyond the neonatal period, the most common cause (90% to 95%) of constipation is voluntary withholding or functional constipation.
5. Most cases can be treated with a diet or a mild stool softener for a short time.

HIRSCHSPRUNG DISEASE

Hirschsprung disease, or congenital aganglionic megacolon, occurs in 1 in 5,000 children and results from the failure of the ganglion cells of the myenteric plexus to migrate down the developing colon. As a result, the abnormally innervated distal colon remains tonically contracted and obstructs the flow of feces. Hirschsprung disease is three times more common among boys and accounts for 20% of cases of neonatal intestinal obstruction. In 75% of cases, the aganglionic segment is limited to the rectosigmoid colon, whereas 15% extend beyond the splenic flexure.

CLINICAL MANIFESTATIONS

The diagnosis should be suspected in any infant who fails to pass meconium within the first 24 hours of life and who requires repeated rectal simulation to induce bowel movements. In the first month of life, the neonate develops evidence of obstruction with poor feeding, bilious vomiting, and abdominal distention. In some cases, particularly those with short segment (less than 5 cm) involvement, the diagnosis goes undetected into childhood. In the older child, failure to thrive may be seen, as well as intermittent bouts of intestinal obstruction, enterocolitis with bloody diarrhea, and, occasionally, bowel perforation, sepsis, and shock.

Stool that is palpable throughout the abdomen and an empty rectum on digital examination are most suggestive of the disease. Abdominal radiograph shows distention of the proximal bowel and no gas or feces in the rectum. Barium enema may demonstrate a transition zone between the narrowed abnormal distal segment and the dilated normal proximal bowel. However, a normal barium enema does not rule out the diagnosis. Anal manometry demonstrates failure of the internal sphincter to relax with balloon distention of the rectum. Rectal biopsy revealing absence of ganglion cells and hypertrophied nerve trunks is necessary for the diagnosis.

TREATMENT

Hirschsprung disease is treated surgically in two stages. The first stage involves the creation of a diverting colostomy with the bowel that contains ganglion cells, thus permitting decompression of the ganglion-containing bowel segment. In the second stage, the aganglionic segment is removed by pulling the ganglionic segment through the rectum. This procedure is postponed until the infant is 12 months of age or delayed for 3 to 6 months when the disease has been diagnosed in an older child. The mortality rate for this disorder is low in the absence of enterocolitis; major complications include anal stenosis (5%–10%) and incontinence (1%–3%).

8-10 KEY POINTS

1. Hirschsprung disease results from the failure of the ganglion cells of the myenteric plexus to migrate down the developing colon. As a result, the abnormally innervated distal colon remains tonically contracted and obstructs the flow of feces.
2. The diagnosis should be suspected in any infant who fails to pass meconium within the first 24 hours of life and who requires repeated rectal simulation to induce bowel movements.
3. In the first month of life, evidence of obstruction includes poor feeding, bilious vomiting, and abdominal distention.
4. Rectal biopsy revealing no ganglion cells and hypertrophied nerve trunks is necessary for the diagnosis.

GASTROINTESTINAL BLEEDING

GI bleeding may be acute or chronic, gross or microscopic, and may manifest itself as hematemesis, hematochezia, or melena. A plethora of disorders in childhood can cause GI bleeding.

Hematemesis refers to the emesis of fresh or old blood from the GI tract. Fresh blood becomes chemically altered to a ground-coffee appearance within 5 minutes of exposure to gastric acid. Hematochezia is the passage of fresh (bright red) or dark maroon blood from the rectum. The source is usually the colon, although upper GI tract bleeding that has a rapid transit time can also result in hematochezia. Melena describes shiny, jet black, tarry stools that are guaiac positive. It usually results from upper GI bleeding; the blood has been chemically altered during passage through the gut.

DIFFERENTIAL DIAGNOSIS

The differential diagnosis for GI bleeding is generally divided into upper and lower GI tract etiologies. Upper GI bleeding occurs at a site proximal to the ligament of Treitz, whereas lower GI bleeding occurs at a site distal to the ligament. Although hematemesis from upper GI bleeding can be seen in critically ill children from esophagitis or gastritis, or in children with portal hypertension from esophageal varices, most GI bleeding in children is from the lower tract and manifests as rectal bleeding. Table 8-3 lists the most common causes of rectal bleeding by age. Minor bleeding presents as stool streaked with blood and is usually caused by an anal fissure or polyp. Inflammatory diseases, such as IBD or infectious enterocolitis, result in diarrheal stool mixed with blood. Causes of hematochezia include IBD, Meckel diverticulum, hemolytic uremic syndrome, HSP, and infectious enterocolitis. Table 8-4 lists the associated signs and symptoms of the major causes of GI bleeding.

CLINICAL MANIFESTATIONS

History

It is important to define the onset and duration of bleeding, color (bright red vs. dark maroon vs. tarry black), rate (brisk vs. gradual), and type of bleeding (hematochezia, hematemesis, melena, blood-streaked stool). Some chronic medical conditions result in GI bleeding, including previous GI surgery, liver disease,

■ TABLE 8-3 Causes of Rectal Bleeding by Age of Patient

Newborn	Infant to 2 Yr	2 Yr to Preschool	Preschool to Adolescence
Most Frequent Causes			
Vitamin K deficiency	Anal fissure	Infectious diarrhea	IBD
Ingested maternal blood	Milk colitis	Polyp	Infectious diarrhea
Cow/soy milk enterocolitis	Infectious diarrhea	Anal fissure	Peptic ulcer
Infectious diarrhea	Intussusception	Meckel diverticulum	Esophageal varices
Necrotizing enterocolitis	Polyp	Intussusception	Polyp
Hirschsprung disease	Meckel diverticulum	HUS	HSP
Less Frequent Causes			
Volvulus	HUS	PUD	Anal fissure
Duplication cyst	Duplication cyst	Esophageal varices	HUS
Vascular malformation	PUD	IBD	HSP
Stress ulcer	Vascular malformation		

IBD, inflammatory bowel disease; HUS, hemolytic uremic syndrome; HSP, Henoch-Schönlein purpura; PUD, peptic ulcer disease.

esophagitis, peptic ulcer disease, IBD, milk colitis, colonic polyps, or coagulopathy.

For upper GI bleeding, questions about forceful vomiting, ingestion of ulcerogenic drugs (salicylates, nonsteroidal anti-inflammatory drugs, steroids), and a family history of liver disease or peptic ulcer disease are helpful. For lower GI tract bleeding, inquire about diarrhea, infectious contacts, foreign travel, antibiotic or chemotherapeutic use, and constipation with large or hard stools and difficult or painful defecation.

A 24- to 48-hour food history is important because multiple episodes of "red" vomitus or diarrhea could result from the ingestion of red fluids or foods (sugared children's drinks, beets, red gelatin, acetaminophen elixir). Black stool is not always caused by blood in the stool; it can occur in children who have ingested iron, bismuth, blackberries, or spinach.

Physical Examination

The immediate priority when examining a child GI bleeding is to determine if hypovolemia exists from an acute bleed. Vital signs should be examined for orthostatic changes or for evidence of shock (tachycardia, tachypnea, hypotension). The earliest sign of significant GI bleeding is a raised resting heart rate. A drop in blood pressure is not seen until at least 40% of the intravascular volume is depleted. Dermatologic

abnormalities such as petechiae and purpura indicate coagulopathy, whereas cool or clammy skin with pallor is suggestive of shock or anemia. On abdominal examination, masses (a right lower quadrant mass may be caused by Crohn disease or intussusception); tenderness (epigastric tenderness suggests peptic ulcer disease, right lower quadrant tenderness may be caused by Crohn disease or infectious enterocolitis); and hepatosplenomegaly and caput of medusa (evidence of portal hypertension and risk of varices) may specify the diagnosis. Capillary refill (thenar eminence in neonates and infants) should be assessed on the extremity examination. On rectal examination, the clinician may assess for anal fissure, which is best seen by spreading the buttocks and everting the anal canal (most fissures are located at the 6 and 12 o'clock positions), perform a stool guaiac examination, feel for hard stool, and look for a dilated rectum in children with chronic constipation or anal fissure.

DIAGNOSTIC EVALUATION

Unless the source of bleeding is clearly from the nasopharynx, an anal fissure, or hemorrhoids, a complete blood count with manual differential, coagulation studies, and a type and cross should be sent.

If the bleeding source is unclear and the patient is unstable, gastric lavage determines whether the

■ **TABLE 8-4** Diagnosis of Gastrointestinal Bleeding

Site	Cause	Signs and Symptoms
Upper	Medications	Ingestion of ASA, other NSAIDs
	Varices	Splenomegaly or evidence of liver disease
	Esophagitis	Dysphagia, vomiting, dyspepsia, irritability in infants
Lower	PUD	Epigastric pain, meal related, may be increased at night; family history
	Fissure	Bright red blood on surface of stool; pain, constipation; fissure often visible on anal eversion
	Colonic polyps	Bright red blood on surface of stool; painless
	Milk colitis	Blood mixed with stool, diarrhea; patient may have hypoproteinemia, edema
	Meckel diverticulum	Painless bleeding, mixed with stool; often a lot of blood
	IBD	Diarrhea, fever, abdominal pain, poor growth, associated systemic signs and symptoms
	Bacterial colitis	Abdominal pain, diarrhea, fever, antibiotics
	HSP	Joint pain, purpura, abdominal pain, nephritis (casts, RBCs in urine)
	HUS	Diarrhea, renal failure, thrombocytopenia, microangiopathic hemolytic anemia
	Intussusception	Intermittent abdominal pain, vomiting, pallor, "red currant jelly" stool, right-sided mass

ASA, acetylsalicylic acid; NSAID, nonsteroidal anti-inflammatory drug; PUD, peptic ulcer disease; IBD, inflammatory bowel disease; HSP, Henoch-Schönlein purpura; HUS, hemolytic uremic syndrome; RBC, red blood cell.

bleeding is from the upper or lower GI tract. A well-lubricated nasogastric or orogastric tube of the largest bore possible should be placed. The stomach is lavaged with room-temperature normal saline until lavage fluid is clear. Iced saline may cause hypothermia and should be avoided. Esophageal varices are not a contraindication to the placement of a nasogastric or orogastric tube. Return of clear lavage fluid makes the diagnosis of upper GI bleeding unlikely, although occasionally duodenal ulcers may bleed only distally. Return of guaiac-positive bright red blood or "coffee grounds" that eventually clear indicates upper GI bleeding that has remitted. Persistent return of bright red blood indicates active bleeding and mandates aggressive intravenous fluid management and a surgical consult.

In the stable patient, a thorough history and physical examination with consideration of the age-related causes usually leads to diagnosis. Gastric lavage is unnecessary in children with minor or nonacute GI bleeding. The precise diagnosis is usually made by upper or lower endoscopy.

If there is bloody diarrhea, stool should be sent for methylene blue staining (to look for white bell cells) and stool culture. In the neonate with bloody stool, necrotizing enterocolitis must be considered, and an abdominal film and evaluation for sepsis should be performed. When swallowed maternal blood is suspected as the cause of GI bleeding, the Apt test is performed on the child's stool or emesis to differentiate maternal blood from the blood of the neonate. If oral blood is noted and there is a worsening pulmonary examination, a chest radiograph may demonstrate pulmonary hemorrhage. A Meckel scan can be performed when Meckel diverticulum is suspected.

TREATMENT

The unstable child with severe bleeding or hypo-volemia is evaluated by primary and secondary surveys as outlined in Chapter 1. A normal hemoglobin or hematocrit does not rule out severe acute bleeding; full hemodilution takes up to 12 hours in the acutely bleeding patient. Intravenous normal saline or Ringer lactate at 20 mL per kg boluses should be given until the patient is stable. Type O-negative whole blood should be reserved for the unstable patient with acute bleeding that cannot quickly be brought under control.

The most common error in management of the child with severe GI bleeding is inadequate volume replacement. Hypotension is a late finding; fluid resuscitation should be governed by the level of tachycardia.

The stable child without heavy bleeding or signs of hypovolemia should be evaluated and treated according to the particular diagnosis.

Figure 8-1 illustrates a useful algorithm for the evaluation and management of GI bleeding. Three common causes of GI bleeding—Meckel diverticulum, ulcerative colitis, and Crohn disease—are discussed in the following sections.

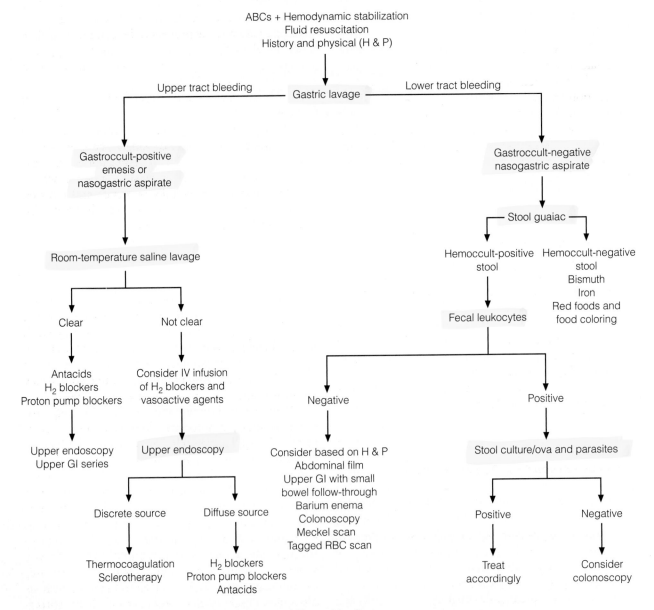

Figure 8-1 • Algorithm for evaluation and management of GI tract bleeding.

1. Upper GI bleeding occurs at a site proximal to the ligament of Treitz, whereas lower GI bleeding occurs distal to the ligament.
2. Most GI bleeding in children is from the lower GI tract and manifests as rectal bleeding.
3. The earliest sign of significant GI bleeding is a raised resting heart rate. A drop in blood pressure is not seen until at least 40% of the intravascular volume is depleted.

MECKEL DIVERTICULUM

Meckel diverticulum, the vestigial remnant of the omphalomesenteric duct, is the most common anomaly of the GI tract. It is present in 2% to 3% of the population and is located within 100 cm of the ileocecal valve in the small intestine. The peak incidence of bleeding from the diverticulum is at 2 years of age. Heterotopic tissue, usually gastric, is ten times more common in symptomatic cases because of acid secretion and ulceration.

Clinical Manifestations

The most common presentation of Meckel diverticulum is painless rectal bleeding. Eighty-five percent of patients with Meckel diverticulum have melena, 10% develop intestinal obstruction from intussusception or volvulus, and 5% suffer from painful diverticulitis mimicking appendicitis. The diagnosis is made by performing a Meckel scan. The technetium-99 pertechnetate scan, preceded by prepentagastrin stimulation or a histamine H_2-receptor antagonist (cimetidine), identifies the ectopic acid-secreting cells creating the hemorrhage in the diverticulum.

Treatment

Definitive treatment is surgical resection.

1. Meckel diverticulum, the vestigial remnant of the omphalomesenteric duct, is the most common anomaly of the GI tract.
2. The most common presentation of Meckel diverticulum is painless rectal bleeding.

INFLAMMATORY BOWEL DISEASE

IBD is a generic term for **Crohn disease** and **ulcerative colitis**, which are chronic inflammatory disorders of the intestines.

Ulcerative colitis produces diffuse superficial colonic ulceration and crypt abscesses. It involves the rectum in 95% of patients, with or without contiguous extension higher in the colon. Ulcerative colitis does not affect the small intestine.

The pathology of Crohn disease involves transmural inflammation in a discontinuous pattern, which results in skip lesions. Crohn disease may involve any part of the GI tract (mouth to anus). In pediatric patients, the process is ileocolonic in 40% of cases, involves the small intestine alone in approximately 30% of cases, and is isolated to the colon in only 20% of cases. Fibrosis is transmural, and strictures are common. Granulomas are observed in up to 30% of patients.

Although the exact etiology of these disorders is not known, a combination of genetic, environmental, psychological, infectious, and immunologic mechanisms are implicated. IBD is most common in whites and Jews and occurs equally in males and females. Most pediatric patients are adolescents, but both diseases have been reported in infancy.

Clinical Manifestations

Crampy abdominal pain, recurrent fever, and weight loss are common manifestations in Crohn disease. Although diarrhea is common, it is not universal. Rectal bleeding is noted in only 35% of cases of Crohn disease. Abdominal pain tends to be more severe in Crohn disease than in ulcerative colitis, may be diffuse, and is frequently worse in the right lower quadrant. Perianal disease may produce skin tags, fissures, fistulas, or abscesses. Anorexia, poor weight gain, and delayed growth occur in 40% of patients.

Most children with ulcerative colitis exhibit bloody mucinous diarrheal stool (100%), abdominal pain (95%), and tenesmus (75%). Ninety percent of patients exhibit mild to moderate disease. Mild disease is defined as less than six stools per day, no fever, no anemia, and no hypoalbuminemia, whereas moderate disease has greater than six stools per day, fever, anemia, and hypoalbuminemia. Severe disease may be fulminant, with high fever, abdominal tenderness, distention, tachycardia, leukocytosis, hemorrhage, severe anemia, and more than eight stools per day.

Toxic megacolon and intestinal perforation are rare complications. After 10 years of disease, there is a cumulative risk of 1% to 2% per year for the development of carcinoma. Table 8-5 compares Crohn disease and ulcerative colitis.

Extraintestinal sequelae, similar in both diseases, may precede or accompany GI symptoms and include polyarticular arthritis, ankylosing spondylitis, primary sclerosing cholangitis, chronic active hepatitis, sacroiliitis, pyoderma gangrenosum, erythema nodosum, aphthous stomatitis, episcleritis, recurrent iritis, and uveitis. Patients with Crohn disease are also at increased risk for nephrolithiasis secondary to ileal disease and abnormal absorption of oxalate.

In the evaluation of suspected IBD in the pediatric patient, a full colonoscopy with ileoscopy is indicated to evaluate all affected areas and to attempt to differentiate between Crohn disease and ulcerative colitis. An upper endoscopy is often performed to assess for any microscopic inflammation in the upper GI tract. Even with a full evaluation, it is sometimes difficult to make a definitive diagnosis in patients with primary colonic disease. Visualization of the mucosa in ulcerative colitis reveals diffuse superficial ulceration and easy bleeding. In Crohn disease, deep ulcerations may be present, and diseased areas may be more focal.

Radiographic examination with a double air contrast barium enema demonstrates diffuse colonic lesions and pseudopolyp formation in ulcerative colitis. This examination should be delayed in patients with severely active disease to avoid precipitating toxic megacolon. Upper GI study with small bowel follow-through in Crohn disease often reveals ileal or proximal small bowel disease with segmental narrowing of the ileum (string sign), and longitudinal ulcers. Barium enema may show colonic involvement with skip lesions, rectal sparing, or strictures.

Anemia is common and usually associated with iron deficiency. Megaloblastic anemia secondary to folate and vitamin B_{12} deficiency may also be present. An elevation of the erythrocyte sedimentation rate is seen in approximately 50% of cases of ulcerative colitis and in 80% of Crohn disease cases. Hypoalbuminemia, caused by poor protein intake, is common in individuals with severe symptoms. Serum aminotransferase levels are increased if hepatic inflammation is a complicating feature. Stool examination reveals blood and fecal leukocytes with a negative stool culture.

Differential Diagnosis

The differential diagnosis of IBD includes chronic bacterial or parasitic causes of diarrhea, appendicitis, hemolytic uremic syndrome, HSP, and radiation enterocolitis. Enteric infections include C. difficile, Campylobacter jejuni, Yersinia enterocolitica, amebiasis, and giardiasis.

Treatment

Treatment of IBD is aimed at control of inflammation and suppression of the immune system. The variety of agents available is quickly increasing. 5-aminosalicylic compounds have long been a mainstay of anti-inflammatory treatment. Antibiotics have a role as anti-inflammatory agents in Crohn disease. Aggressive nutritional support (including tube feeding) is important for growth but also seems to have anti-inflammatory effects and improves symptom control in Crohn disease. Corticosteroids have both anti-inflammatory and immunosuppressive effects, and they remain a mainstay of management. Pure immunosuppressives include 6-mercaptopurine, azathioprine, and methotrexate.

As a general rule, therapy is chosen in an effort to achieve maximum symptom control with minimum side effects. As a result, immunosuppressive agents

TABLE 8-5 Comparison of Crohn Disease and Ulcerative Colitis

Feature	Crohn Disease	Ulcerative Colitis
Malaise, fever, weight loss	Common	Common
Rectal bleeding	Sometimes	Usual
Abdominal mass	Common	Rare
Abdominal pain	Common	Common
Perianal disease	Common	Rare
Ileal involvement	Common	None (backwash ileitis)
Strictures	Common	Unusual
Fistula	Common	Unusual
Skip lesions	Common	Not present
Transmural involvement	Usual	Not present
Granulomas	Common	Not present
Risk of cancer	Increased	Greatly Increased

are reserved for more severe illness but may be necessary to decrease long-term steroid use. New biologic agents are being developed and evaluated that are aimed at very specific components of the inflammatory cascade. Infliximab is an example of a genetically engineered antibody directed against tumor necrosis factor-α, and it shows promise in the control of significant Crohn disease.

Because anorexia and increased nutrient losses in the stool are common in children with IBD, adequate calories and protein are essential. Oral supplements, nasogastric tube feedings, and, in some severe cases, central venous hyperalimentation are necessary. Vitamin and mineral supplementation, especially iron, may be required.

Patients with ulcerative colitis for more than 10 years need annual colonoscopy and rectal biopsy because of the high risk of colon cancer development. Studies have shown that patients with long-standing Crohn colitis are at a similar risk for development of neoplasia.

Surgery is eventually needed in 25% of patients with ulcerative colitis and 70% of children with Crohn disease. Surgery is indicated in ulcerative colitis when there is fulminant colitis with severe blood loss or toxic megacolon, intractable disease with a high-dose steroid requirement, steroid toxicity, growth failure, or colonic dysplasia. Because ulcerative colitis is restricted to the colon, colectomy is curative. Surgery is performed in Crohn disease when hemorrhage, obstruction, perforation, severe fistula formation, or ureteral obstruction is present. In general, conservative management is warranted because removal of the diseased bowel is not curative in Crohn disease. Recurrence rates of up to 50% have been reported after segmental resection.

8-13 KEY POINTS

1. Ulcerative colitis produces diffuse superficial colonic ulceration and crypt abscesses. It involves the rectum in 95% of patients, with or without contiguous extension higher in the colon. Ulcerative colitis does not affect the small intestine.
2. Radiographic examination with a double air contrast barium enema demonstrates diffuse colonic lesions and pseudopolyp formation in ulcerative colitis.
3. Ulcerative colitis places the child at high risk for the development of colon cancer.
4. The pathology of Crohn disease involves transmural inflammation in a discontinuous pattern, which results in skip lesions. Crohn disease may involve any part of the GI tract (mouth to anus).
5. Radiographic examination with a double air contrast barium enema in Crohn disease demonstrates ileal and/or colonic involvement with skip lesions, rectal sparing, segmental narrowing of the ileum (string sign), and longitudinal ulcers.
6. Therapy for inflammatory bowel disease (IBD) is aimed at achieving maximum symptom control with minimum side effects.

Additional Suggested Reading

Baldassano R, Piccoli DA. Inflammatory bowel disease in pediatric and adolescent patients. *Gastoenterol Clin.* 1999;28:445–458.

Braganza SF, Adam M. Gastroesophageal reflux. *Pediatr Rev.* 2005;26:304–305.

Chelimsky G, Czinn S. Peptic ulcer disease in children. *Pediatr Rev.* 2001;22:349–355.

Lasche J, Duggan C. Managing acute diarrhea: what every pediatrician needs to know. *Contemp Pediatr.* 1999;2:16(2):71–82.

Pietzak MM, Thomas DW. Childhood malabsorption. *Pediatr Rev.* 2003;24:195–206.

Squires RH. Gastrointestinal bleeding. *Pediatr Rev.* 1999;20:95–101.

Genetic Disorders

Structural birth defects are categorized as minor or major. Minor birth defects such as skin tags, inner epicanthal folds, and rudimentary polydactyly are of little physiologic significance. Approximately 15% of newborn infants have at least one minor anomaly; 0.5% of infants have three or more minor anomalies. In contrast, major birth defects such as cleft palate, myelomeningocele, and congenital heart disease have an adverse effect on the infant. Major birth defects occur in 2% to 3% of all newborns. The probability of having a major birth defect increases as the number of minor anomalies present increases (Table 9-1). Birth defects can be caused by environmental or genetic factors. Genetic defects may be chromosomal, single gene, imprinting, cytogenetic, or multifactorial disorders.

ENVIRONMENTAL FACTORS

Environmental factors are known to cause at least 10% of all birth defects. **Teratogens** are environmental agents that cause congenital developmental anomalies by interfering with embryonic or fetal organogenesis or growth. Exposure to a teratogen before implantation (days 7 to 10 postconception) can either have no effect or can result in loss of the embryo. To disrupt organogenesis, a teratogenic exposure typically occurs before 12 weeks' gestation. Any teratogenic exposure after 12 weeks' gestation predominantly affects growth and central nervous system development.

Teratogens include intrauterine infections (Chapter 13), high-dose radiation, maternal metabolic disorders (Chapter 13), mechanical forces, and drugs. The most common maternal metabolic disorder that has teratogenic potential is diabetes mellitus; 10% of infants of diabetic mothers have a birth defect. Abnormal intrauterine forces such as uterine fibroids

or oligohydramnios may cause fetal constraint, resulting in clubfoot or hip dysplasia. Table 9-2 lists the most common teratogenic drugs and their effects.

🔑 9-1 KEY POINTS

1. Environmental factors cause 10% of birth defects.
2. Infectious agents, high-dose radiation, maternal metabolic disorders, mechanical forces, and drugs can all serve as teratogens.
3. A teratogenic exposure before 12 weeks' gestation affects organogenesis and tissue morphogenesis, whereas an exposure thereafter usually retards fetal growth and affects central nervous system development.

GENETIC FACTORS

Genetic disorders can be classified as disorders of single genes, chromosomes, imprinting, and molecular cytogenetics. Advances in molecular genetics have blurred the distinction among these categories.

SINGLE-GENE DISORDERS

Normal human cells have 46 chromosomes (22 pairs of autosomes and 1 pair of sex chromosomes). Chromosomes contain genes, which occur in pairs at a single locus or site on specific chromosomes. These paired genes, called **alleles**, determine the genotype of an individual at that locus. If the genes at a specific locus are identical, the individual is **homozygous**; if they are different, the individual is **heterozygous**. More than 3,000 different single-gene disorders have been

TABLE 9-1 Incidence of Major Anomalies in the Presence of Minor Anomalies

Number of Minor Anomalies	Incidence of Major Anomalies (%)
0	<1
1	1
2	3
3	20

When a spontaneous mutation has occurred in a fetus, the risk of recurrence in a subsequent pregnancy is the same as the chance of the spontaneous mutation occurring de novo. Autosomal dominant genes often cause conditions that manifest themselves with varying degrees of severity among affected individuals, a phenomenon known as **variable expressivity** or **variable penetrance**. Table 9-3 lists some important autosomal dominant diseases. Other chapters discuss some of these diseases in detail.

described and are classified by their mode of inheritance (autosomal dominant, autosomal recessive, or X-linked).

Autosomal Dominant Disorders

Autosomal dominant disorders are expressed after alteration of only one gene in the pair (often coding for a structural protein). Homozygous' disease states of autosomal dominant disorders are rare and usually severe or lethal. A mutant gene can be inherited from one parent with the same condition. The risk for the affected parents' offspring is 50% for each pregnancy. Sometimes an individual is the first person in a family to display a trait because of spontaneous mutation.

Autosomal Recessive Disorders

Autosomal recessive disorders are only expressed after alteration of both the maternal and paternal genes of a gene pair (often coding for an enzyme). Because half of the normal enzyme activity is adequate under most circumstances, a person with only one mutant gene is not affected, whereas individuals who are homozygous for a defective gene have the disorder. Both parents of a child with an autosomal recessive disorder are usually heterozygous for that gene, and each child of such a couple has a 25% risk of inheriting the disorder. Table 9-4 lists the more common autosomal recessive disorders.

Most inborn errors of metabolism, with the exception of ornithine transcarbamylase (OTC) deficiency,

TABLE 9-2 Common Teratogenic Drugs

Drug	Results
Warfarin (Coumadin)	Hypoplastic nasal bridge, chondrodysplasia punctata
Ethanol	Fetal alcohol syndrome, microcephaly, CHD (septal defects, patent ductus arteriosus)
Isotretinoin (Accutane)	Facial and ear anomalies, congenital heart disease
Lithium	CHD (Ebstein anomaly, atrial septal defect)
Penicillamine	Cutis laxa syndrome
Phenytoin (Dilantin)	Hypoplastic nails, intrauterine growth retardation, cleft lip and palate
Radioactive iodine	Congenital goiter, hypothyroidism
Diethylstilbestrol	Vaginal adenocarcinoma during adolescence
Streptomycin	Deafness
Testosteronelike drugs	Virilization of female
Tetracycline	Dental enamel hypoplasia, altered bone growth
Thalidomide	Phocomelia, CHD (tetralogy of Fallot, septal defects)
Trimethadione	Typical facies, CHD (tetralogy of Fallot, transposition of the great arteries, hypoplastic left heart)
Valproate	Spina bifida

CHD, congenital heart disease.

■ TABLE 9-3 Examples of Autosomal Dominant Diseases

Autosomal Dominant Disease	Frequency	Chromosome	Gene	Comments
Achondroplasia	1:25,000	4p	FGFR3	80% new mutations; proximal limb shortening
Adult polycystic kidney disease	1:1,200	16p	PKD1/PKD2	Renal cysts, intracranial aneurysm
Hereditary angioedema	1:10,000	11q	CIN4	Deficiency of C1 esterase inhibitor; episodic edema
Hereditary spherocytosis	1:5,000	8p, 14q	ANK1	See Chapter 10; some variants autosomal recessive
Marfan's syndrome	1:20,000	15q	Fibrillin-1	Aortic root dilatation, tall stature
Neurofibromatosis	1:3,000	17q	NF1/NF2	50% new mutations; café-au-lait spots
Protein C deficiency	1:15,000	2q,17q, 22q	multiple genes	Hypercoagulable state
Tuberous sclerosis	1:30,000	9q, 16p	TSC1, TSC2, TSC3, TSC4	"Ash-leaf" spots; seizures
von Willebrand's disease	1:100	12p	Multiple genes	See Chapter 10

p, short arm of chromosome; q, long arm of chromosome.

■ TABLE 9-4 Examples of Autosomal Recessive Diseases

Autosomal Recessive Disease	Frequency	Chrom	Gene	Comments
Congenital adrenal hyperplasia	1:5,000–1:15,000; 1:700 in Yupik Eskimos	6p	CYP21A2, CYP11A1, CYP17, ACTHR	See Chapter 6
Cystic fibrosis	1:2,000 (Caucasians)	7q	CFTR	See Chapter 20
Galactosemia	1:60,000	9p	GALT	Carbohydrate metabolism disorder
Gaucher's disease	1:2,500 (Ashkenazi Jews)	1q	GBA	Lysosomal storage disorder
Infantile polycystic kidney	1:14,000	6p	PKD3	Renal and hepatic cysts, hypertension
Phenylketonuria	1:14,000	12q	PAH	Amino acid metabolism disorder
Sickle cell disease	1:625 (African Americans)	11p	HBB	See Chapter 10
Tay-Sachs' disease	1:3,000 (Ashkenazi Jews)	15q	HEXA	Lysosomal storage disorder
Wilson's disease	1:200,000	13q	ATP7B	Defective copper excretion

p, short arm of chromosome; q, long arm of chromosome; Chrom, Chromosome.

are autosomal recessive disorders. Inborn errors of metabolism are discussed later in this chapter.

X-Linked Disorders

X-linked disorders, which are usually recessive, occur when a male inherits a mutant gene on the X chromosome from his mother. The affected male, termed **hemizygous** for the gene, has only a single X chromosome and, therefore, a single set of X-linked genes. The mother of the affected individual is heterozygous for that gene because she has both a normal X chromosome and a mutant one. She may be asymptomatic or demonstrate mild symptoms of the disorder because of lyonization, in which only one X chromosome is transcriptionally active in each cell. Recurrence risk for X-linked disorders differs depending on which parent has the abnormal gene. An affected father will pass the defective X chromosome on to his daughters, who are carriers for the disorder; his sons will not be affected. A mother with an abnormal X chromosome is a carrier, and there is a 50% chance she will pass the abnormal chromosome to her progeny. Daughters who receive the abnormal X chromosome will be carriers for the disease, and sons will have the disease. Table 9-5 lists the most common X-linked disorders.

9-2 KEY POINTS

1. Single-gene defects are classified by their mode of inheritance into autosomal dominant, autosomal recessive, and X-linked disorders.
2. In autosomal dominant disorders, the phenomenon of incomplete penetrance results in variable expression of the defective gene.
3. Defective genes in autosomal dominant disorders typically code for structural proteins, whereas those in autosomal recessive disorders code for enzymes.
4. Most inborn errors of metabolism (with the noted exception of ornithine transcarbamylase deficiency [OTC] and some mitochondrial disorders) are autosomal recessive disorders.

CHROMOSOMAL DISORDERS

Chromosomal disorders are responsible for pregnancy loss, congenital malformation, and mental retardation. Although more than 50% of first-trimester pregnancy losses are caused by chromosomal imbalances, only 0.6% of newborn infants have chromosomal abnormalities. Most chromosomal defects arise de novo during gametogenesis, so that an infant can be conceived with a chromosomal abnormality without any prior family history. Chromosomal abnormalities can also be passed from parent to offspring. In such cases, there is often a family history of multiple spontaneous abortions or a higher than chance frequency of children with chromosomal problems. Disorders of chromosome number may involve autosomes or sex chromosomes. Birth defects caused by autosomal abnormalities are generally more severe than those caused by sex chromosome abnormalities. Numeric defects of the autosomes include trisomy of chromosomes 21, 18, and 13. Examples of sex chromosome numerical abnormalities are Turner syndrome and Klinefelter's syndrome.

Indications for obtaining chromosomal studies include confirmation of a suspected chromosomal syndrome, multiple organ system malformations, significant developmental delay or mental retardation without an alternate explanation, short stature or extremely delayed menarche in girls, infertility or a history of multiple spontaneous abortions, ambiguous genitalia, or advanced maternal age. Fetal karyotyping may be accomplished through amniocentesis or chorionic villus sampling.

Autosomal Trisomies

Trisomy 21 (Down Syndrome)

Trisomy 21 is the most common autosomal chromosomal abnormality in humans, with an incidence of 1 per 700 live births. The risk of Down syndrome increases with advancing maternal age; it is 1 in 365 for mothers 35 years of age and 1 in 50 for those 45 years or older. Of children with Down syndrome, 95% have three number 21 chromosomes (47 total chromosomes), which results typically from chromosomal nondisjunction during maternal meiosis. Four percent have translocation of a third number 21 chromosome to another chromosome (46 total chromosomes). A third of translocation cases are familial, meaning one of the parents has a balanced translocation involving one number 21 chromosome and another chromosome. One percent of children with Down syndrome have chromosome mosaicism, with some cells having two number 21 chromosomes (46 total chromosomes) and some cells having three number 21 chromosomes (47 total chromosomes). The mosaicism results from a mitotic division error that occurred during embryonic development.

TABLE 9-5 X-Linked Diseases

X-Linked Disease	Frequency	Comments
Bruton agammaglobulinemia	1:100,000	Absence of immunoglobulins; recurrent infections
Chronic granulomatous disease	1:1,000,000	Defective killing by phagocytes; recurrent infections
Color blindness	1:100,000	
Duchenne muscular dystrophy	1:3600	Proximal muscle weakness; Gower sign
Glucose-6-phosphate dehydrogenase	1:10 (African Americans)	Oxidant-induced hemolytic anemia deficiency
Hemophilias A and B	1:10,000	See Chapter 10
Lesch-Nyhan's syndrome	1:100,000	Purine metabolism disorder; self-mutilation
Ornithine transcarbamylase deficiency	—	Urea cycle disorder; hyperammonemia

Common dysmorphic facial features include brachycephaly (flat occiput), flat facial profile, up-slanted palpebral fissures, small ears, flat nasal bridge with epicanthal folds, and a small mouth with a protruding tongue. Anomalies of the hand include single palmar creases (simian creases), short, broad hands (brachydactyly) with an incurved fifth finger (clinodactyly) and hypoplastic middle phalanx, and an excessive gap between the first and second toes ("sandal sign"). Other features include short stature, generalized hypotonia, cardiac defects (endocardial cushion defects and septal defects are seen in 50% of cases), gastrointestinal anomalies (duodenal atresia and Hirschsprung's disease), hypothyroidism, and mental retardation (IQ range: 35 to 65). Leukemia is 20 times more common in children with trisomy 21 than in the general population. During the third and fourth decades, an Alzheimerlike dementia can develop. With improved medical, educational, and vocational management, life expectancy for patients with Down syndrome now extends well into adulthood.

Trisomy 18 (Edwards)

Trisomy 18 occurs in 1 per 8,000 live births. Eighty percent of cases are the result of meiotic nondisjunction, which is associated with advanced maternal age. The remaining 20% may be partial (involving only a portion of the chromosome) or mosaic, caused by mitotic nondisjunction in the zygote. Chromosome translocation as the cause of trisomy 18 is extremely rare, and its presence should prompt karyotyping of the parents to exclude an inherited defect. Table 9-6 shows the clinical manifestations of trisomy 18. The prognosis for

TABLE 9-6 Key Features of Trisomy 13 and Trisomy 18

	Trisomy 13	Trisomy 18
Head and neck	Microcephaly with sloping forehead	Prominent occiput
	Cutis aplasia of scalp	Narrow bifrontal diameter of forehead
	Microphthalmia	Low-set, malformed ears
	Cleft lip and palate	Micrognathia
Chest and abdomen	Congenital heart disease (VSD, ASD, PDA)	Congenital heart disease (VSD, ASD, PDA)
	Omphalocele	Short sternum
Extremities	Clenched hands with overlapping fingers	Clenched hands with overlapping fingers
	Polydactyly	Rocker-bottom feet
	Polycystic kidney or other renal defects	Horseshoe kidney
Other	Cryptorchidism	Lack of subcutaneous fat
	Agenesis of corpus callosum	

VSD, ventricular septal defect; ASD, atrial septal defect; PDA, patent ductus arteriosus.

patients with trisomy 18 is extremely poor: 30% die before reaching 1 month of age, and 90% die by 1 year of age.

Trisomy 13 (Patau)

Trisomy 13 occurs in 1 per 10,000 live births but constitutes 1% of all spontaneous abortions. Approximately 75% of surviving cases are the result of meiotic nondisjunction, although the increased risk with advanced maternal age is much less than that for trisomy 21. Twenty percent of children with trisomy 13 have a translocation of a third chromosome 13 to another chromosome. A quarter of translocation cases are familial, meaning that one of the parents has a balanced translocation involving one chromosome 13 and another chromosome. The remaining 5% of children with trisomy 13 have mosaicism; some cells have 46 chromosomes with two number 13 chromosomes, and some cells have 47 chromosomes with three number 13 chromosomes. The mosaicism results from a mitotic division error that occurs during embryonic development. Table 9-6 shows the clinical manifestations of trisomy 13. Prognosis for patients with trisomy 13 is extremely poor: 50% die before reaching 1 month of age, and 90% die by 1 year of age.

Sex Chromosome Abnormalities

Sex chromosome anomalies involve abnormalities in the number or structure of the X or Y chromosomes or both.

Turner Syndrome

Turner syndrome occurs in 1 per 5,000 live births. Approximately 98% of fetuses with Turner syndrome expire in utero; only 2% are born. Therefore, the recurrence risk for parents who have a child with Turner syndrome is no higher than that of the general population.

Several genotypes can cause the Turner phenotype. In 60% of cases, the karyotype is 45,XO, in which the female lacks an X chromosome. Another 15% of individuals are mosaics with a genotype of 45,XO/46,XX; 45,XO/46,XX/47,XXX; or 45,XO/46,XY. Mosaic individuals may have fewer physical stigmata of Turner syndrome. In the remaining 25% of cases, there are two X chromosomes but the short (p) arm of one of the X chromosomes is missing.

Clinical Manifestations

Dysmorphic features include lymphedema of the hands and feet, a shield-shaped chest, widely spaced hypoplastic nipples, a webbed neck, low hairline, cubitus valgus (increased carrying angle), short stature, and multiple pigmented nevi. Additional abnormalities include gonadal dysgenesis, gonadoblastoma, renal anomalies, congenital heart disease, autoimmune thyroiditis, and learning disabilities. Gonadal dysgenesis, present in 100% of patients, is associated with primary amenorrhea and lack of pubertal development because of loss of ovarian hormones. The gonads are appropriately infantile at birth but regress during childhood and develop into "streak" ovaries by puberty. In mosaics with a Y chromosome in one of their cell lines, gonadoblastoma is common. Therefore, prophylactic gonadectomy is necessary in these patients. Renal anomalies, usually duplicated collecting system or horseshoe kidney, occur in 40% of those with Turner syndrome. Congenital heart disease occurs in 20% of patients; common defects include coarctation of the aorta, aortic stenosis, and bicuspid aortic valve. As a consequence of having only one functional X chromosome, females with Turner syndrome display the same frequency of sex-linked disorders as males. The diagnosis is made by karyotype and fluorescent in situ hybridization. Because of their mosaicism, some girls suspected of having Turner syndrome have a 46,XX karyotype in the peripheral blood, and a skin biopsy may be necessary to make the diagnosis.

Short stature has been successfully treated using human growth hormone. Secondary sexual characteristics develop after estrogen and progesterone administration. As mentioned earlier, gonadectomy is indicated in patients with dysgenetic gonads and the presence of a Y chromosome. With the rare exception of a few mosaics, women with Turner syndrome cannot become pregnant.

Klinefelter's Syndrome

Klinefelter's syndrome, caused by an extra X chromosome, affects 1 in 1,000 newborn males, 20% of aspermic adult men, and 1 in 250 men over 6 feet tall. The karyotype is XXY in 80% of cases and mosaic (XY/XXY) in 20%. Recurrence risk is the same as the initial risk in the general population.

Clinical Manifestations

The physical stigmata of Klinefelter's syndrome are not obvious until puberty, at which time males are incompletely masculinized. They have a female body habitus with decreased body hair, gynecomastia, and small phallus and testes. Infertility results from hypospermia or aspermia. Affected males are usually taller than average relative to their families, and their arm span can be greater than their height. There is an increased incidence of learning difficulties, but the average IQ is 98. Gonadotropin levels are usually elevated because of inadequate testosterone levels.

Testosterone therapy during adolescence may improve secondary sexual characteristics and prevent gynecomastia.

IMPRINTING DISORDERS

Imprinting refers to different phenotypes resulting from the same genotype, depending on whether the abnormal chromosome is inherited from the mother or father. **Uniparental disomy** is the term used when both chromosomes of a pair have been inherited from only one parent. Prader-Willi and Angelman's syndromes are examples of imprinting, and some cases are also examples of uniparental disomy.

Prader-Willi's Syndrome

Prader-Willi's syndrome occurs in 1 per 15,000 newborns and is associated with an interstitial deletion of the long arm of chromosome 15 (deletion of 15q11–13). Approximately 70% of those affected have a chromosome deletion in the paternally derived chromosome 15 and a normal maternal chromosome 15. The remaining 20% to 25% have a normal-appearing chromosome complement with two copies of maternal chromosome 15. This is known as **uniparental maternal disomy**, and the syndrome results from the lack of a paternal copy of chromosome 15. The remainder abnormalities of imprinting are caused by translocations narrowing the region. The recurrent risk for parents of an affected child is 1 in 100, unless the chromosome 15 deletion results from a parental translocation, which is extremely rare. The disorder is sporadic.

Clinical Manifestations

Dysmorphisms include narrow bifrontal diameter, almond-shaped eyes, a down-turned mouth, and small hands and feet. Short stature and hypogonadotropic hypogonadism with small genitalia and incomplete puberty are seen. These children suffer from severe hypotonia, which is associated with feeding difficulties and failure to thrive in infancy. By several years of age, these children develop an uncontrollable appetite that leads to severe central obesity. These children eat constantly unless food is locked away. Obesity-related obstructive sleep apnea and cardiorespiratory complications (Pickwickian's syndrome) may develop. There is mild mental retardation with characteristic impulse control problems.

For the average patient, strict dietary control is attempted but difficult to enforce. Although those affected can live normal life spans, complications of obesity such as obstructive sleep apnea and diabetes mellitus often lead to earlier death.

Angelman's Syndrome

Approximately 60% of patients with Angelman's syndrome have a microdeletion on the maternal chromosome 15 (deletion of 15q11–13) and a normal paternal chromosome 15. Five percent of cases result from **uniparental paternal disomy**, where two normal copies of paternally derived chromosome 15 are inherited. Five percent result from imprinting, and 5% are caused by a single gene mutation (UBE3A). Ten to twenty-five percent result from small subtelomeric deletions or translocations or are of unknown etiology.

Clinical Manifestations

Dysmorphisms seen in Angelman's syndrome include maxillary hypoplasia, large mouth, prognathism, and short stature. Patients are severely mentally retarded, with impaired or absent speech and inappropriate paroxysms of laughter. Jerky arm movements, ataxic gait, and tiptoe walk result in marionettelike movements, leading to its designation as the "happy puppet" syndrome. Many patients have seizures.

MOLECULAR CYTOGENIC DISORDERS

FRAGILE X SYNDROME

Fragile X, an X-linked form of mental retardation that occurs in 1 in 1,000 males, is an example of a trinucleotide repeat disorder. The gene involved, called FMR-1, is active in brain and sperm. In normal individuals, the DNA trinucleotide CGG is repeated approximately 30 times at the start of this gene. Those affected with fragile X have more than 200 CGG repeats. The disorder received its name because a cytogenetically detectable breakage occurs at a specific fragile site on the X chromosome. Currently, Southern blot analysis and polymerase chain reaction (PCR) are used to determine the number of CGG repeats. Clinical manifestations may include macrosomia at birth, macroorchidism because of testicular edema, dysmorphic facial features (large jaw and large ears), perseverative speech, and mental retardation (90% of affected males have an IQ between 20 and 49). Some males with fragile X syndrome have mental retardation as the sole manifestation. Female carriers of the fragile X chromosome may have a subnormal IQ. Autism occurs more commonly in children with the fragile X chromosome than in the general population. There is no treatment for the syndrome.

CHROMOSOME 22Q11 DELETION SYNDROME

Microdeletion of 22q11.2 has been found in 90% of children with DiGeorge's syndrome, in 70% of children with velocardiofacial syndrome, and in 15% of children with isolated conotruncal cardiac defects. Although the names just mentioned are still in use, the more general term **22q11.2 deletion syndrome** more appropriately encompasses the spectrum of abnormalities found in these children. Its prevalence in the general population is 1 per 4,000 live births. The deletion can be inherited (8% to 28% of cases), but it more typically occurs as a de novo event. However, if a parent has the deletion, the risk to each child is 50%. The microdeletion can be detected using fluorescent in situ hybridization (FISH) probes. Classic cardiac features of this spectrum of disorders include conotruncal defects such as tetralogy of Fallot, interrupted aortic arch, and vascular rings. Other common findings are absent thymus, hypocalcemic hypoparathyroidism, T-cell-mediated immune deficiency, and palate abnormalities. These children usually have feeding difficulties, cognitive disabilities, and behavioral and speech disorders.

OTHER MALFORMATIONS AND ASSOCIATIONS

Some syndromes without a detectable chromosomal abnormality have clinical features that suggest a chromosomal disorder. These syndromes often enter into the differential diagnosis of a suspected genetic disorder. CHARGE is an acronym for a nonrandom association of features including coloboma of the retina or iris; heart abnormalities; atresia of the choanae; retarded growth; genital hypoplasia in males; and ear abnormalities that can include deafness. CHARGE syndrome was found to result from a point mutation at gene CH7. VATER refers to the nonrandom association of vertebral and anal anomalies, tracheoesophageal fistula with esophageal atresia, and radial or renal abnormalities. Exposure to significant levels of serum alcohol results in a constellation of clinical features referred to as **fetal alcohol syndrome**. Typical findings include short palpebral fissures, smooth philtrum, and thin upper lip. Affected infants may also have hypotonia, poor growth, developmental delay, congenital heart disease, and renal anomalies.

9-3 KEY POINTS

1. Approximately 50% of first-trimester spontaneous abortions have chromosomal abnormalities.
2. Birth defects caused by autosomal anomalies are generally more severe than those caused by sex chromosome abnormalities.
3. Indications for obtaining chromosomal studies include confirmation of a suspected chromosomal syndrome, multiple organ system malformations, significant developmental delay or mental retardation not otherwise explained, short stature or extremely delayed menarche in girls, infertility or a history of multiple spontaneous abortions, ambiguous genitalia, or advanced maternal age.

METABOLIC DISORDERS

APPROACH TO METABOLIC DISORDERS

Although individual metabolic disorders are rare, collectively they are responsible for significant morbidity and mortality. Inborn errors of metabolism are genetic diseases that occur when a defective protein disrupts a metabolic pathway at a specific step. Precursors and toxic metabolites of excess precursors accumulate, and products needed for normal metabolism are deficient. Certain ethnic groups are at increased risk for specific metabolic errors.

Clinical presentation and age at onset vary. Urea cycle defects and organic acidemias present early in life with acute metabolic decompensation. Fatty acid oxidation and carbohydrate metabolism disorders usually present with lethargy, encephalopathy, and hypoglycemia after low carbohydrate intake or fasting. Lysosomal storage disorders are characterized by progressive hepatomegaly, splenomegaly, and, occasionally, neurologic deterioration. Findings that should increase suspicion for an inborn error of metabolism include emesis and acidosis after initiation of feeding, unusual odor of urine or sweat, hepatosplenomegaly, hyperammonemia, early infant death, failure to thrive, developmental regression, mental retardation, and seizures. Several important disorders are discussed here.

CARBOHYDRATE METABOLISM DISORDERS

Galactosemia

Galactosemia, the most common error of carbohydrate metabolism, is caused by a deficiency of the enzyme galactose-1-phosphate uridyltransferase, resulting in impaired conversion of galactose-1-phosphate to glucose-1-phosphate (which can undergo glycolysis). Galactose-1-phosphate accumulates in the liver, kidneys, and brain. The disorder occurs in 1 of 40,000 live births, and inheritance is autosomal recessive.

Clinical Manifestations

Clinical manifestations are noted within a few days to weeks after birth. Initial symptoms include evidence of liver failure (hepatomegaly, direct hyperbilirubinemia, disordered coagulation), renal dysfunction (acidosis, glycosuria, aminoaciduria), emesis, anorexia, and poor growth. Cataracts may develop by 2 months of age in untreated children. Infants with galactosemia are at an increased risk of *Escherichia coli* sepsis. Older children can have severe learning disabilities, whether or not they were treated in infancy. Affected females have a high incidence of premature ovarian failure. Detecting reduced levels of erythrocyte galactose-1-phosphate uridyltransferase is diagnostic. Laboratory findings include a direct hyperbilirubinemia, elevated serum aminotransferases, prolonged prothrombin and partial thromboplastin times, hypoglycemia, and aminoaciduria. Galactose in the urine is detected by a positive reaction for reducing substances and no reaction with glucose oxidase on urine test strips.

Treatment

All formulas and foods containing galactose (including lactose-containing formulas and breast milk) must be eliminated from the child's diet.

Glycogen Storage Diseases

Glycogen is a highly branched polymer of glucose that is stored in liver and muscle. Glycogen storage diseases (GSDs) are a group of conditions that result from a deficiency of enzymes involved in glycogen synthesis or breakdown. Because many different enzymes are involved in glycogen metabolism, the clinical manifestations of the GSDs are variable. Typical manifestations include growth failure, hepatomegaly, and fasting hypoglycemia. The most common GSDs are **type I, von Gierke's disease; type II, Pompe's disease; and type V, McArdle's disease.** All are autosomal recessive disorders. Treatment is designed to prevent hypoglycemia while avoiding storage of even more glycogen in the liver.

AMINO ACID METABOLISM DISORDERS

Phenylketonuria

Phenylketonuria (PKU), the most common of these disorders, occurs in 1 in 10,000 live births. PKU results from a deficiency of phenylalanine hydroxylase, the enzyme that converts phenylalanine to tyrosine. With normal phenylalanine intake, patients develop high serum concentrations of toxic metabolites such as phenylacetic acid and phenyllactic acid.

Clinical Manifestations

Unlike most amino acid disorders, symptoms of untreated PKU develop in childhood rather than early infancy. Neurologic manifestations include moderate to severe mental retardation, hypertonia, tremors, and behavioral problems. Tyrosine is needed for the production of melanin, so the block in the conversion of phenylalanine to tyrosine results in a light complexion. The patient's urine smells mouselike.

Treatment

Prevention of mental retardation in PKU is achieved by early and lifelong dietary restriction of phenylalanine. Most states include PKU detection on their mandatory neonatal screens. Pregnant women with PKU who do not restrict phenylalanine intake dramatically increase the risk of having a child with microcephaly, mental retardation, and congenital heart disease.

Homocystinuria

Homocystinuria is caused by a defect in the amino acid metabolic pathway that converts methionine to cysteine and serine. The incidence of the cystathionine synthase deficiency is 1 in 100,000 live births. The neonatal screen used by most states detects increased methionine levels in the blood.

Clinical Manifestations

No symptoms are apparent in infancy. Clinical manifestations observed during childhood include a Marfanlike body habitus (long thin limbs and digits, scoliosis, sternal deformities, and osteoporosis), dislocated eye lenses, mild to moderate mental retardation, and vascular thromboses that result in childhood stroke or myocardial infarction.

Treatment

Dietary management is extremely difficult because restriction of sulfhydryl groups leads to a very low-protein, foul-tasting diet. Approximately 50% of patients respond to large doses of pyridoxine.

Ornithine Transcarbamylase Deficiency

OTC deficiency, a urea cycle defect, is one of the few inborn errors of metabolism with X-linked inheritance. Amino acid catabolism produces free ammonia that is detoxified to urea through a series of reactions known as the **urea cycle**. In the urea cycle, ornithine joins with carbamoylphosphate through the action of OTC to form citrulline within the mitochondria. When OTC levels are less than 20% of normal, the nitrogen-containing moiety in ornithine cannot be quickly converted to urea for excretion and, instead, forms ammonia, which results in severe hyperammonemia when the patient consumes protein. Milder forms of the condition are seen in heterozygous females and in some affected males.

Clinical Manifestations

Within 24 to 48 hours after the initiation of protein-containing feedings, the newborn becomes progressively lethargic and may develop coma or seizures as the serum ammonia level rises. Female carriers may develop headaches and emesis after protein meals and manifest mental retardation and learning disabilities. Diagnosis is aided by measuring the level of orotic acid, a by-product of carbamoylphosphate metabolism, in the urine.

Treatment

Treatment centers on an extremely low-protein diet and the exploitation of alternative pathways for nitrogen excretion using benzoic acid and phenylacetate. Early intervention may minimize deleterious effects, but management is complex and extremely difficult for parents to maintain.

LYSOSOMAL STORAGE DISORDERS

Deficiency of a lysosomal enzyme causes its substrate to accumulate in lysosomes of tissues that degrade it, creating a characteristic clinical picture. These storage diseases are classified as mucopolysaccharidoses (e.g., Hurler, Hunter, and Sanfilippo's syndromes), lipidoses (e.g., Niemann-Pick, Krabbe, Gaucher, and Tay-Sachs' diseases), or mucolipidoses (e.g., fucosidosis and mannosidosis), depending on the nature of the stored material.

Hurler's Syndrome

Deficiency of α-iduronidase leads to accumulation of the dermatan and heparan sulfates in tissues and their excretion in urine. Typical features include coarse facies, corneal clouding, exaggerated kyphosis, hepatosplenomegaly, umbilical hernia, and congenital heart disease. Developmental regression begins in the first year of life. Most children with Hurler's syndrome die in early adolescence.

Gaucher's Disease

Gaucher's disease is caused by deficiency of the enzyme β-glucosidase, leading to the accumulation of glucocerebroside. The classic form does not involve the central nervous system. Patients characteristically have hepatomegaly and splenomegaly. Storage of glucocerebroside in the bone marrow leads to anemia, leukopenia, thrombocytopenia, and recurrent episodes of bone pain. Radiologic changes include an Erlenmeyer flask shape of the distal femur. A low enzyme level in the white blood cells confirms the diagnosis. Recombinant enzyme therapy improves most symptoms.

Additional Suggested Reading

American Academy of Pediatrics: Molecular genetic testing in pediatric practice. A subject review. *Pediatrics.* 2000;106:1494.

Brent R. Addressing environmentally caused human birth defects. *Pediatr Rev.* 2001;22:153–165.

Siegal B, Milunsky J. When should the possibility of a genetic disorder cross your radar screen? *Contemp Pediatr.* 2004;21(5):30–95.

Hematology

ANEMIA

Anemia, defined as a hemoglobin concentration (or hematocrit) two or more standard deviations below the mean value for age and sex, is not a disease but rather a symptom of another disorder. The hemoglobin concentration is relatively high in the newborn but then declines, reaching a nadir known as **physiologic anemia** of infancy. This nadir occurs at approximately 6 weeks of age in the premature infant and 2 to 3 months of age in the term infant. Thereafter, the hemoglobin concentration rises gradually during childhood, reaching adult values after puberty.

DIFFERENTIAL DIAGNOSIS

Anemia results from decreased red cell production, increased red cell destruction, or blood loss. Decreased red cell production is caused by either deficiency of hematopoietic precursors or bone marrow failure. Increased red cell destruction results from hemolytic disease, which may be caused by extracorpuscular or intracorpuscular defects. Blood loss may be acute or chronic. Table 10-1 outlines the most common causes of anemia.

The adjusted reticulocyte count (ARC) is used to determine whether there has been an adequate erythropoietic response to the given anemia. The ARC is calculated as follows:

$$ARC = (\text{Measured Hematocrit/Expected Hematocrit}) \times \text{Reticulocyte Count}$$

An ARC less than 2 in an anemic patient signifies ineffective erythropoiesis. An ARC greater than 2 signifies effective erythropoiesis, suggesting hemolysis or chronic blood loss.

CLINICAL MANIFESTATIONS

History

In the young infant, perinatal history may reveal twin-to-twin or fetomaternal transfusion. In the older child, the dietary history may suggest risk factors for iron, vitamin B_{12}, or folate deficiency anemia. Both iron deficiency anemia and lead poisoning can manifest as pica. Signs of overt or occult bleeding include melena, hematochezia, hematuria, hematemesis, abnormal menses, or epistaxis. The patient's race/ethnicity and a family history of splenectomy or cholecystectomy may suggest an inherited hemolytic anemia. Poor weight gain should prompt consideration of anemia of chronic disease. Medications can cause either bone marrow suppression or hemolysis. Other questions should attempt to elicit a history of fever, weight loss, fatigue, rash, bruising, jaundice, and cough.

Physical Examination

A careful examination often suggests the severity of anemia. Important findings include pallor (skin, conjunctiva, mucosa) and loss of palmar crease pigmentation. Comparing the complexion of the patient and parents is also useful. Tachycardia and postural changes in heart rate and blood pressure are seen with acute blood loss. Other findings may provide evidence of congestive heart failure (hepatosplenomegaly, lower extremity edema, tachycardia); pancytopenia (petechiae, purpura); blood loss (positive stool guaiac or gastroccult, gross hematuria); hemolysis (scleral icterus, jaundice, urobilinogen in the urine); or infiltrative disorders (lymphadenopathy, hepatosplenomegaly). Table 10-2 lists physical findings that suggest a specific cause of anemia.

■ TABLE 10-1 Differential Diagnosis of Common Anemias Defined by Mean Corpuscular Volume

Anemia	Differential Diagnosis
Microcytic Anemias	Iron deficiency
	Severe lead poisoning
	Thalassemia's syndromes
	Sideroblastic anemia
	Chronic disease
Macrocytic Anemias	
Megaloblastic	Vitamin B_{12} deficiency
	Folate deficiency
	Orotic aciduria
Nonmegaloblastic	Aplastic anemia
	Diamond-Blackfan anemia
	Bone marrow infiltration
	Hypothyroidism
	Fanconi anemia
	Liver disease
Inherited hemolytic anemias	Abnormal hemoglobins
	Sickle cell disease
	Thalassemia
	Red blood cell enzyme disorders
	G6PD deficiency
	Pyruvate kinase deficiency
	Red blood cell membrane disorders
	Hereditary spherocytosis, elliptocytosis
Acquired hemolytic anemias	Antibody-mediated anemias
	Autoimmune hemolytic anemias
	Isoimmune hemolytic anemias
	Microangiopathic hemolytic anemias
	Hemolytic uremic syndrome
	Disseminated intravascular coagulation
	Paroxysmal nocturnal hemoglobinuria
Normocytic Anemias	
Chronic inflammation[a]	
Acute blood loss	

(Continued)

■ TABLE 10-1 Differential Diagnosis of Common Anemias Defined by Mean Corpuscular Volume (*continued*)

Anemia	Differential Diagnosis
Splenic sequestration	
Transient erythroblastopenia of childhood	
Chronic renal disease	

[a]Seventy-five percent of anemias of chronic illness are normocytic; 25% are microcytic.

DIAGNOSTIC EVALUATION

The goal of testing is to determine whether the anemia results from decreased production, increased destruction, or blood loss. Initial laboratory tests needed to evaluate anemia include a complete blood count with manual differential and red blood cell indexes, reticulocyte count, and peripheral blood smear.

The mean corpuscular volume (MCV) and adjusted reticulocyte count categorize the disorder as microcytic, normocytic, or macrocytic anemia, with adequate or inadequate red blood cell production. Peripheral blood smear is used to assess the red and white blood cell morphology and the platelet number and size. If hemolysis is suspected, electrolytes, lactate dehydrogenase, bilirubin, Coombs test (indirect and direct), and serum haptoglobin should be obtained. Urobilinogen may be detected on urinalysis. A glucose-6-phosphate dehydrogenase (G6PD) assay should be performed in African American and Mediterranean populations who present with hemolytic anemia. Hemoglobin electrophoresis is used to diagnose suspected hemoglobinopathies. If iron deficiency anemia is high on the differential, serum iron level, total iron-binding capacity, and serum ferritin level are needed for analysis. A lead level is indicated if lead poisoning is contemplated. Free erythrocyte protoporphyrin (FEP) levels can be obtained quickly and with a small amount of blood. Elevated FEP levels suggest the disordered heme incorporation seen with iron deficiency and lead poisoning. The erythrocyte sedimentation rate (ESR) is generally elevated in anemia of chronic disease. Positive heme tests of stool or gastric contents indicate gastrointestinal bleeding. If a macrocytic anemia is found, both vitamin B_{12} and red blood cell folate levels are needed.

■ TABLE 10-2 Physical Findings in the Evaluation of Anemia

System	Observation	Significance
Skin	Hyperpigmentation	Fanconi anemia, dyskeratosis congenita
	Café-au-lait spots	Fanconi anemia
	Vitiligo	Vitamin B_{12} deficiency
	Partial oculocutaneous albinism	Chédiak-Higashi's syndrome
	Jaundice	Hemolysis
	Petechiae, purpura	Bone marrow infiltration, autoimmune hemolysis with autoimmune thrombocytopenia, hemolytic uremic syndrome
	Erythematous rash	Parvovirus, Epstein-Barr virus
	Butterfly rash	Systemic lupus erythematosus
Head	Frontal bossing	Thalassemia major, severe iron deficiency, chronic subdural hematoma
	Microcephaly	Fanconi anemia
Eyes	Microphthalmia	Fanconi anemia
	Retinopathy	Sickle cell disease
	Optic atrophy	Osteopetrosis
	Blocked lacrimal gland	Dyskeratosis congenita
	Kayser-Fleischer ring	Wilson's disease
	Blue sclera	Iron deficiency
Ears	Deafness	Osteopetrosis
Mouth	Glossitis	B_{12} deficiency, iron deficiency
	Angular stomatitis	Iron deficiency
	Cleft lip	Diamond-Blackfan's syndrome
	Pigmentation	Peutz-Jeghers' syndrome (intestinal blood loss)
	Telangiectasia	Osler-Weber-Rendu's syndrome (blood loss)
	Leukoplakia	Dyskeratosis congenita
Chest	Shield chest or widespread nipples	Diamond-Blackfan's syndrome
	Murmur	Endocarditis: prosthetic valve hemolysis
Abdomen	Hepatomegaly	Hemolysis, infiltrative tumor, chronic disease, hemangioma, cholecystitis
	Splenomegaly	Hemolysis, sickle cell disease, (early) thalassemia, malaria,
	Nephromegaly	lymphoma, Epstein-Barr virus, portal hypertension
	Absent kidney	Fanconi anemia
Extremities	Absent thumbs	Fanconi anemia
	Triphalangeal thumb	Diamond-Blackfan's syndrome
	Spoon nails	Iron deficiency
	Beau line (nails)	Heavy metal intoxication, severe illness
	Dystrophic nails	Dyskeratosis congenita
Rectal	Hemorrhoids	Portal hypertension
	Heme-positive stool	Intestinal hemorrhage
Nerves	Irritable, apathy	Iron deficiency
	Peripheral neuropathy	Deficiency of vitamins B_1, B_{12}, and E, lead poisoning
	Dementia	Deficiency of vitamins B_{12} and, E Vitamin B_{12} deficiency
	Ataxia, posterior column signs Stroke	Sickle cell disease, paroxysmal nocturnal hemoglobinuria

TREATMENT

Treatment varies depending on the cause of the anemia.

> ### 🔑 10-1 KEY POINTS
>
> 1. Anemia is not a disease but rather a symptom of another disorder.
> 2. Anemia results from decreased red cell production, increased red cell destruction, or blood loss.
> 3. The mean corpuscular volume and adjusted reticulocyte count categorize the disorder into a microcytic, normocytic, or macrocytic anemia, with adequate or inadequate red blood cell production.

MICROCYTIC ANEMIAS WITH DECREASED RED BLOOD CELL PRODUCTION

Hypochromic microcytic red blood cells indicate impaired synthesis of the heme or globin components of hemoglobin. Defective heme synthesis may be the result of iron deficiency, lead poisoning, chronic inflammatory disease, pyridoxine deficiency, or copper deficiency. Defective globin synthesis is characteristic of the thalassemia syndromes. Iron deficiency anemia, the thalassemia syndromes, and anemia of chronic disease are the most common causes of hypochromic microcytic anemias. Lead poisoning, which may cause a mild hypochromic microcytic anemia, is discussed in detail in Chapter 2.

IRON DEFICIENCY ANEMIA

Iron deficiency, the most common cause of anemia during childhood, is usually seen between 6 and 24 months of age. Nutritional iron deficiency develops when rapid growth and an expanding blood volume put excessive demands on iron stores. Dietary risk factors include extended exclusive breast-feeding (more than 6 months) without iron supplementation, consumption of low-iron formula preparations, early institution of low-iron solids, excessive whole-milk intake, and the absence of iron supplements. The iron present in breast milk is much more bioavailable than the iron in cow milk. Ascorbic acid enhances the absorption of nonheme iron, whereas tea decreases its absorption.

Iron deficiency anemia can occur as early as 3 months of age in the premature infant who has inadequate iron stores at birth. It can occur in the infant or toddler who receives a diet exclusively composed of milk or low-iron formula. Nutritional iron deficiency can also occur during adolescence when a rapid growth spurt coincides with a diet with suboptimal iron content. This is a particular problem in adolescent females because of iron loss during menses.

Iron deficiency caused by blood loss can also occur in young children. Prenatal iron loss can occur from fetomaternal transfusion or from twin-to-twin transfusion. Perinatal bleeding may result from obstetric complications such as placental abruption or placenta previa. Postnatal blood loss may occur from obvious sources such as surgery or trauma or may be occult, as occurs with idiopathic pulmonary hemosiderosis, parasitic infestations, and inflammatory bowel disease.

Clinical Manifestations

Mild iron deficiency is usually asymptomatic. With moderate iron deficiency (hemoglobin: 6 to 8 g per dL), the infant develops anorexia, irritability, apathy, and easy fatigability. On physical examination, the anemic infant may have skin and mucous membrane pallor, glossitis, angular stomatitis, and koilonychia (spoon nails). The child may also have tachycardia and a systolic ejection murmur at the left upper sternal border. The infant with severe anemia (hemoglobin less than 3g per dL) shows signs of congestive heart failure, which include tachycardia, an S_3, cardiomegaly, hepatomegaly, distended neck veins, and pulmonary rales.

Table 10-3 lists the laboratory findings typical for the microcytic anemias. Bone marrow examination is not clinically indicated to confirm the diagnosis but when performed, it demonstrates micronormoblastic hyperplasia of the erythroid line.

Treatment

Mild to moderate iron deficiency anemia without evidence of congestive heart failure is treated with 3 to 6 mg/kg/day of elemental iron. The reticulocyte count increases within 2 to 3 days, and the hemoglobin increases at a rate of approximately 0.3g/dL/day after 4 to 5 days. Therapy is continued for 8 weeks after the hemoglobin has returned to normal to replenish tissue stores. If the hemoglobin has not increased substantially after 1 month of therapy and compliance has been established, other causes of hypochromic microcytic anemia must be considered. Although infants can tolerate remarkable degrees of anemia, especially if the decline in hemoglobin is gradual, infants with severe anemia must be transfused very slowly with

■ **TABLE 10-3** Laboratory Findings for the Common Microcytic Anemias

	Iron Deficiency	Thalassemia Trait	Thalassemia Major	Plumbism Chronic Disease	
RDW	↑	NL	↑	↑	NL
MCV	↓	↓	↓	↓	NL ↓
RBC no.	↓	NL	↓	↓	↓
FEP	↑	NL	NL	↑↑	↑
Hib A$_2$	↓	β-↑	β-↑	NL	NL
α-NL	α-NL				
Iron	↓	NL	↑	NL	↓
TIBC	NL ↑	NL	NL ↑	NL	NL ↓
% saturation	↓	NL	↑	NL	↓
Ferritin	↓	NL	↑	NL	NL

FEP, free erythrocyte protoporphyrin; hgb, hemoglobin; TIBC, total iron-binding capacity; ↑, increased; ↓, decreased; NL, normal; MCV, mean corpuscular volume; RDW, red blood cell distribution width.

small (3 to 5 mL per kg) aliquots of packed red blood cells to avoid causing cardiac decompensation.

🔑 10-2 KEY POINTS

1. Iron deficiency anemia, the thalassemia syndromes, and anemia of chronic disease are the most common causes of hypochromic microcytic anemias.
2. Iron deficiency is by far the most common cause of anemia during childhood and most often seen between 6 and 24 months of age.
3. Mild to moderate iron deficiency anemia is treated with 3 to 6 mg/kg/day of elemental iron. If the hemoglobin has not increased substantially after 1 month of therapy, other causes of hypochromic microcytic anemia should be considered.

α- AND β-THALASSEMIA

Pathogenesis and Clinical Manifestations

The thalassemias are hereditary hemolytic anemias characterized by decreased or absent synthesis of one or more globin subunits of the hemoglobin molecule. α-Thalassemia, caused by deletion of one or more of the four α-globin genes, leads to reduced synthesis of α-globin chains. β-Thalassemia is caused by errors in the transcription or translation of β-globin mRNA and leads to reduced synthesis of β-globin chains. Table 10-4 compares the thalassemia syndromes.

The number of deleted α-globin genes determines the hematologic consequences of α-thalassemia. These deletions can be *cis* or *trans*. *Cis* deletions occur when two α-globin genes are deleted from one chromosome, whereas *trans* deletions signify a single α-globin gene deletion on each of the two chromosomes. Different races and ethnicities have varying rates of both *cis* and *trans* deletions of α-globin genes in their population.

Homozygous α-thalassemia, or hemoglobin Bart's disease, occurs when all four α-globin genes are deleted. Failure to produce any α-globin chains results in γ-globin tetramers (hemoglobin Bart). Hemoglobin Bart has a high affinity for oxygen and does not release it to the tissue. The result is severe anemia, tissue anoxia, heart failure, hepatosplenomegaly, generalized edema, and death in utero because of hydrops fetalis. The *cis* deletion is most prevalent in Southeast Asians.

Hemoglobin H disease results from deletion of three α-globin genes. γ-Globin chains are only produced in utero. In normal infants, fetal hemoglobin (which consists of two α-globin chains and two γ-globin chains) usually predominates at birth. In newborn infants with hemoglobin H disease, the dearth of α-globin leads to the formation of hemoglobin Bart, which accounts for 10% to 40% of the total hemoglobin. With the cessation of γ-globin synthesis and the onset of β-globin synthesis at birth, hemoglobin Bart diminishes and hemoglobin H (which consists of a β-globin tetramer) predominates after the first few months of life. Hemoglobin H eventually accounts for 30% to 40% of the total hemoglobin, and normal

■ **TABLE 10-4** Comparison of the Thalassemia's Syndromes

Genetic Abnormality	Percentage Hemoglobin (Hb)			
	Hb A	Hb A_2	Hb F	Other
Normal $\alpha\beta$	90–98	2–3	2–3	—
β-Thalassemias				
Thalassemia major				
β-thal^0 β-thal^0	0	2–5	95	—
β-thal$^+$ β-thal$^+$	Very low	2–5	20–80	—
Thalassemia intermedia (varied genetic globin abnormalities)	Overlaps with thalassemia major			
Thalassemia minor				
β β-thal^0 or β β-thal$^+$	90–95	5–7	2–10	
α-Thalassemias				
Homozygous α-Thalassemia — —/— —	—	—	—	Hb H (β4) Hb Bart (γ4)
Hemoglobin H disease — —/— α	60–70	2–5	2–5	Hb H 30–40
α-Thalassemia minor — α/— α or α α/— —	90–98	2–3	2–3	
Silent carrier — α/α α	90–98	2–3	2–3	

hemoglobin A accounts for approximately 60% to 70% of the total hemoglobin. This diagnosis is most common in children with Southeast Asian ancestry.

α-Thalassemia trait, also known as α-thalassemia minor, results from deletion of two α-globin genes. This defect manifests with mild anemia, hypochromia, and microcytosis. The α-thalassemia trait, present in 3% of U.S. blacks, is often confused with mild iron deficiency. The hemoglobin electrophoresis is normal in these children, and the diagnosis is one of exclusion confirmed by documenting parental microcytosis.

Those with deletion of only one α-globin gene are considered silent carriers for α-thalassemia because they have a normal hemoglobin concentration and normal red blood cell indexes. The condition can be measured only by quantitative measurement of globin chain synthesis or by gene analysis. A carrier can produce offspring with α-thalassemia trait or hemoglobin H disease. β-Thalassemia can be subdivided into homozygous (β-thalassemia major) and heterozygous forms (β-thalassemia minor). β-Thalassemia major results either from complete absence of β-globin synthesis (B0/B0 genotype) because of defective transcription of mRNA or from partial reduction of gene product (B$^+$/B$^+$ genotype) because of translational errors. The child with β-thalassemia minor, the heterozygous form, has one normal β-globin gene and one abnormal β-globin gene.

Children with β-thalassemia major have severe hemolytic anemia and splenomegaly during the first year of life. If untreated, bone marrow hyperplasia and extramedullary hematopoiesis produce characteristic features such as tower skull, frontal bossing, maxillary hypertrophy with prominent cheekbones, and an overbite. Failure to thrive is prominent. Death occurs within the first few years of life because of progressive congestive heart failure if the patient is not supported with blood transfusions. Despite severe anemia, there is reticulocytopenia, reflecting ineffective hematopoiesis. Peripheral blood smear reveals marked hypochromia, microcytosis, anisocytosis, and poikilocytosis. On hemoglobin electrophoresis, hemoglobin A is either markedly decreased (B^+/B^+ or $B^+/B0$) or totally absent ($B0/B0$). On quantitative hemoglobin electrophoresis, hemoglobin F accounts for 95% in the B0/B0 genotype and 20% to 80% in the B^+/B^+ genotype. If the diagnosis is in question or the child's hemoglobin electrophoresis is equivocal, the parental complete blood count, smears, and hemoglobin electrophoresis may clarify the diagnosis.

Children with β-thalassemia minor have only a mild hemolytic anemia. On blood smear, the hypochromia, microcytosis, and anisocytosis are disproportionately severe given the degree of anemia. Hemoglobin electrophoresis shows elevation of the hemoglobin A_2 level and sometimes a mild elevation of hemoglobin F.

Epidemiology

α-Thalassemia is most common in African, Southeast Asian, Mediterranean, and Middle Eastern populations. The most severe forms of α-thalassemia, three- and four-gene deletions, are seen in the Southeast Asian population because of the high prevalence of *cis* deletions. β-thalassemia is most often found in populations originating from the Mediterranean, Middle East, and India.

Treatment

Therapy for children with β-thalassemia major consists of frequent packed red blood cell transfusions to ameliorate the anemia and prevent congestive heart failure. These children require 10 to 20 mL per kg of leucodepleted red blood cells every 3 to 5 weeks to maintain the hemoglobin above 10 g per dL. This regimen eliminates an increased erythropoietic drive, allowing normal linear growth and bone development. Suppression of erythropoiesis also limits the stimulus for increased iron absorption, which helps minimize iron overload.

Splenectomy is considered when transfusion requirements exceed 250 mL/kg/year. Iron overload develops in children with β-thalassemia, whether they are transfused or not, because of hyperabsorption of dietary iron. When the bone marrow storage capacity for iron is exceeded, iron accumulates in the liver, heart, pancreas, gonads, and skin, producing symptoms of hemochromatosis. As a result, many thalassemic patients develop cardiomyopathy and congestive heart failure in their late teens. To minimize the morbidity associated with iron overload, patients are treated with chelating agents such as desferrioxamine. Because of the constant state of increased erythropoiesis, folic acid supplementation is recommended for patients not maintained on chronic transfusion therapy in order to prevent folate deficiency and megaloblastic anemia. Bone marrow transplantation is curative, but because of its associated morbidity and mortality, this procedure is performed in only a few centers using HLA-matched sibling donors.

Principles of therapy for hemoglobin H disease are the same as those for β-thalassemia major. The need for transfusion and chelation therapy depends on the severity of the anemia.

No treatment is necessary for α- or β-thalassemia minor. Genetic counselling is recommended. Because the smear of iron deficiency anemia and α- and β-thalassemia minor are quite similar, the child with presumed iron deficiency anemia who does not respond to oral iron therapy and is believed to be compliant should have a hemoglobin electrophoresis to rule out β-thalassemia minor. The child with α-thalassemia trait has a normal hemoglobin electrophoresis (outside the neonatal period), whereas the electrophoresis of the child with β-thalassemia minor may show an elevated hemoglobin A_2 and hemoglobin F.

⚒ 10-3 KEY POINTS

1. The severity of symptoms of α- and β-thalassemia depends on the level of α- or β-globin chain synthesis.
2. Hemoglobin H disease and β-thalassemia major are treated with red blood cell transfusions, iron chelation, and/or folate supplementation, depending on the severity of the disease. α- and β-Thalassemia minor usually do not require treatment but may be mistaken for iron deficiency anemia.

ANEMIA OF CHRONIC DISEASE

Anemia of chronic disease can result from chronic inflammatory diseases, such as inflammatory bowel disease and juvenile rheumatoid arthritis; chronic infections, such as tuberculosis; and malignancy. Typically, anemia of chronic disease is normocytic; 25% of cases of anemia of chronic disease have microcytosis. Anemia of chronic disease results from an inability to mobilize iron from its storage sites in macrophages. The chronic inflammatory state triggers cytokines that result in reticuloendothelial blockade within the marrow. A modest decrease in the survival time of red blood cells and a relatively limited erythropoietin response also contribute to the anemia.

Clinical Manifestations

The anemia is mild in degree (hemoglobin: 8–10 g per dL). Table 10-3 notes the laboratory findings typical for anemia of chronic disease. As in iron deficiency anemia, the serum iron level is reduced; in contrast to iron deficiency anemia, the total iron-binding capacity is low, and the serum ferritin level is normal or increased. Bone marrow examination shows micronormoblastic hyperplasia and an increase in storage iron but a decrease in the number of iron-containing erythroblasts.

Treatment

The anemia resolves when the underlying condition is treated adequately. Therapy with iron supplements is unnecessary unless true iron deficiency is also present.

✎ 10-4 KEY POINTS

1. Anemia of chronic disease can result from chronic inflammatory diseases, chronic infections, and malignancy.
2. Anemia of chronic disease typically is normocytic; 25% of cases of anemia of chronic disease are microcytic.
3. Anemia of chronic disease results from an inability to mobilize iron from its storage sites in macrophages.

NORMOCYTIC ANEMIAS WITH DECREASED RED CELL PRODUCTION

Normocytic anemias result from the failure of the bone marrow to produce adequate numbers of red blood cells because of systemic illness. Bone marrow function can be impaired by fibrosis, malignant infiltration, transient marrow failure, or failure to synthesize erythropoietin (chronic renal disease). Transient marrow failure states include transient erythroblastopenia of childhood, parvovirus B19–induced aplastic crisis, and drug toxicity from myelosuppressive agents. A normocytic anemia also occurs with acute blood loss. Re-equilibration of the total blood volume before erythropoiesis results in the anemia. Chronic inflammatory states result in anemia of chronic disease, which can be normocytic (75%) or microcytic (25%), as noted earlier.

TRANSIENT ERYTHROBLASTOPENIA OF CHILDHOOD

Transient erythroblastopenia of childhood (TEC) is an acquired pure red cell aplasia caused by transient bone marrow suppression. The resulting anemia is normocytic. Although a specific etiology has not been identified, TEC is usually preceded by a viral infection. TEC occurs between the 6 months and 5 years of age, with a peak incidence at 2 years of age. In contrast to Diamond-Blackfan's syndrome, which is a congenital macrocytic pure red cell aplasia, 85% of cases of TEC occur after 1 year of age, there are no other associated anomalies, and fetal hemoglobin and i antigen are not present.

Clinical Manifestations

The history and physical examination are unremarkable except for the gradual onset of pallor over the course of weeks. Peripheral smear is normal other than reticulocytopenia. Bone marrow examination reveals few erythroid precursors and normal myeloid and platelet precursors.

Treatment

The hemoglobin is usually at its nadir at the time of diagnosis. Spontaneous recovery occurs within 1 to

2 months of diagnosis. Red blood cell transfusions are necessary only if the patient has signs or symptoms of congestive heart failure.

🔑 10-5 KEY POINTS

1. Transient erythroblastopenia of childhood, a normocytic anemia caused by bone marrow suppression, is an acquired pure red cell aplasia with a peak incidence at 2 years of age.
2. Viral infection usually precedes transient erythroblastopenia of childhood (TEC), but no specific etiology has been identified.
3. Recovery from TEC is spontaneous.

NORMOCYTIC ANEMIAS WITH INCREASED RED CELL PRODUCTION

HEMOLYTIC ANEMIA

Normocytic anemias with increased red cell production are most commonly caused by hemolytic anemias. The red blood cell destruction and anemia are sensed by the kidneys, which release erythropoietin to stimulate bone marrow erythropoiesis. Hemolytic anemias are caused by factors extrinsic to the red cell (extracorpuscular) or by defects intrinsic to the red cell (intracorpuscular). In general, extrinsic defects are acquired and intrinsic defects are hereditary.

Extracorpuscular anomalies are divided into isoimmune, autoimmune, and nonimmune hemolytic anemias. Isoimmune hemolytic anemia results from antibodies produced by one individual against the red blood cells of another individual of the same species. ABO or minor antigen incompatibility is an example of isoimmune hemolytic anemia (see Chapter 13). In autoimmune hemolytic anemia, abnormal antibodies directed against red blood cells are produced by the patient. Autoimmune hemolytic anemias can be idiopathic, postinfectious (*Mycoplasma pneumoniae*, Epstein-Barr virus), drug induced (penicillin, quinidine, α-methyldopa), or may result from a chronic autoimmune disease (systemic lupus erythematosus) or malignancy (non-Hodgkin lymphoma). Therapy for autoimmune hemolytic anemia varies depending on the etiology of the hemolysis and the clinical condition of the patient. In general, treatment is supportive, with the careful use of packed red blood cell transfusions and corticosteroids. Autoantibodies react with virtually all red blood cells, making crossmatching difficult. In some severe chronic cases, intravenous immunoglobulin, immunosuppressive pharmacotherapy, and splenectomy may be indicated.

The antibodies that cause isoimmune and autoimmune hemolytic anemias may be of the IgG or IgM classes. IgG antibodies tend to be **warm reactive** (maximal activity at 37°C) and are considered incomplete antibodies. They coat the surface of the red blood cells and fix early complement components but cannot agglutinate red blood cells or activate the complement cascade through the entire hemolytic sequence. Hemolysis occurs extravascularly because of trapping of the opsonized red blood cells by macrophages in the reticuloendothelial system. IgG antibodies are associated with autoimmune diseases, lymphomas, and viral infections. These antibodies are identified by the direct Coombs test. IgM antibodies are usually **cold reactive** (maximal activity at low temperatures) and are deemed complete antibodies. They agglutinate red blood cells and activate the complement sequence through C9, causing lysis of red blood cells. Hemolysis occurs intravascularly. IgM antibodies are associated with *Mycoplasma pneumoniae*, Epstein-Barr virus, and transfusion reactions.

Nonimmune hemolytic anemias can be microangiopathic (disseminated intravascular coagulation, thrombotic thrombocytopenic purpura, hemolytic uremic syndrome, malignant hypertension, giant hemangioma, preeclampsia, renal graft rejection) or can be caused by damage from nonendothelialized surfaces (artificial heart valve, arteriovenous malformation, Kasabach-Merritt's syndrome), hypersplenism, abetalipoproteinemia, toxins (snake venom, copper, arsenic), malaria, or burns.

Intracorpuscular defects include intrinsic membrane defects such as hereditary spherocytosis, hereditary elliptocytosis, hereditary stomatocytosis, and paroxysmal nocturnal hemoglobinuria (PNH). PNH is the only intracorpuscular disorder that is not inherited. Hemoglobinopathies (sickle cell disorders) and enzyme disorders (G6PD deficiency, pyruvate kinase deficiency) are also intracorpuscular disorders. Following are discussions of hereditary spherocytosis, sickle cell anemia, and G6PD deficiency, three of the most common intracorpuscular defects.

HEREDITARY SPHEROCYTOSIS

Hereditary spherocytosis is caused by a defect in red blood cell membrane-supporting proteins (spectrin, ankyrin, or band 3 protein). The defect leads to a loss of membrane fragments without a proportional loss of volume. Therefore, microspherocytes (small spherical red blood cells with a high volume-to-surface ratio) form. Microspherocytes are less deformable than normal red blood cells, so they are trapped and destroyed in the microvasculature of the spleen. Inheritance is usually autosomal dominant, but 25% of cases are caused by new mutations or autosomal recessive forms.

Clinical Manifestations

Hereditary spherocytosis varies greatly in clinical severity, ranging from an asymptomatic, well-compensated, mild hemolytic anemia discovered incidentally to a severe hemolytic anemia with growth failure, splenomegaly, and chronic transfusion requirements in infancy necessitating early splenectomy. The newborn with this disorder may present with severe unconjugated hyperbilirubinemia caused by hemolysis. Occasionally, patients present with aplastic crisis after parvovirus B19 infection. Because of chronic hemolysis, teenagers develop gallstones and cholecystitis. Physical examination reveals pallor, scleral icterus, and mild to moderate splenomegaly. Laboratory studies demonstrate mild normocytic anemia, reticulocytosis, and indirect hyperbilirubinemia. During an aplastic crisis, the anemia becomes severe and reticulocytopenia occurs. Diagnosis is confirmed by a positive **osmotic fragility test**.

Treatment

Treatment includes folic acid supplementation to meet the needs of increased red blood cell turnover and red blood cell transfusions during an aplastic crisis. Splenectomy alleviates anemia, reticulocytosis, and scleral icterus, although microspherocytes persist. Splenectomy should be deferred until after 6 years of age because of the higher the risk of sepsis from encapsulated organisms in young children.

SICKLE CELL DISEASE

Pathogenesis

Sickle cell disease is an autosomal recessive disorder that results from a valine-for-glutamine substitution in the sixth amino acid position of the β-globin chain. This substitution alters the structure of the hemoglobin molecule, which, under conditions of deoxygenation, promotes aggregation of hemoglobin into long polymers that distort the red blood cell into a sickle shape. Sickling shortens red blood cell survival time and results in a chronic hemolytic anemia. Sickled cells also cause microvascular obstruction, which leads to tissue ischemia and infarction. The sickling phenomenon is accentuated by hypoxia, acidosis, increased or decreased temperature, and dehydration. If only one of the two β-globin genes is affected, the individual has **sickle cell trait**, which is the heterozygous state without clinical consequence. If both β-globin genes have the genetic substitution, the patient is homozygous for hemoglobin S and has **sickle cell disease**. Sickling disorders of varying severity also result from hemoglobin S existing in combination with other abnormal hemoglobins (hemoglobin C, $D_{Los\ Angeles}$, O_{Arab}) or thalassemias (B^+ or B0 thalassemia).

Epidemiology

Sickle cell disease affects 1 in 625 African Americans, making it the most common autosomal recessive disorder in that population. It also occurs in those of Greek, Italian, and Saudi Arabian descent.

Clinical Manifestations and Management

Children with sickle cell trait are generally asymptomatic. Rarely, an individual exhibits painless hematuria and inability to properly concentrate the urine (isosthenuria). Patients with sickle cell trait occasionally have sickle cells on peripheral blood smear, but hemoglobin electrophoresis provides the definitive diagnosis. Typically, hemoglobin electrophoresis reveals 55% to 60% hemoglobin A, 40% to 45% hemoglobin S, and 2% to 3% hemoglobin A_2. It is important to detect the trait for genetic counseling.

Unlike sickle cell trait, sickle cell disease causes severe morbidity and mortality. Quantitative hemoglobin electrophoresis shows 0% hemoglobin A, 80% to 95% hemoglobin S, 2% to 3% hemoglobin A_2, and up to 15%. In most cases, diagnosis is made from newborn screening tests. The highly variable clinical manifestations of sickle cell disease result from anemia, infection, and vaso-occlusion (Table 10-5).

At approximately 4 months of age, when the percentage of hemoglobin F diminishes and the percentage of hemoglobin S rises, the child with sickle cell disease develops a progressive hemolytic anemia. The anemia of sickle cell disease is a chronic, well-compensated, severe anemia that is rarely transfusion dependent. Common manifestations of the anemia include pallor, jaundice, splenomegaly in infancy, a systolic ejection murmur, and delayed sexual development and growth. Splenic sequestration, aplastic crisis, and hyperhemolytic crisis all superimpose acute life-threatening declines in hemoglobin concentration on the chronic compensated anemia of sickle cell disease. In splenic sequestration, rapid splenic engorgement caused by trapping of red blood cells may lead to hypovolemic shock. Sequestration typically occurs between 6 months and 2 years of age. Viral suppression of red blood cell precursors in the bone marrow, most often by parvovirus B19, precipitates aplastic crisis. Exposure of a patient with sickle cell disease and concomitant G6PD deficiency to an oxidative stress results in acute hemolysis superimposed on a chronic hemolytic anemia (hyperhemolytic crisis). Medications or infection usually cause the acute hemolysis. Splenic sequestration, aplastic crisis, and hyperhemolytic crisis are

■ **TABLE 10-5** Clinical Manifestations of Sickle Cell Anemia[a]

Manifestation	Comments
Anemia	Chronic, onset 3–4 mo of age; requires folate therapy for chronic hemolysis
Aplastic crisis	Parvovirus infection; may require transfusion
Sequestration crisis	Massive splenomegaly, shock; treat with transfusion
Hemolytic crisis	May be associated with G6PD deficiency
Dactylitis	Hand/foot swelling in early infancy
Pain crisis	Microvascular painful vasoocclusive infarcts of muscle, bone, lung, intestines
Cerebral vascular accidents	Large- and small-vessel sickling and thrombosis (stroke); requires chronic transfusion
Acute chest syndrome	Infection and/or infarction, severe hypoxemia, infiltrate, dyspnea, rales
Chronic lung disease	Pulmonary fibrosis, restrictive lung disease, cor pulmonale
Priapism	May cause eventual impotence; treat with pseudoephedrine, venous drainage, transfusion, oxygen, or corpora cavernosa-to-spongiosa shunt
Ocular	Retinopathy
Gallbladder's disease	Bilirubin stones; cholecystitis
Renal	Hematuria, papillary necrosis, renal-concentrating deficit; nephropathy
Cardiomyopathy	Heart failure (fibrosis)
Infections	Functional asplenia; increased risk of invasive infection because of encapsulated bacteria such as *Streptococcus pneumoniae*, *Haemophilus influenzae*, and *Neisseria meningitidis*; *Salmonella* and *Staphylococcus aureus* osteomyelitis; severe *Mycoplasma* pneumonia; transfusion-acquired infections
Growth failure, delayed puberty	May respond to nutritional supplements

[a]Clinical manifestations with sickle cell trait are rare but include renal papillary necrosis (hematuria), sudden death on exertion, intraocular hyphema extension, and sickling in unpressurized airplanes.
G6PD, glucose-6-phosphate dehydrogenase.

often treated with red blood cell transfusion. Because of the presence of chronic hemolytic anemia, gallstone formation and cholecystitis are common during adolescence.

As the sickled cells traverse the spleen, they cause microvascular obstruction, infarction, and fibrosis of the spleen. This process, known as **autoinfarction,** causes the spleen to regress in size gradually; by 4 years of age, the spleen is no longer palpable. More important, autoinfarction diminishes the capability of the spleen to filter encapsulated bacterial organisms and places the infant at great risk for overwhelming infection from *Streptococcus pneumoniae* or *Haemophilus influenzae.* Any infant or child who has sickle cell disease and fever (temperature greater than 38.5°C) must be evaluated immediately. Although the child likely has a benign viral infection, invasive bacterial infection must be excluded. To minimize the risk of life-threatening infection, children with sickle cell disease start penicillin prophylaxis at approximately 4 months of age and receive vaccinations. Both the *H. influenzae* type b (Hib) and heptavalent pneumococcal conjugate (Prevnar) vaccines are given at the 2-, 4-, and 6-month visits and then again between 12 months and 15 months of age. The 23-valent pneumococcal polysaccharide vaccine (PPV) should be administered at 2 years of age and then again at 4 to 6 years of age. Penicillin prophylaxis is continued until at least 5 years of age.

Vaso-occlusive crises result from microvascular infarcts, may occur in any organ or tissue of the body, and are commonly precipitated by infection, cold exposure, dehydration, venous stasis, and acidosis. Dactylitis, or hand-foot syndrome, is symmetrical painful swelling of the dorsal surface of the hands and feet caused by avascular necrosis of the metacarpal and metatarsal bones. Dactylitis occurs at 4 to 6 months of age and is the earliest clinical manifestation of vaso-occlusive disease in the sickle cell patient. In older children, pain crises most often localize to the long bones of the arms and legs, vertebral column, and sternum. Pain crises last from 2 to 7 days and are treated with nonsteroidal anti-inflammatory drugs and narcotics. Hydroxyurea maintenance therapy decreases the number and severity of vaso-occlusive crises. Avascular necrosis of the femoral head, another vaso-occlusive manifestation in bone, typically occurs in the adolescent population.

Microvascular obstructive disease can also occur in the lungs, central nervous system, penis, myocardium, and intestine. Acute chest syndrome, a vaso-occlusive crisis within the lungs, is often caused by pulmonary infection and infarction. Patients present with hypoxia, respiratory distress, and pulmonary infiltrates. Oxygen, analgesia, antibiotics, and exchange transfusion are used to maximize respiratory status and minimize further pulmonary damage. Similarly, occlusion of the large cerebral vessels results in stroke. Patients present with mental status changes, seizures, and focal paralysis. Because of the high risk of recurrence, children who have had a stroke are placed on chronic red blood cell transfusion protocols to minimize the risk of future stroke. Priapism typically occurs in males between 6 and 20 years of age. The child develops sudden painful engorgement of the penis that will not subside. Acute chest syndrome, stroke, and priapism are treated by exchange transfusion to decrease the percentage of hemoglobin S to below 30% in an attempt to minimize vaso-occlusion.

By adolescence, the effects of chronic myocardial microvascular obstruction and infarction are evident by an enlarged hypertrophic heart. Many adults eventually succumb to congestive heart failure from progressive myocardial damage. Abdominal crisis results from microvascular obstruction of the intestinal circulation. Patients present with ileus and rebound tenderness, mimicking an acute abdomen. The pain may be familiar to the patient and readily recognized as "crisis pain." Abdominal pain consistent with the child's normal pain constellation during crisis may warrant a period of observation with hydration and analgesic administration. If the abdominal pain is not typical for the patient during a vaso-occlusive crisis, surgical consultation should be obtained.

🔑 10-8 KEY POINTS

1. Sickle cell disease is an autosomal recessive disorder that results from an amino acid substitution on the β-globin chain. This substitution results in an alteration of the structure of the hemoglobin molecule, which, under conditions of deoxygenation, promotes aggregation of hemoglobin into long polymers that distort the red blood cell into a sickle shape.
2. Sickling shortens red blood cell survival time and results in a chronic hemolytic anemia.
3. The clinical manifestations of sickle cell anemia result from anemia, infection, and vaso-occlusion.

GLUCOSE-6-PHOSPHATE DEHYDROGENASE DEFICIENCY

G6PD deficiency, the most common red blood cell enzyme defect, is transmitted as an X-linked recessive trait. The lack of this enzyme in the hexose monophosphate shunt pathway results in depletion of nicotinamide adenine dinucleotide phosphate (NADPH) and the inability to regenerate reduced glutathione, which is needed to protect the red blood cell from oxidative stress.

The most common forms of G6PD deficiency are the A+ and Mediterranean variants. The A+ variant, found in approximately 10% of African Americans in the United States, is associated with an isoenzyme that deteriorates rapidly, with a half-life of 13 days. The Mediterranean variant occurs predominantly in persons of Greek and Italian descent; its isoenzyme is extremely unstable, with a half-life of several hours.

When there is an oxidative stress on the red blood cell, exposed sulfhydryl groups on the hemoglobin are oxidized, leading to dissociation of heme and globin moieties, with the globin precipitating as **Heinz bodies**. Damaged red cells are removed from circulation by the reticuloendothelial system; severely damaged cells may lyse intravascularly. Known oxidants include sulfonamides, nitrofurantoin, primaquine, and dimercaprol. Hemolysis may also be precipitated by fava beans and infection.

Clinical Manifestations

The classic course of G6PD deficiency is episodic stress- or drug-induced hemolytic anemia. Patients with the A− variant have a limited hemolysis confined to the older red blood cell population. Recovery occurs as young red blood cells with enzyme activity sufficient to resist oxidative stress emerge from the bone marrow. Hemolysis is most common in males who possess a single abnormal X chromosome. Heterozygous females who have randomly inactivated a higher percentage of the normal gene may become symptomatic, as may homozygous females with the A− variant. One percent of African American females are A− variant homozygous. Patients with the Mediterranean variant have hemolysis that destroys most of their red cells and may require transfusions until the drug is eliminated from their bodies. The neutrophils of patients with the most severe degrees of G6PD deficiency demonstrate defective oxidative killing because of the depletion of NADPH, which serves as an electron donor to the membrane-bound oxidase that produces bactericidal oxygen species.

On peripheral blood smear, the red cells appear to have "bites" taken out of them (blister cells). The bitten areas result from phagocytosis of Heinz bodies by splenic macrophages. During hemolytic episodes, physical examination reveals jaundice and dark urine (caused by hemoglobinuria and high levels of urobilinogen). Laboratory tests reveal elevated indirect bilirubin and lactate dehydrogenase and low haptoglobin. Initially, the hemolysis exceeds the ability of the bone marrow to compensate, so the reticulocyte count may be low for the first 3 to 4 days.

The diagnosis of G6PD deficiency is made by finding deficient NADPH formation on G6PD assay. G6PD levels may be normal in the setting of acute, severe hemolysis because most of the deficient cells have been destroyed. Repeating the test at a later time when the patient is in a steady-state condition, testing the mother of males with suspected G6PD deficiency, and performing electrophoresis to identify the precise variant facilitate diagnosis.

Treatment

Patients with G6PD deficiency associated with acute severe hemolysis need to avoid drugs that initiate hemolysis. Treatment is supportive, including packed red blood cell transfusion during significant cardiovascular compromise and vigorous hydration and urine alkalinization to protect the kidneys against damage from precipitated free hemoglobin.

🔑 10-9 KEY POINTS

1. Glucose-6-phosphate dehydrogenase (G6PD) deficiency, the most common red blood cell enzyme defect, is transmitted as an X-linked recessive trait.
2. The lack of this enzyme in the hexose monophosphate shunt pathway results in a depletion of nicotinamide adenine dinucleotide phosphate (NADPH) and an inability to regenerate reduced glutathione, which is needed to protect the red blood cell from oxidative stress.

MACROCYTIC ANEMIAS WITH DECREASED RED CELL PRODUCTION

Macrocytic anemias are subdivided according to the presence or absence of megaloblastosis, a marker of ineffective DNA synthesis within a red blood cell precursor. Causes of megaloblastic anemia include vitamin

B_{12} and folate deficiency, drugs that interfere with folate metabolism (phenytoin, methotrexate, trimethoprim), and metabolic disorders (orotic aciduria, methylmalonic aciduria, Lesch-Nyhan's syndrome). Macrocytic anemias without megaloblastosis result from bone marrow failure and include bone marrow failure syndromes (Diamond-Blackfan's syndrome, Fanconi anemia, idiopathic aplastic anemia, preleukemia); drug-induced anemias (azidothymidine, valproic acid, carbamazepine); chronic liver disease, and hypothyroidism.

MEGALOBLASTIC MACROCYTIC ANEMIAS

Vitamin B_{12} Deficiency

Vitamin B_{12}, a coenzyme for 5-methyl-tetrahydrofolate formation, is needed for DNA synthesis. It is found in meat, fish, cheese, and eggs. Dietary vitamin B_{12} deficiency is rare in developed countries except in the breast-fed infant whose mother is a vegan with poor attention to dietary sources of vitamin B_{12}. Another cause of vitamin B_{12} deficiency is selective or generalized malabsorption. Vitamin B_{12} combines with intrinsic factor, which is produced by gastric parietal cells and absorbed in the terminal ileum. Transcobalamin II then transports vitamin B_{12} to the liver for storage. The availability of vitamin B_{12} is reduced by any condition that alters intrinsic factor production, interferes with intestinal absorption, or reduces transcobalamin II levels. Disorders such as congenital pernicious anemia (absent intrinsic factor), juvenile pernicious anemia (autoimmune destruction of intrinsic factor), and transcobalamin II deficiency result in vitamin B_{12} deficiency. Other causes include ileal resection, small bowel bacterial overgrowth, and infection with the fish tapeworm *Diphyllobothrium latum*.

Clinical Manifestations

The effects of vitamin B_{12} deficiency include glossitis, diarrhea, and weight loss. Neurologic sequelae include paresthesias, peripheral neuropathies, and, in the most severe cases, dementia, ataxia, and/or posterior column spinal degeneration. Vitiligo is the main dermatologic manifestation.

Megaloblastic changes on peripheral blood smear include ovalocytosis, neutrophils with hypersegmented nuclei (more than four per cell), nucleated red blood cells, basophilic stippling, and Howell-Jolly bodies. The mean corpuscular volume is usually greater than 100 fL. Intramarrow hemolysis results in elevated levels of serum lactate dehydrogenase, indirect bilirubin, and serum iron. In severe cases, megaloblastic anemia may be accompanied by leukopenia and thrombocytopenia.

Diagnosis is confirmed by a subnormal serum level of vitamin B_{12}. In nondietary deficiency, the **Schilling test** helps delineate pernicious anemia from bacterial overgrowth. In this test, an oral dose of radiolabeled vitamin B_{12} is given, and its absorption is checked by urinary excretion. If urinary excretion is minimal, an oral dose of intrinsic factor is given. Normal urinary excretion after intrinsic factor confirms the diagnosis of pernicious anemia. Inadequate urinary excretion after intrinsic factor suggests bacterial overgrowth. Antibiotics are given, and if vitamin B_{12} urinary excretion then increases, the patient has bacterial overgrowth.

Treatment

Treatment for most forms of vitamin B_{12} deficiency, with the exception of bacterial overgrowth and fish tapeworm, is monthly intramuscular vitamin B_{12}. The erythropoietic response is rapid, with marrow megaloblastosis improving within hours, reticulocytosis appearing by day 3 of therapy, and anemia resolving within 1 to 2 months.

Folate Deficiency

Folate is found in liver, green vegetables, cereals, and cheese and converted to tetrahydrofolate, which is required for DNA synthesis. Because folate stores are relatively small, deficiency may develop within 1 month and anemia within 4 months of deprivation. Etiologies include inadequate dietary intake, impaired absorption of folate, increased demand for folate, and abnormal folate metabolism. Dietary deficiency of folic acid is unusual in developed countries. Children at risk are infants fed goat milk, evaporated milk, or heat-sterilized milk or formula; each has inadequate folate content. Malabsorptive states of the jejunum, such as inflammatory bowel disease and celiac sprue, can cause folate deficiency. Increased demand for folate occurs with an increased rate of red blood cell turnover (hyperthyroidism, pregnancy, chronic hemolysis, malignancy). Relative folate deficiency may develop if the diet does not provide adequate folate to meet these needs. Certain anticonvulsant drugs (phenytoin, phenobarbital) interfere with folate metabolism.

Clinical Manifestations

Specific symptoms are often absent, although pallor, glossitis, malaise, anorexia, poor growth, and recurrent infection may be seen. Unlike vitamin B_{12} deficiency, neurologic disease is not associated with folate deficiency.

Laboratory findings include low red blood cell folate and normal serum vitamin B_{12} levels. Megaloblastic changes on peripheral blood smear and bone marrow aspirate are the same as those noted with vitamin B_{12} deficiency.

Treatment

It is imperative not to misdiagnose B_{12} deficiency as folate deficiency because treatment with folate may result in hematologic improvement and allow for progressive neurologic deterioration. Treatment with 1 mg of folate given orally each day for 1 to 2 months treats the anemia and replenishes body stores. Clinical response is rapid, following a time course similar to that of vitamin B_{12} replacement therapy. Children with chronic hemolytic conditions require continued folate supplementation.

🔑 10-10 KEY POINTS

1. Megaloblastic macrocytic anemias reflect ineffective DNA synthesis and can result from vitamin B_{12} or folate deficiency, drugs that interfere with folate metabolism, and some rare metabolic disorders.
2. Vitamin B_{12} is a coenzyme needed for DNA synthesis. Dietary vitamin B_{12} deficiency is rare in developed countries because vitamin B_{12} stores are large. The usual cause of vitamin B_{12} deficiency is malabsorption.
3. Folate is converted to tetrahydrofolate, which is required for DNA synthesis. Because folate stores are relatively small, deficiency may develop within 1 month and anemia within 4 months of deprivation.
4. Neurologic sequelae of vitamin B_{12} deficiency include paresthesias, peripheral neuropathies, and, in the most severe cases, dementia, ataxia, and posterior column spinal degeneration.
5. Misdiagnosis and treatment of vitamin B_{12} deficiency as folate deficiency may result in hematologic improvement while allowing progressive neurologic deterioration.

NONMEGALOBLASTIC MACROCYTIC ANEMIAS

Diamond-Blackfan's Syndrome

Diamond-Blackfan's syndrome is a congenital, pure red cell aplasia. Both autosomal dominant and recessive patterns are reported. Twenty-five percent of patients have a mutation in the ribosomal protein S19 gene (RPS19).

Clinical Manifestations

The anemia develops shortly after birth but is not usually detected until later, when symptoms develop; 90% of cases are observed within the first year of life. Infants present with mild macrocytosis and reticulocytopenia. On hemoglobin electrophoresis, there is an elevated hemoglobin F, and fetal i antigen is present on the red cells. Twenty-five percent of patients have associated congenital anomalies that include short stature, web neck, cleft lip, shield chest, and triphalangeal thumb. These children are at high risk for leukemia later in life.

Treatment

Seventy-five percent of patients respond to high-dose corticosteroids but must receive therapy indefinitely. Those who do not respond to steroid treatment are transfusion dependent and at risk for the complications of iron overload. Bone marrow transplantation with a matched sibling donor is an option for some patients.

Severe Aplastic Anemia

Severe aplastic anemia is an acquired failure of the hematopoietic stem cells that results in pancytopenia. The disorder may result from exposure to chemicals (benzene, phenylbutazone), drugs (chloramphenicol, sulfonamides), infectious agents (hepatitis virus), or ionizing radiation. Often an etiologic agent is not identified, and the case is classified as idiopathic.

Clinical Manifestations

These patients suffer from pancytopenia, and bone marrow aspirate reveals a hypocellular marrow.

Treatment

The treatment of choice is a bone marrow transplant with a matched sibling donor. In patients who do not have a donor, antithymocyte or antilymphocyte globulin in combination with corticosteroids and growth factors (G-CSF) may be effective. Cyclosporin A and high-dose cyclophosphamide have also been used. Without treatment, 80% of patients die within 3 months of diagnosis from bleeding or infection. If transplantation is considered, it is important to minimize transfusions to reduce exposure to potentially sensitizing blood products. Neutropenic patients are at risk for serious bacterial infection and usually require antibiotics when they develop fever.

Fanconi Anemia

Fanconi anemia is an autosomal recessive disorder that results in pancytopenia. Commonly associated conditions include pigmentary changes and skeletal, renal, and developmental abnormalities. The disorder results from defective DNA repair mechanisms that lead to excessive chromosomal breaks and recombinations. These chromosomal anomalies are found in all cells of the body, not just the hematopoietic stem cells. The mean age at onset of pancytopenia is 8 years.

Clinical Manifestations

Common signs include hyperpigmentation and café-au-lait spots, microcephaly, microphthalmia, short stature, horseshoe or absent kidney, and absent thumbs. Hematologic manifestations include progressive pancytopenia. Macrocytosis is universal even before the onset of anemia, and hemoglobin F is seen on hemoglobin electrophoresis. Approximately 10% of children with Fanconi anemia develop leukemia during adolescence.

Diagnosis is confirmed by demonstrating increased chromosomal breakage with exposure to diepoxybutane or other agents that damage DNA.

Treatment

Patients frequently require red blood cell transfusions and antibiotics to treat anemia and infections. Some patients transiently respond to androgens. Corticosteroids are often given with the androgens to counterbalance androgen-induced growth acceleration. Bone marrow transplantation is the treatment of choice if an HLA-matched donor can be found. Because of chromosomal sensitivity, the preparative radiation and chemotherapeutic regimen must be modified because normal protocols result in severe morbidity and mortality.

🔑 10-11 KEY POINTS

1. Macrocytic anemias without megaloblastosis result from bone marrow failure and include bone marrow failure syndromes (Diamond-Blackfan's syndrome, Fanconi anemia, idiopathic aplastic anemia, preleukemia), drug-induced anemias, chronic liver disease, and hypothyroidism.
2. Diamond-Blackfan's syndrome is an inherited pure red cell aplasia. Associated anomalies include short stature, web neck, cleft lip, shield chest, and triphalangeal thumb.
3. Idiopathic aplastic anemia is an acquired failure of the hematopoietic stem cells that results in pancytopenia.
4. Fanconi anemia is an autosomal recessive disorder that results in pancytopenia and pigmentary, skeletal, renal, and developmental abnormalities.

DISORDERS OF HEMOSTASIS

Normal hemostasis requires the integrity of the blood vessels, platelets, and soluble clotting factors. Bleeding derangements can result from abnormal hemostatic plug formation, which occurs in platelet disorders; aberrant clot formation, which is noted in defects of the coagulation cascade; or with vascular abnormalities.

Examples of vascular anomalies that result in bleeding include hereditary defects of collagen synthesis (Ehlers-Danlos's syndrome), acquired disorders of collagen production (vitamin C deficiency, scurvy), and vasculitis (Henoch-Schönlein purpura, or HSP). HSP is associated with abdominal pain, arthritis, nephritis, and purpura, classically distributed over the buttocks and lower extremities.

PLATELET DISORDERS

Platelet disorders can be either quantitative or qualitative and result in abnormal hemostatic plug formation. Quantitative abnormalities are detected by the platelet count or platelet estimate on peripheral blood smear, whereas qualitative disorders are detected by the bleeding time or platelet aggregation studies. **Thrombocytopenia**, defined as a platelet count below $150,000/\text{mm}^3$, is the most common cause of abnormal bleeding. A low platelet count can result from inadequate production or increased destruction of platelets. Platelet production is evaluated by assessing the number of megakaryocytes in the bone marrow aspirate.

Decreased platelet production can result from failure of the bone marrow or bone marrow suppression. Bone marrow failure states causing thrombocytopenia include disorders resulting in pancytopenia (Fanconi anemia, idiopathic aplastic anemia, leukemia); thrombocytopenia-absent radius (TAR) syndrome; and Wiskott-Aldrich's syndrome. TAR syndrome, also known as congenital megakaryocytic hypoplasia, is an autosomal recessive disorder in which thrombocytopenia develops in the first few months of life and then resolves spontaneously after 1 year of age. Transient leukocytosis is common and often suggests leukemia. Deformity of the radii is pathognomonic. Wiskott-Aldrich's syndrome is an X-linked disorder characterized by hypogammaglobulinemia, eczema, and thrombocytopenia. Bone marrow transplantation is curative. Etiologies of thrombocytopenia caused by bone marrow suppression include chemotherapeutic agents; acquired viral infections (human immunodeficiency virus [HIV], Epstein-Barr virus, measles); congenital infections, including toxoplasmosis, syphilis, rubella, cytomegalovirus, and parvovirus B19; and certain drugs (anticonvulsants, sulfonamides, quinidine, quinine, and thiazide diuretics). Acquired postnatal infections (with the exception of HIV) and drug reactions usually cause transient thrombocytopenia, whereas congenital infections may produce prolonged suppression of bone marrow function.

Thrombocytopenia caused by shortened platelet survival is much more common than thrombocytopenia caused by inadequate production. Platelet destruction is most commonly immune mediated. Thrombocytopenia in the newborn can result from isoimmune or autoimmune antibodies. Isoimmune IgG antibodies are produced against the fetal platelets when the fetal platelet crosses the placenta and presents itself to the maternal immune system. If there is an antigen on the fetal platelet that does not exist on the maternal platelet, it is recognized as foreign and isoimmune antibodies are created against the antigen. Maternal antiplatelet antibodies then cross the placenta, causing destruction of the fetal platelet. This disorder is known as **neonatal isoimmune thrombocytopenic purpura**. The maternal antiplatelet antibody does not produce maternal thrombocytopenia. Autoimmune IgG antibodies are transferred to the fetus through the placenta when the mother has idiopathic thrombocytopenic purpura, systemic lupus erythematosus, or drug-induced thrombocytopenia. In all three cases, maternal autoantibodies cross the placenta and attack the fetal platelets. In contrast to isoimmune antibodies, autoimmune antibodies also result in maternal thrombocytopenia. After birth, infants with severe isoimmune or autoimmune thrombocytopenia may be treated with corticosteroids or intravenous immunoglobulin until the maternal antiplatelet antibodies dissipate. A detailed discussion of childhood idiopathic thrombocytopenia purpura (ITP) appears later in this chapter.

Microangiopathic hemolytic anemias also cause thrombocytopenia by decreasing platelet survival. Microangiopathic disorders include disseminated intravascular coagulation (DIC), hemolytic-uremic syndrome (HUS), and thrombotic thrombocytopenic purpura (TTP). DIC is discussed later. HUS, characterized by a microangiopathic hemolytic anemia, renal cortical injury, and thrombocytopenia, is a major cause of acute renal failure in children. Verotoxin-producing gram-negative organisms (such as *Escherichia coli* O157:H7) that bind to endothelial cells cause HUS. Because of endothelial cell injury, there is localized clotting and platelet activation. Microangiopathic hemolytic anemia results from mechanical injury to red cells as they pass through the injured vascular endothelium, and thrombocytopenia results from platelet adhesion to the damaged endothelium. An estimated 60% to 80% of patients with HUS transiently require dialysis. Most children survive the acute phase and recover normal renal function. In TTP, platelet consumption precipitated by a plasma factor or the lack of an inhibitory factor appears to be the primary process. There is moderate deposition of fibrin, which causes red cell destruction.

Diminished platelet survival can also result from platelet trapping, as seen with giant hemangiomas and hypersplenism. Hypersplenism most commonly occurs secondary to sickle cell anemia, thalassemia syndromes, Gaucher's disease, and portal hypertension. Table 10-6 lists the common causes of thrombocytopenia during the neonatal, infant, and childhood periods.

🔑 10-12 KEY POINTS

1. Abnormal hemostatic plug formation occurs in platelet disorders.
2. Platelet disorders can be either quantitative or qualitative.
3. Thrombocytopenia is the most common cause of abnormal bleeding in children.
4. Thrombocytopenia caused by shortened platelet survival is much more common than thrombocytopenia caused by inadequate production and is caused by isoimmune antibodies, autoimmune antibodies, and microangiopathic hemolytic anemias.

Idiopathic Thrombocytopenic Purpura

ITP refers to a thrombocytopenia for which a cause is not apparent. ITP results from the development of antiplatelet antibodies that bind to the platelet membrane. These antibody-coated platelets are then destroyed in the reticuloendothelial system. Rarely, ITP may be the presenting symptom of an autoimmune disease, such as systemic lupus erythematosus or HIV infection.

Clinical Manifestations

Children typically present 1 to 4 weeks after a viral illness with abrupt onset of petechiae and ecchymoses on the skin and bleeding of the mucous membranes. Severe bleeding occurs after trauma. Spontaneous internal hemorrhage, although rare, has been noted with platelet counts below 10,000/mm³.

■ TABLE 10-6 Causes of Thrombocytopenia

Neonate

Maternal ITP,[a] SLE, drugs, preeclampsia

Isoimmune[a]

Congenital megakaryocytic hypoplasia (thrombocytopenia absent radius)

Giant hemangioma

Sepsis[a]

DIC

Congenital infections

Infant

Wiskott-Aldrich's syndrome

Viral infections[a]

Medications

Malignancies (leukemia, neuroblastoma)

Hemolytic-uremic's syndrome

Sepsis

ITP

Childhood

ITP[a]

Medications[a]

Aplastic anemia

Leukemia[a]

Hypersplenism (thalassemia, Gaucher disease, portal hypertension)

Sepsis

SLE

Virus-induced hemophagocytic syndrome

ITP with autoimmune hemolytic anemia (Evan's syndrome)

AIDS

[a]Common.
SLE, systemic lupus erythematosus; DIC, disseminated intravascular coagulation; ITP, idiopathic thrombocytopenic purpura.

myeloid and erythroid elements and an increased number of megakaryocytes.

Treatment

Approximately 80% of the cases of acute ITP resolve spontaneously within 6 months. Some cases, however, become relapsing or chronic.

Clinically significant bleeding or severe thrombocytopenia (platelet count less than 20,000) is treated with high-dose steroids, intravenous immunoglobulins (IVIG), or anti-D immune globulin (in Rh-positive children). These measures all decrease the duration of severe thrombocytopenia by decreasing the rate of clearance of antibody-coated platelets in the reticuloendothelial system but do not diminish the production of antiplatelet antibodies. None of these measures affects the long-term outcome of ITP.

Chronic ITP, defined as thrombocytopenia continuing for more than 6 months after an acute ITP episode, is treated with IVIG and/or splenectomy. Repeated treatments with IVIG have been effective in delaying splenectomy. Splenectomy induces remission in 70% to 80% of cases of chronic ITP. Rituximab (anti-CD20 antibody) may also be effective. In refractory cases, immunosuppression with azathioprine or cyclophosphamide and plasmapheresis may be indicated. Aminocaproic acid (Amicar), a drug that inhibits fibrinolysis, may be helpful for oral bleeding.

🔑 10-13 KEY POINTS

1. Idiopathic thrombocytopenic purpura (ITP) results from autoimmune antibody formation against host platelets.
2. Approximately 80% of cases of acute ITP resolve spontaneously within 6 months. Some cases, however, become relapsing or chronic.
3. Clinically significant bleeding or severe thrombocytopenia (platelet count less than 20,000) is treated with high-dose steroids, intravenous immunoglobulins, and anti-D globulin.
4. Chronic ITP is treated with intravenous immunoglobulins and/or splenectomy. Splenectomy induces remission in 70% to 80% of the cases of chronic ITP.

Disseminated Intravascular Coagulation

Normal homeostasis is a balance between hemorrhage and thrombosis. In DIC, this balance is altered by severe illness so the patient has activation of both coagulation (thrombin) and fibrinolysis (plasmin). Endothelial injury,

Other than thrombocytopenia, the complete blood count is normal. Large platelets are seen on peripheral blood smear, and serology reveals antiplatelet antibodies. Diagnosis of ITP does not require a bone marrow aspirate. However, if there are atypical findings on either the complete blood count or the peripheral blood smear, marrow examination is indicated to exclude leukemia and idiopathic aplastic anemia. In ITP, bone marrow aspiration reveals normal release of thromboplastic procoagulant factors into the circulation, and impairment of clearance of activated clotting factors directly activate the coagulation cascade. Intravascular activation of the coagulation cascade leads to fibrin deposition in the small blood vessels, tissue ischemia, release of tissue thromboplastin, consumption of clotting factors, and activation of the fibrinolytic system. Coagulation elements, especially platelets, fibrinogen, and clotting factors II, V, and VIII, are consumed, as are the anticoagulant proteins, especially antithrombin III, protein C, and plasminogen. Acute and chronic conditions associated with DIC include sepsis, burns, trauma, asphyxia, malignancy, and cirrhosis.

Clinical Manifestations

The bleeding diathesis is diffuse, with bleeding from venipuncture sites and around indwelling catheters. Gastrointestinal and pulmonary bleeding can be severe, and hematuria is common. Thrombotic lesions affect the extremities, skin, kidneys, and brain. Both ischemic and hemorrhagic strokes can occur.

The diagnosis of DIC is a clinical one bolstered by laboratory evidence. Thrombocytopenia is evident, along with prolonged prothrombin time (PT) and partial thromboplastin time (PTT). Fibrin split products and d-dimers are elevated. Fibrinogen and factor V and VIII levels are low. The peripheral blood smear reveals schistocytes, which are classically seen with microangiopathic disease.

Treatment

The treatment of DIC is supportive. The disorder that caused DIC must be treated, and hypoxia, acidosis, and perfusion abnormalities need to be corrected. If bleeding persists, the child should be treated with platelets and fresh-frozen plasma, which replaces depleted clotting factors. Heparin may be useful in the presence of significant arterial or venous thrombotic disease unless sites of life-threatening bleeding coexist.

🔑 10-14 KEY POINTS

1. Disseminated intravascular coagulation (DIC) results from severe illness, causing activation of both coagulation (thrombin) and fibrinolysis (plasmin).
2. Intravascular activation of the coagulation cascade leads to fibrin deposition in the small blood vessels, tissue ischemia, release of tissue thromboplastin, consumption of clotting factors, and activation of the fibrinolytic system.

DEFECTS OF THE COAGULATION CASCADE

Coagulation disorders can be inherited or acquired. The most common inherited defects are hemophilia A and B and von Willebrand's disease, whereas vitamin K deficiency is an important acquired coagulation defect.

Hemophilia A and B

Hemophilia A is caused by deficiency of **factor VIII** and occurs in 1 in 5,000 males, whereas hemophilia B results from **factor IX** deficiency and is found in 1 in 25,000 males. Both are X-linked recessive disorders. All other clotting factors are coded on autosomal chromosomes and are therefore inherited in an autosomal fashion. The lack of factor VIII or IX causes a delay in the production of thrombin, which catalyzes the formation of the primary fibrin clot by the conversion of fibrinogen to fibrin and stabilizes the fibrin by activating factor XIII.

Clinical Manifestations

Other than their factor replacement regimens, hemophilia A and B are indistinguishable clinically, and the severity of each disorder is determined by the degree of factor deficiency. Children with mild hemophilia (5% to 49% of normal factor) require significant trauma to induce bleeding, and spontaneous bleeding does not occur. Patients with moderate hemophilia (1% to 5% of normal factor) require moderate trauma to induce bleeding episodes. Severe hemophiliacs (children with less than 1% of normal factor) may have spontaneous bleeding and bleed with very minor trauma. Mild hemophilia may go undiagnosed for many years, whereas severe hemophilia manifests itself during infancy. Hemophilia is characterized by spontaneous or traumatic hemorrhages, which can be subcutaneous, intramuscular, or within joints (hemarthroses). Life-threatening internal hemorrhage may follow trauma or surgery. In newborns with hemophilia, there may be intracranial bleeding secondary to traumatic delivery or after circumcision; otherwise, bleeding complications are uncommon in the first year of life. Circumcision should be avoided in boys with a family history of hemophilia.

In both forms of hemophilia, the PTT is prolonged. In hemophilia A, factor VIII coagulant activity (VIII:c) is low, whereas in hemophilia B, factor IX activity is low. Table 10-7 compares hemophilia A, hemophilia B, and von Willebrand's disease.

■ **TABLE 10-7** Comparison of Hemophilia A, Hemophilia B, and von Willebrand Disease

	Hemophilia A	Hemophilia B	von Willebrand Disease
Inheritance	X-linked	X-linked	Autosomal dominant
Factor deficiency	Factor VIII	Factor IX	vWF and VIII:C
Bleeding site(s)	Muscle, joint, surgical	Muscle, joint, surgical	Mucous membranes, skin, surgical, menstrual
PT	Normal	Normal	Normal
aPTT	Prolonged	Prolonged	Prolonged or normal
Bleeding time	Normal	Normal	Prolonged or normal
Factor VIII coagulant activity (VIII:C)	Low	Normal	Low or normal
vWF:Ag	Normal	Normal	Low
vWF:Act	Normal	Normal	Low
Factor IX	Normal	Low	Nomal
Ristocetin-induced platelet agglutination	Normal	Normal	Normal or low
Platelet aggregation	Normal	Normal	Normal

VWF, von Willebrand factor; PT, prothrombin time; aPTT, activated partial thromboplastin time; vWF:Ag, von Willebrand antigen; vWF:Act, von Willebrand activity.

Treatment

The goal of therapy is to prevent long-term crippling orthopedic injuries caused by hemarthroses. Most patients require periodic infusions of factor VIII or IX to raise their factor levels high enough to stop the bleeding. Many patients with severe hemophilia receive regular infusions of factor to prevent bleeding episodes (prophylaxis). Whereas plasma-derived factors were used in the past, recombinant factors VIII and IX are now available. For mild to moderate bleeding episodes, such as hemarthroses, a 40% factor level is appropriate. For life-threatening bleeding, levels of 80% to 100% of normal factors VIII and IX are necessary. Desmopressin acetate (DDAVP), a synthetic vasopressin analogue, releases factor VIII from endothelial cells. When administered, it triples or quadruples the initial factor VIII level of a patient with hemophilia A but has no effect on factor IX levels. If adequate hemostatic levels of factor VIII can be achieved with DDAVP, it is the initial treatment of bleeding for those afflicted with mild to moderate hemophilia A. Because DDAVP is an antidiuretic hormone analogue, hemophiliacs who frequently use DDAVP should be monitored for hyponatremia caused by water retention. Mild acute bleeding episodes can be treated in the home once the patient has attained the appropriate age and the parents have learned how to administer recombinant factor VIII or

IX or DDAVP. Bleeding associated with surgery, trauma, or dental extraction can be anticipated, and excessive bleeding can be prevented with appropriate replacement therapy. Aminocaproic acid (Amicar), an inhibitor of fibrinolysis, may help treat oral bleeding after a dental procedure. It is generally given before and after the procedure.

Testing of blood products for HIV and hepatitis viruses did not begin until the mid-1980s, and as a result, many hemophiliacs contracted the viruses. Between 1979 and 1984, 90% of hemophiliacs who received plasma-derived factor products became HIV seropositive. Acquired immunodeficiency syndrome (AIDS) is the most common cause of death in older patients with hemophilia. Newer pooled concentrates are safer, and all recombinant preparations are safe from viral agents.

Another significant complication of therapy is the formation of inhibitors, which are IgG antibodies directed against transfusion factors VIII and IX. Inhibitors arise during therapy in 15% of patients with factor VIII deficiency and in 1% of those with factor IX deficiency. The treatment of bleeding patients with an inhibitor is difficult. For low-titer inhibitors, options include continuous factor VIII infusions or administration of porcine factor VIII. For high-titer inhibitors, it usually is necessary to administer a product that bypasses the inhibitor, such as activated prothrombin complex concentrates or recombinant factor VIIa. The use of frequent high doses of prothrombin complex concentrates, and especially of the activated products, paradoxically increases the risks of thrombosis, which has resulted in fatal myocardial infarction and stroke in adults. Induction of immune tolerance with continuous antigen exposure with or without immunosuppression may be beneficial.

🔑 10-15 KEY POINTS

1. Hemophilia A results from a deficiency of factor VIII, and hemophilia B results from a lack of factor IX. Both disorders are inherited in an X-linked recessive fashion.
2. Other than their factor replacement regimens, hemophilia A and B are indistinguishable clinically, and the severity of each disorder is determined by the degree of factor deficiency.
3. Hemophilia is characterized by spontaneous or traumatic hemorrhages, which can be subcutaneous, intramuscular, or within joints (hemarthroses). Life-threatening internal hemorrhage may follow trauma or surgery.

---

von Willebrand's Disease

von Willebrand's disease is caused by deficiency of von Willebrand factor (vWF), an adhesive protein that connects subendothelial collagen to activated platelets and also binds to circulating factor VIII, protecting it from rapid clearance. Von Willebrand's disease is classified on the basis of whether vWF is quantitatively reduced but not absent (type 1), qualitatively abnormal (type 2; dysproteinemia), or absent (type 3).

Clinical Manifestations

The clinical manifestations of von Willebrand's disease are similar to those of thrombocytopenia and include mucocutaneous bleeding, epistaxis, gingival bleeding, cutaneous bruising, and menorrhagia. In severe von Willebrand's disease, factor VIII deficiency may be profound and the patient may also have manifestations similar to those of hemophilia A. If there is little or no vWF in the blood to bind factor VIII, factor VIII is cleared quickly from the circulation, resulting in factor VIII deficiency. Approximately 85% of patients with von Willebrand's disease have classic type 1 disease, which results in mild to moderate deficiency of vWF.

Laboratory testing includes measurement of the amount of protein, usually accomplished by immuno-logic detection of vWF antigen (vWF:Ag) and vWF activity (vWF:Act). vWF activity is measured functionally by the ristocetin cofactor assay (vWF:RCoF), which uses the antibiotic ristocetin to induce vWF to bind to platelets. The patient typically has a prolonged bleeding time because of the effect of vWF deficiency on platelet activity, and a prolonged PTT, which results from the effect of vWF deficiency on factor VIII activity. Table 10-7 compares the findings in classic von Willebrand's disease with those in hemophilia A and B.

Treatment

The treatment of von Willebrand's disease depends on the severity of bleeding. DDAVP, which stimulates the release of vWF from endothelial cells, is the treatment of choice for bleeding episodes in most patients with type I vWD. Patients with type 3 disease (who have no vWF to release) or with severe bleeding not responding to DDAVP can be treated with a virally attenuated vWF-containing concentrate (Humate P). Cryoprecipitate may also be used, but it cannot be virally attenuated. Hepatitis B vaccine should be given before exposure to plasma-derived products. As in all bleeding disorders, medications that alter platelet function, such as aspirin, should be avoided.

🔑 10-16 KEY POINTS

1. Von Willebrand disease is caused by deficiency of vWF, an adhesive protein that connects subendothelial collagen to activated platelets and also binds to circulating factor VIII, protecting it from rapid clearance.
2. The clinical manifestations of mild to moderate von Willebrand disease are similar to those of thrombocytopenia and include mucocutaneous bleeding, epistaxis, gingival bleeding, cutaneous bruising, and menorrhagia.
3. In severe von Willebrand disease, factor VIII deficiency may be profound, and the patient may also have manifestations similar to hemophilia A.
4. Desmopressin acetate (DDAVP) is the treatment of choice for the majority of bleeding episodes in patients.

Vitamin K Deficiency

Coagulation factors (factors II, VII, IX, and X) and antithrombotic factors (protein C and protein S) are synthesized in the liver and depend on vitamin K for their activity. When vitamin K is deficient, coagulation is impaired. Vitamin K deficiency often occurs because of malabsorption, especially with cystic fibrosis and with antibiotic-induced suppression of intestinal bacteria that produce vitamin K. Overdose of Coumadin, a drug that interferes with vitamin K metabolism, causes deficiency of vitamin K–dependent factors. Similarly, maternal use of Coumadin or anticonvulsant therapy (phenobarbital, phenytoin) may also result in vitamin K deficiency in the newborn. The most common disorder resulting from vitamin K deficiency is hemorrhagic disease of the newborn, which occurs in neonates who do not receive intramuscular vitamin K at birth.

Clinical Manifestations

Although most newborn infants are born with reduced levels of vitamin K–dependent factors, only a few develop hemorrhagic complications. Because breast milk is a poor source of vitamin K, breast-fed infants who do not receive prophylactic vitamin K on the first day of life are at the highest risk for hemorrhagic disease. Peak incidence is at 2 to 10 days of life. The recommended preventive dose of vitamin K is 1.0 mg given intramuscularly. The disorder is marked by generalized ecchymoses, gastrointestinal hemorrhage, and bleeding from the circumcision site and umbilical stump. Affected neonates are at risk for intracranial hemorrhage.

Both the PTT and PT are prolonged in vitamin K deficiency because factors of both extrinsic and intrinsic pathways are affected. Prolongation of the PT is a more sensitive test for vitamin K deficiency because most infants have transient prolongation of the PTT at birth. The coagulopathy seen with hemorrhagic disease may be confused with liver disease or DIC, both of which have a prolonged PT and decreased factor VII level. Table 10-8 differentiates vitamin K deficiency, liver disease, and DIC by laboratory data.

Treatment

Nutritional disorders and malabsorptive states respond to parenteral administration of vitamin K. Fresh-frozen plasma or prothrombin complex concentrate, which is a mixture of coagulation factors II, VII, IX, and X, is indicated for severe bleeding.

🦴 10-17 KEY POINTS

1. Coagulation factors II, VII, IX, and X and antithrombotic factors protein C and protein S are synthesized in the liver and depend on vitamin K for their activity.
2. The most common disorder resulting from vitamin K deficiency is hemorrhagic disease of the newborn, which occurs in neonates who do not receive vitamin K at birth.
3. The coagulopathy seen with hemorrhagic disease may be confused with liver disease or disseminated intravascular coagulation (DIC), both of which have a prolonged prothrombin time (PT) and decreased factor VII level.

■ **TABLE 10-8** Differentiation of Vitamin K Deficiency, Liver Disease, and Disseminated Intravascular Coagulation (DIC)

Laboratory Test	Vitamin K Deficiency	Liver Disease	DIC
PT	↑	↑	↑
Platelets	NL	↓ to NL	↓
Fibrinogen	NL	↓↓	
Factor VIII	NL	NL to ↑	↓
Fibrinogen degradation products	NL	NL to ↑	↓
Factor VII	↓	↓	↓ to NL
Factor V	NL	Low	Low

PT, prothrombin time; NL, normal.

Additional Suggested Reading

Cines DB, BlanchetteVS. Immune thrombocytopenic purpura. *N Engl J Med.* 2002;346:995–1008.

Journeycake JM, Buchanan GR. Coagulation disorders. *Pediatr Rev.* 2003;24:83–91.

Mannucci PM, Tuddenham E. The hemophiliac—from royal genes to gene therapy. *N Engl J Med.* 2001;44:1773–1779.

Sackey K. Hemolytic anemia: Part 1. *Pediatr Rev.* 1999;20:152–159.

Sackey K. Hemolytic anemia: Part 2. *Pediatr Rev.* 1999;20:204–208.

Segal GB, Hirsh MG, Feig SA. Managing anemia in pediatric office practice: Part 1. *Pediatr Rev.* 2002;23:75–84.

Segal GB, Hirsh MG, Feig SA. Managing anemia in pediatric office practice: Part 2. *Pediatr Rev.* 2002;23:111–122.

Immunology, Allergy, and Rheumatology

IMMUNOLOGY

The immune system, composed of specialized cells and molecules, is responsible for recognizing and neutralizing foreign antigens. Specific complex interactions produce adaptive inflammatory responses and defend against infection. **Immunodeficiency's syndromes** increase susceptibility to infection, malignancy, and autoimmune disorders (Table 11-1). Table 11-2 lists clinical criteria that should prompt an evaluation for immunodeficiency.

DISORDERS OF HUMORAL IMMUNITY

B cells produce antibodies, the primary effectors of humoral immunity. Antibodies are a vital component of the immune system, particularly in defense against extracellular pathogens such as encapsulated bacteria. A variety of antibodies activate complement, serves as opsonins, inhibits microbial adherence to mucous membranes, and neutralizes various toxins and viruses. As a group, **antibody (humoral) deficiency syndromes** are the most common immunodeficiency diseases encountered in pediatric practice.

Clinical Manifestations

History and Physical Examination

A history of recurrent infections with **encapsulated** organisms such as *Haemophilus influenzae* and *Streptococcus pneumoniae* and failure to respond to appropriate antibiotic therapy is suggestive of a primary B-cell deficiency. In addition, there is often a history of frequent upper respiratory tract infections beginning after 6 months of age, including otitis media, sinusitis, and pneumonia.

Differential Diagnosis

X-linked agammaglobulinemia (XLA; also termed Bruton tyrosine kinase deficiency or Bruton disease) occurs in boys and appears after 6 months of age as maternally-derived antibody levels fall. These patients do not produce antibodies and have virtually no mature B cells. In addition to their susceptibility to encapsulated organisms, individuals with this disorder are prone to severe, often life-threatening enterovirus infections.

Common variable immunodeficiency is an inherited disorder of hypogammaglobulinemia (particularly IgG and IgA) with equal distribution between the genders. In addition, antibody formation may be defective. Infections are usually less severe; however, the incidences of lymphoma and autoimmune disease are increased in these patients.

Selective IgA deficiency is the mildest and most common immunodeficiency syndrome. Serum levels of the other antibody classes are usually normal. Patients react normally to viral infections but are more susceptible to bacterial infections of the respiratory, gastrointestinal, and urinary tracts.

Diagnostic Evaluation

Quantitative measurement of total and fractionated serum immunoglobulin levels is an important screening test for specific deficiencies and for panhypogammaglobulinemia. Antibody titers generated against tetanus, diphtheria, and pneumococci after immunization assess B-cell *function*.

■ TABLE 11-1 Causes, Characteristics, and Evaluation of Immune Component Deficiencies

Condition	Mechanism	Sequelae	Laboratory Tests
Disorders of humoral immunity	Impaired opsonization Inability to lyse, agglutinate bacteria Inability to neutralize bacterial toxins	Frequent, recurrent pyogenic infections with extracellular encapsulated organisms Frequent bacterial otitis media, sinusitis, and pneumonia infections	Quantitative total, fractionated immunoglobulin levels Vaccination antibody titers
Disorders of cell-mediated immunity	Inability of T cells to direct B-cell antibody synthesis to T-cell-specific antigens	Frequent, recurrent infections with opportunistic/low-grade organisms and viruses Increased incidence of autoimmune disorders and malignancies Anergy	Absolute lymphocyte count (ALC) Abnormal mitogen stimulation response Delayed hypersensitivity skin testing
Phagocytic disorders (neutropenia)	Insufficient number of neutrophils	Cellulitis, skin abscesses, furunculosis Stomatitis, gingivitis, rectal inflammation Pneumonia, sepsis	Absolute neutrophil count Blood smear examination for blasts Antineutrophil antibodies
Phagocytic disorders (chronic granulomatous disease)	Inability to kill intracellular bacteria secondary to failure to generate oxygen metabolites such as the superoxide anion	Increased susceptibility to infections with catalase-positive bacteria and fungi Chronic lymphadenitis, abscesses, granulomas, osteomyelitis	Nitroblue tetrazolium test DHR (dihydrorhodamine reduction) conversion test
Complement disorders	Impaired opsonization	Recurrent bacterial infections with encapsulated, extracellular organisms Increased susceptibility to meningococcal, gonococcal disease Increased incidence of autoimmune disease	Total hemolytic complement (CH_{50}) Assays of the classical and alternative pathways

Treatment

The mainstays of therapy are appropriate antibiotic use and periodic gammaglobulin administration. **Intravenous immunoglobulin** (IVIG) and/or intramuscular gammaglobulin provide antibody replacement and have revolutionized the treatment of humoral immunodeficiency syndromes.

TRANSIENT HYPOGAMMAGLOBULINEMIA OF INFANCY

Although maternal IgG is actively transported across the placenta and is protective throughout the first few months of life, neonates are considered relatively immunocompromised hosts. All serum immunoglobulin

TABLE 11-2 Clinical Criteria for Evaluation for Immunodeficiency Syndromes

More than two serious/systemic bacterial infections within 1 yr (any bacterial or fungal infection that recurs despite treatment or does not respond to appropriate therapy)

Infection by an unusual[a] or opportunistic pathogen

Infection at an unusual site (e.g., brain or liver abscess)

Chronic gingivitis

[a]Including *Aspergillus, Serratia marcescens, Nocardia* species, and *Burkholderia cepacia.*

classes are present at birth, but most do not reach adult levels until early to middle childhood. Over the first 6 to 8 weeks of life, maternally derived immunoglobulins decrease and are replaced by the child's growing production. Thus, infants are particularly susceptible to infection at 6 to 12 weeks, their immunologic nadir.

Transient hypogammaglobulinemia of infancy is a recognized disorder in which acquisition of normal infant immunoglobulin levels is delayed. Although some of these patients are subsequently diagnosed with other primary immunodeficiencies, most eventually develop normal immunity.

11-1 KEY POINTS

1. Humoral immunodeficiency syndromes are the most common immunodeficiency diseases encountered in pediatrics.
2. Humoral immunodeficiency predisposes patients to infection with encapsulated organisms. Common infections include otitis media, pneumonia, and sinusitis.
3. Quantitative immunoglobulin studies and antibody titers against vaccine antigens are abnormal in patients with humoral immune dysfunction.
4. Gammaglobulin therapy (intravenous or intramuscular) provides antibodies to patients with humoral immunodeficiency.

DISORDERS OF CELL-MEDIATED IMMUNITY

T cells modulate most immune responses, primarily through the secretion of interleukins. In addition, they are major effectors of cell-mediated immunity,

important in the defense against intracellular and opportunistic infections. Certain subclasses are capable of killing tumor and viral-infected cells. Patients with dysfunctional T cells are at increased risk for autoimmune disorders. T-cell diseases generally impart significantly greater morbidity and mortality to their victims than humoral disorders alone. Chromosome 22q11 deletion (DiGeorge) syndrome, a congenital disorder, and human immunodeficiency virus, an acquired one, both represent **T-cell immunodeficiencies**.

Clinical Manifestations

History and Physical Examination

T-cell abnormalities predispose patients to infections with intracellular infections, including viruses and mycobacteria. Patients with near-total thymic hypoplasia are highly susceptible to opportunistic infections from organisms such as fungi and *Pneumocystis carinii.*

Children with DiGeorge's syndrome present early in infancy with disease unrelated to the immune system (e.g., congenital heart disease, hypocalcemic tetany from thymic hypoplasia). Other structures and organs derived from the branchial pouches during embryogenesis may be malformed as well, including the ears and face. The severity of the immunodeficiency is extremely variable.

Diagnostic Evaluation

Absolute lymphocyte counts are normal or moderately decreased. T-cell function, measured by in vitro mitogen stimulation and intradermal delayed hypersensitivity testing, is absent or significantly compromised. No thymic shadow is seen on chest radiograph in patients with DiGeorge's syndrome. Fluorescent in situ hybridization (FISH) testing of chromosome 22 detects the 22q11.2 deletion.

Treatment

The immunodeficiency of chromosome 22q11.2 deletion (DiGeorge) syndrome has been successfully treated with both thymic and bone marrow transplantation. Initial therapy should be aimed at repairing associated congenital heart defects and maintaining normocalcemia.

Chapter 12 discusses human immunodeficiency virus (HIV) in detail.

COMBINED IMMUNODEFICIENCY SYNDROMES

Combined humoral and cell-mediated immunodeficiencies tend to be inherited and manifest a wide range of clinical severity. Affected patients display increased susceptibility to both traditionally virulent and opportunistic infections.

Severe combined immunodeficiency disease (SCID) is a particularly devastating disorder characterized by substantial deficits in both humoral and cell-mediated immunity. The disease may be X linked, autosomal recessive, or occur as a spontaneous genetic mutation. Patients are susceptible to a wide range of infections and usually present with multiple illnesses (pneumonia, sepsis, meningitis) in the first few months of life. An absolute lymphocyte count, noted on a routine complete blood count (CBC), is less than 2,800. T-cell response to stimulation is abnormal, and immunoglobulin levels are extremely low. Bone marrow and cord blood transplantation have been curative; gene therapy is now being studied as a possible alternative treatment.

Ataxia telangiectasia is an extremely rare autosomal recessive disorder characterized by variable humoral and cell-mediated immune deficits, cerebellar ataxia, and oculocutaneous telangiectasia (small dilated vessels easily visible along the bulbar conjunctiva and skin surface). The incidence of malignancy, especially non-Hodgkin lymphoma and gastric carcinoma, is increased. No specific therapy is available; most patients are wheelchair bound by puberty and die prematurely.

Wiskott-Aldrich's syndrome is an X-linked recessive disorder of (primarily) B- and (usually) T-cell immunity, atopic dermatitis, and thrombocytopenia. Specifically, the host's antibodies do not respond normally to carbohydrate antigens. Survival to adulthood is rare because of bleeding, infections, and associated malignancies.

DISORDERS OF PHAGOCYTIC IMMUNITY

Phagocytes are responsible for removing particulate matter from the blood and tissues by ingesting and destroying microorganisms. These cells must be able to adhere to the endothelium, move through the tissues to their site of action, engulf the harmful matter, and kill it intracellularly. Phagocytic's disorders are caused by an insufficient number of normal neutrophils (neutropenia) or by phagocytic cell dysfunction. **Neutropenia** may result from infection (particularly viruses); medication administration (e.g., penicillin, sulfonamides, phenothiazine, and some anticonvulsants); circulating antineutrophil antibodies; malignancy in the bone marrow; or aplastic anemia. **Chronic granulomatous disease** (CGD), the most common inherited disorder of phagocytic immunity, occurs when neutrophils and monocytes are unable to kill certain organisms after ingesting them.

Clinical Manifestations

History and Physical Examination

Patients with neutropenia generally do not experience serious or life-threatening infections unless the neutropenia is both *severe* (absolute neutrophil count (ANC) $<0.5 \times 10^3$ per μL) and *chronic* (lasting longer than 2 to 3 months). Typical complaints include gingivitis, skin infections, rectal inflammation, otitis media, pneumonia, and sepsis. Patients are often infected with *Staphylococcus aureus* and gram-negative organisms. Of note, patients with neutropenia are unable to mount a sufficient inflammatory response, so typical signs of infection such as erythema, warmth, and swelling may be absent even in the presence of significant involvement.

CGD is characterized by chronic or recurrent pyogenic infections caused by bacterial and fungal pathogens that produce catalase (including *Staphylococcus aureus*, *Candida albicans*, *Aspergillus*, and most gram-negative enteric bacteria).

Both X-linked and autosomal inheritance occur. Abscesses and granuloma formation occur in the lymph nodes, liver, spleen, lungs, skin, and gastrointestinal tract. Failure to thrive, chronic diarrhea, and persistent candidiasis of the mouth and diaper area are common. Affected individuals are also at increased risk for opportunistic infections, disseminated viral illnesses, and inflammatory bowel disease.

Diagnostic Evaluation

Severe neutropenia is defined as an ANC $< 0.5 \times 10^3$ per µL. Serial complete blood counts reveal a leukoerythroblastic response unless the condition is chronic. Bone marrow examination is required if malignancy or aplastic anemia is a consideration.

In CGD, the white blood cell count typically ranges between 10,000 and 20,000 per µL with 60% to 80% polymorphonuclear cells. Leukocyte chemotaxis is normal. The hallmark abnormality is the inability of affected cells to produce an oxidative burst resulting in hydrogen peroxide. The **nitroblue tetrazolium test** (NBT) and the dihydrorhodamine reduction (DHR) test are laboratory studies performed to detect this reduction reaction.

Treatment

Children with acute neutropenia need no special treatment. Patients with chronic neutropenia and those with infectious complications may respond to recombinant human granulocyte colony-stimulating factor (rhG-CSF) injections. All patients with CGD should receive prophylactic trimethoprim-sulfamethoxazole and interferon gamma therapy. Judicious antibiotic therapy during infections is critical. Bone marrow transplantation is not as successful as in other immunodeficiency syndromes. Gene therapy is a promising area of research.

11-3 KEY POINTS

1. Severe neutropenia, defined as an absolute neutrophil count (ANC) $<0.5 \times 10^3$ per µL, may result from infection, certain medications, circulating antineutrophil antibodies, malignancy, or bone marrow dysfunction.
2. Typical signs of infection (erythema, warmth, swelling) are often absent in the presence of neutropenia.
3. Chronic granulomatous disease (CGD) is characterized by chronic or recurrent infections caused by catalase-producing bacteria or fungi. In particular, patients develop frequent skin infections and abscesses.
4. The nitroblue tetrazolium test and the dihydrorhodamine reduction (DHR) test are laboratory studies that are useful for detecting CGD.
5. Patients with CGD should receive daily prophylactic trimethoprim-sulfamethoxazole and -interferon gamma.

DISORDERS OF COMPLEMENT IMMUNITY

Although quantitative deficiencies of virtually all complement components have been described, they are less common than the immunodeficiencies mentioned earlier. The primary mechanism of disease is impaired opsonization. Patients with **complement disorders** have increased susceptibility to bacterial infections and a higher incidence of rheumatologic disease. In particular, deficiencies of the terminal complement components C5 to C8 increase the likelihood of *Neisseria meningitidis* infections.

ALLERGY

An **allergic reaction** is an undesirable immune-mediated response to an environmental stimulus. Allergies have been implicated as a contributing factor in anaphylaxis, asthma, allergic rhinitis, and atopic dermatitis. Allergic reactions range from mild to life-threatening and are *never* considered adaptive.

The **allergic triad** of atopic disease consists of allergic rhinitis, asthma, and atopic dermatitis (eczema). Children with one known atopic disease are likely to suffer from a second atopic condition.

ALLERGIC RHINITIS

Pathogenesis

Allergic rhinitis is a type 1 hypersensitivity immune response to environmental allergens including airborne pollens, animal dander, dust mites, and molds. The offending allergen binds to IgE on mast cells in the upper respiratory tract, with subsequent release of inflammatory mediators. This localized inflammation results in nasal congestion, rhinorrhea and/or postnasal drainage, sneezing, and occasionally itching. Allergic rhinitis is the most frequent cause of chronic or recurrent clear rhinorrhea in the pediatric population.

Epidemiology

An estimated 40% of children are affected by allergic rhinitis by the time they are 6 years of age. Seasonal allergic rhinitis, or **hay fever**, limited to months of pollination, is uncommon before 5 years of age. Tree pollens are common during early spring, followed by grass pollens, which are detected until the early summer. Ragweed season starts in the late summer and persists until the first frost. Perennial's disease persists year round, usually in response to household allergens (molds, dust mites).

Risk Factors

Atopy and genetic predisposition are the major risk factors. Maternal smoking in the first year of life also increases the likelihood of subsequent disease. Paradoxically, heavy exposure to animal dander early in life may reduce the risk of subsequent atopic disease.

Clinical Manifestations

History

Patients with allergic rhinitis are plagued with nasal congestion, profuse watery rhinorrhea, and sneezing. Associated allergic conjunctivitis is common. Unrelenting postnasal drip produces frequent coughing or throat clearing. Patients may also complain of being drowsy because of recurrent brief awakenings at night. As a group, children with untreated allergic rhinitis have decreased school performance when compared with their peers.

Physical Examination

On examination, the nasal mucosa appears boggy and bluish. Two characteristic features of allergic rhinitis are **allergic shiners** (dark circles that develop under the eyes secondary to venous congestion) and the **allergic salute** (a horizontal crease across the middle of the nose caused by a constant upward wiping motion with the hand). Because of the severe congestion, patients may become obligate mouth breathers, and a gaping mouth and palatal arching may be seen on physical examination. Children with allergic rhinitis are also prone to recurrent sinusitis and otitis media with effusion.

Differential Diagnosis

Infectious rhinitis, much more common than allergic rhinitis in infants and toddlers, is often mucopurulent. *Sinusitis* causes chronic rhinorrhea and postnasal drip associated with facial tenderness, cough, and/or headache. When a *nasal foreign body* is present, the discharge is usually unilateral, thick, and foul smelling. Other possible diagnoses include *vasomotor* (idiopathic nonallergic) *rhinitis*, which appears to be caused by an exaggerated vascular response to irritants, and *rhinitis medicamentosa*, which results from overuse of topical decongestants.

Diagnostic Evaluation

A careful history usually confirms the diagnosis. Patients who do not respond favorably to a trial of second-generation (nonsedating) antihistamines may require further workup. Elevated nasopharyngeal eosinophil levels may support the diagnosis; however, a serum radioallergosorbent test (RAST) or direct skin testing is the preferred method for specific allergy testing.

Treatment

The most effective treatment for any allergic condition is **allergen avoidance**. Switching to air-conditioning in the summer (rather than keeping the windows open) affords some protection to patients with pollen allergies. Limiting the amount of humidity in the home can decrease the presence of dust mites and various fungi. Eliminating animal dander and limiting exposure to cigarette smoke are also helpful.

Pharmacotherapy is an important adjunct if avoidance is not possible. **H$_1$-histamine blockers** (oral or intranasal) are the mainstay of treatment. They are now available in nonsedating formulations approved for use in children older than 2 years. Intranasal cromolyn is helpful as a preventive medication if taken prior to the onset of symptoms. Nasal topical steroids are very effective treatments with minimal side effects.

Oral leukotriene receptor antagonists may be beneficial in some patients. Topical and inhaled sympathomimetics (the most popular being pseudoephedrine) are useful for short-term therapy only and, if taken improperly, may result in severe rebound congestion. Allergy immunotherapy (i.e., injections) is painful, time consuming, and expensive; it is indicated only for severe symptoms not controlled with conventional pharmacotherapy.

Studies now suggest that children with seasonal allergies who are appropriately treated at a young age have a lower risk of developing subsequent atopic disease than those who are left untreated.

🔑 11-4 KEY POINTS

1. Allergic rhinitis may be seasonal or perennial.
2. Allergic rhinitis should be considered in any child with chronic or recurrent rhinorrhea and upper respiratory tract symptoms.
3. "Allergic shiners" and the "allergic salute" are characteristic physical features of allergic rhinitis.
4. Nonsedating H_1-histamine blockers and nasal topical steroids are the mainstays of treatment.

ASTHMA

Chapter 20 discusses asthma in detail. A significant proportion of asthma cases are allergic in nature. Allergens frequently associated with asthma exacerbations include mold, dust mites, and pet dander. Allergen avoidance is the first step in effective treatment. Other therapies are discussed in Chapter 20.

ATOPIC DERMATITIS

Atopic dermatitis is a chronic, relapsing and remitting inflammatory skin reaction to specific allergens, including specific foods and environmental allergens. Eczema usually appears in infancy and affects upward of 10% of the pediatric population. Genetic predilection is the highest risk factor. Approximately half of patients with atopic dermatitis later develop asthma.

Clinical Manifestations

The typical rash consists of a pruritic, erythematous, weeping papulovesicular reaction that progresses to scaling, hypertrophy, and lichenification. In infants younger than 2 years, the eruption involves the extensor surfaces of the arms and legs, the wrists, the face, and the scalp; the diaper area is invariably spared. Flexor areas predominate in older age groups, as well as the neck, wrists, and ankles. The diagnosis of atopic dermatitis is primarily clinical, based on history, physical examination, and response to treatment. The differential diagnosis includes contact dermatitis and psoriasis, a chronic nonallergic skin disorder (Chapter 5).

Treatment

The goal of treatment is termination of the "itch-scratch-itch" cycle. Patients should try to keep their skin well hydrated by avoiding hot water and strong or fragrant soaps. Tight clothing and heat may precipitate exacerbations. Moisturizers are the mainstay of treatment, followed by the use of **topical corticosteroids** for areas of inflammation. Pimecrolimus cream, a cytokine blocker, is now approved for patients older than 24 months who cannot tolerate topical steroids or have resistant disease. Topical tacrolimus is another immunomodulator that may be used in more severe cases. Severe chronic eczema may be complicated by bacterial superinfection.

URTICARIA AND ANGIOEDEMA

Urticaria and angioedema are classic type 1 hypersensitivity reactions. **Urticaria** describes the typical raised edematous hives on the skin or mucous membranes resulting from vascular dilation and increased permeability. The lesions itch, blanch, and generally resolve within a few hours to days. **Angioedema** is a similar process confined to the lower dermis and subcutaneous areas; the depth results in a well-demarcated area of swelling devoid of pruritus, erythema, or warmth. Although acute urticaria and angioedema occur frequently in the pediatric population, chronic forms are rare.

Clinical Manifestations

The diagnosis is based on a detailed history of recent exposures or changes in the patient's environment. The multiple allergens and conditions associated with urticaria and angioedema include foods, medications, infections, and some systemic illnesses. Clinical manifestations may be delayed as long as 48 hours after the initial encounter. Hereditary forms exist; patients with hereditary angioedema have an inherited **C1 esterase** inhibitor deficiency. Greater than 50% of the time, the inciting trigger remains a mystery.

Treatment

Treatment depends on severity, which ranges from mild to life-threatening (i.e., swelling around the airway). Subcutaneous epinephrine is the treatment of choice in emergency situations, followed by intravenous diphenhydramine and steroids. Oral antihistamines, sympathomimetics, and occasionally oral steroids are appropriate in milder cases.

FOOD ALLERGIES

Pathogenesis

Food allergy is an immune-mediated response to a specific food protein. It is important to distinguish between food intolerance (an undesirable nonimmunologic reaction) and true food hypersensitivity, which is mediated by immune mechanisms. Examples of nonimmunologic adverse food reaction include caffeine-induced tachycardia and lactose intolerance.

Epidemiology

Eighty percent of all food allergies present during the first year of life. The overall prevalence of food allergies is also higher in children (5% to 8%) than in adults (1% to 2%). Relatively few foods are represented; **peanuts, eggs, milk proteins, soy, wheat**, and **fish** account for more than 90% of reported cases. Exclusive breast-feeding may delay presentation unless the mother is ingesting the offending proteins regularly. A third of patients with atopic dermatitis and 10% of those with asthma also have a food allergy.

Clinical Manifestations

History and Physical Examination

A detailed history, including daily records of intake and symptoms, is essential for the diagnosis. True food allergies can present with isolated cutaneous reactions, gastrointestinal symptoms, respiratory symptoms, and life-threatening anaphylaxis. Symptoms that develop during weaning are particularly suggestive of food allergies.

Diagnostic Evaluation

Skin testing has a low positive predictive value; it is more helpful for ruling out specific food proteins as causative IgE triggers. A RAST identifies IgE antibodies to specific foods in the serum. The **double-blind,** **placebo challenge–food challenge** is the current gold standard. Several foods are eliminated from the patient's diet for a period before testing. Then the foods are disguised and tested, alternating with placebos, over several days. A challenge is considered positive if signs and symptoms recur after ingestion. Such testing must be performed in a hospital setting because anaphylaxis is a possible complication.

Treatment

Treatment entails eliminating the offending food from the diet. Patients and their caregivers should be educated in the use of an auto-injectable epinephrine pen. In children with severe, widespread allergies, elemental hypoallergenic formulas are available. Cow milk, soy, egg, and wheat allergies are usually outgrown after avoidance of the offending food. Oral challenges can be conducted safely to reintroduce the food. However, nut and fish allergies usually persist. Breast-feeding coupled with delay in the introduction of solid foods until after 4 to 6 months of age may prevent the development of certain food allergies.

🔑 11-5 KEY POINTS

1. Peanuts, eggs, milk, soy, wheat, and fish account for the overwhelming majority of food allergies.
2. Signs and symptoms of food allergy in infants include irritability, diarrhea, and failure to thrive.
3. The double-blind, placebo challenge–food challenge is the gold standard of diagnosis.

RHEUMATOLOGY

Rheumatology involves the diagnosis and treatment of a variety of loosely related chronic, recurrent, arthritic, and connective tissue disorders. Most are thought to result from misdirected host defense mechanisms; the immune system fails to recognize "self" antigens and initiates an inappropriate inflammatory response against the host. Usually, autoantibodies are produced and may be recovered from plasma or tissue samples, assisting with diagnosis.

JUVENILE RHEUMATOID ARTHRITIS

Pathogenesis

Juvenile rheumatoid arthritis (JRA) consists of a group of immunologic disorders characterized by chronic synovitis. The American College of Rheumatology has established the following criteria for the diagnosis of JRA:

- Age younger than 16 years.
- Arthritis in at least one joint for 6 consecutive weeks.
- Arthritis as defined by the presence of limitation of range of motion, tenderness or pain on motion, or increased warmth.
- Exclusion of other causes of arthritis.

Epidemiology

JRA, as is true of most rheumatologic conditions, occurs more commonly in girls. Patients may be afflicted early or late in childhood or in adolescence.

Risk Factors

Many patients have a positive family history for other rheumatologic disorders. Certain HLA types also have been associated with increased risk of disease (e.g., HLA-DR5 with pauciarticular JRA, HLA-DR4 with rheumatoid factor-positive polyarticular JRA).

Clinical Manifestations

History and Physical Examination

Table 11-3 lists the noteworthy clinical manifestations.

■ TABLE 11-3 Signs and Symptoms in Juvenile Rheumatoid Arthritis (JRA)

Joint-Related Symptoms	Systemic Manifestations
Morning stiffness	Asymptomatic uveitis (pauciarticular and polyarticular JRA)
Gelling (stiffness after inactivity)	
Guarding	Fatigue
Deformity	Anorexia
	Failure to thrive
	Rash
	Irritability
	Lymphadenopathy
	Hepatosplenomegaly
	Pericarditis

Systemic-onset JRA constitutes approximately 10% to 20% of all cases and occurs equally in boys and girls. It presents with high spiking fevers and a salmon-colored, evanescent rash prior to the onset of joint symptoms. These children appear quite ill during a febrile episode. Lymphadenopathy and hepatosplenomegaly are often present on exam; 30% have pericarditis. Elevated white blood cell and platelet counts, anemia, and a high sedimentation rate are characteristic. Tests for antinuclear antibody (ANA) and rheumatoid factor are generally negative. These patients do not develop chronic uveitis. Approximately half experience complete resolution, and half develop very destructive arthritis even though their systemic systems abate.

Pauciarticular JRA presents in 50% to 60% of children with JRA. Girls outnumber boys 4:1. In pauciarticular JRA, the patient may have involvement in up to four joints, typically large joints such as knees and ankles. Seventy percent of these patients have a positive ANA, which indicates an increased risk factor for the development of asymptomatic uveitis. Approximately 70% go into remission after several years of active arthritis.

Polyarticular JRA, seen in 30% to 40% of children with JRA, involves five or more joints. Girls predominate, with a ratio of 3:1. Joint involvement may include small and large joints as well as the temporomandibular joint and cervical vertebrae. Rheumatoid factor may be present, usually in adolescents, who go on to develop disease similar to adult rheumatoid arthritis. Fewer patients have a positive ANA, but those that do are at risk for asymptomatic uveitis. Those without rheumatoid factor tend to do better; half eventually go into remission.

Uveitis (also called iritis or iridocyclitis) is an inflammation of the anterior chamber and initially leads to synechiae (an adhesion between the iris and either cornea or lens, manifested by an irregular pupil). Uveitis is entirely asymptomatic and can lead to visual loss. But if discovered early by slit-lamp examination, it is usually controlled by steroid eye drops and mydriatics. Systemic therapy, such as methotrexate, occasionally is required.

Differential Diagnosis

Virtually any rheumatologic disorder can present initially with isolated arthritis. Other conditions to consider include septic arthritis, toxic synovitis, Lyme's disease, spondyloarthropathy, and reactive arthritis. Chapter 19 discusses noninflammatory causes of limb and joint pain in detail.

Diagnostic Evaluation

Synovial fluid analysis typically reveals a white blood cell count of 5,000 to 30,000 per µL and elevated protein. Radiographs show soft-tissue swelling early; later, narrowing of the joint spaces and, finally, bony erosions develop.

Treatment

Treatment consists of medical management with inflammatory-suppressive drugs (nonsteroidal anti-inflammatory drugs; intra-articular corticosteroids; immunosuppressive drugs, especially methotrexate and anti–tumor necrosis factor agents; steroids, etc.) and physical therapy. Surgery, rarely required, is generally delayed until growth is complete.

Most patients with JRA experience little permanent disability and remain in remission for long periods. Severe involvement often leads to joint destruction and deformity and may result in a leg length discrepancy. Children with pauciarticular (and less commonly polyarticular) disease may develop uveitis and vision loss, so ophthalmologic surveillance is needed every 3 to 4 months for several years.

🔑 11-6 KEY POINTS

1. Juvenile rheumatoid arthritis (JRA) is characterized by chronic synovitis and classified according to degree of involvement (systemic, pauciarticular, polyarticular).
2. Patients with a positive antinuclear antibody (ANA) titer are at increased risk for the development of uveitis.
3. Anti-inflammatory drugs and physical therapy are the mainstays of treatment.

SYSTEMIC LUPUS ERYTHEMATOSUS

Pathogenesis

Systemic lupus erythematosus (SLE) is characterized by widespread connective tissue inflammation and arteriolar vasculitis. SLE develops when the immune system somehow begins to recognize "self" nuclear proteins, cytoplasmic contents, and connective tissue as "foreign" and attempts to neutralize or remove them. Antigen-antibody immune complexes become deposited in the walls of small arteries, resulting in inflammation and necrosis. This immune complex vasculitis is the basic pathologic lesion responsible for the extensive clinical manifestations.

Epidemiology

SLE usually appears in late childhood or adolescence and is far more common in females. African American and Hispanic patients tend to have more severe disease.

Clinical Manifestations

History and Physical Examination

The diagnosis of SLE is based on clinical criteria; 4 of the 11 criteria are required to classify a patient as having lupus (Table 11-4). The onset may be precipitous and rapidly progressive or insidious with a slow, steady course. Fever, malaise, and weight loss are frequent constitutional complaints. Arthritis of the hands, wrists, elbows, shoulders, knees, and ankles produces pain out of proportion to the physical signs; in fact, the arthritis of SLE is neither erosive nor deforming. Central nervous system (CNS) involvement may present at any time over the course of the disease.

Lupus nephritis, the most common clinical manifestation, is often present at diagnosis. The World Health Organization classifies renal involvement as normal (type I, 6%, renal failure extremely rare), mesangial

---

■ TABLE 11-4 Diagnostic Criteria[a] for Systemic Lupus Erythematosus

Malar (butterfly) rash

Discoid lupus rash

Photosensitivity

Painless oral or nasal mucocutaneous ulcerations

Nonerosive arthritis

Renal disease (nephritic or nephrotic)

Encephalopathy (seizures or psychosis)

Polyserositis (pleuritis or pericarditis)

Cytopenia (low white blood count, lymphopenia, thrombocytopenia, or hemolytic anemia)

Positive immunoserology (anti-dsDNA, anti-Smith, or anticardiolipin antibodies)

Positive antinuclear antibody test

[a]Four of 11 are required to be classified as SLE.

(type II, 20%, renal failure rare), focal proliferative (type III, 23%, renal failure uncommon), diffuse proliferative (type IV, 40%, progressive renal failure common, high mortality), and membranous disease (type V, renal failure uncommon).

Diagnostic Evaluation

Anemia, leukopenia (with a predominance of neutrophils), and thrombocytopenia are characteristic. Complement levels, including C3, C4, and CH50, are generally depressed or falling, especially during active disease. A positive **ANA test** is very sensitive but not specific. Elevation in **double-stranded DNA** antibodies parallels disease severity, especially renal disease. Other autoantibodies, including antiphospholipid and anticardiolipin antibodies, may be present. **Anti-Smith** is very specific for lupus but only is present in 30% of affected patients. Circulating anti-Ro and anti-La antibodies in an SLE-affected mother may cause congenital heart block in her fetus.

Treatment

Treatment is long term and multifactorial. Careful attention must be paid to nutritional status and fluid balance. Limiting sun exposure and using appropriate sunblock improves skin problems. Aggressive characterization and treatment of kidney disease, including biopsy and frequent imaging, are invaluable in minimizing renal morbidity. Hypertension is a relatively common complication that is usually well controlled with conventional therapy.

Anti-inflammatory therapy remains the mainstay of pharmacologic treatment. Oral prednisone is prescribed as needed for maintenance therapy; high-dose oral or intravenous pulse therapy is preferable during acute exacerbations. Other immunosuppressants, such as cyclophosphamide, are helpful in treating lupus nephritis. Hydroxychloroquine may be used to treat mucocutaneous symptoms. Other frequently used agents include mycophenolate mofetil and azathioprine.

Overall, prognosis and quality of life are improving, and more than 90% of patients have good long-term survival and normal function. Renal's disease produces the most significant morbidity; renal failure is the leading cause of death after infection. **Libman-Sacks endocarditis** is a serious cardiac complication. CNS disease, when present, is associated with slow deterioration in mental capacity.

🔑 11-7 KEY POINTS

1. Systemic lupus erythematosus (SLE) consists of widespread connective tissue inflammation and vasculitis.
2. The diagnosis of SLE is clinical.
3. Lupus nephritis is the most common clinical manifestation, resulting in significant morbidity.
4. Typical laboratory findings include falling complement levels, a positive antinuclear antibody (ANA) titer, and a positive double-stranded DNA antibody titer.
5. The disease usually responds to immunosuppressant therapy.

DERMATOMYOSITIS

Pathogenesis

Dermatomyositis is an inflammatory disease involving the small vessels of the skin, striated muscle, and occasionally the gastrointestinal tract. Immune complexes are deposited in the walls of arterioles, capillaries, and venules, leading to inflammation, ulceration, bleeding, and fibrinous repair. Polymyositis, a similar inflammatory muscular condition without skin findings, occurs less frequently in the pediatric population.

Epidemiology

Onset is typically between 2 and 10 years of age with a peak at 7 years of age. Like most rheumatologic conditions, dermatomyositis is more common in females.

Risk Factors

Predisposition is heritable; HLA B8/DR3 and HLA DQalpha1*0501 occur more often in these children. The condition seems to be associated with viral illnesses in some cases.

Clinical Manifestations

History and Physical Examination

Patients report a history of malaise, fatigue, weight loss, and intermittent fevers. Progressive proximal muscle weakness accompanied by the characteristic **violaceous** dermatitis of the eyelids (heliotrope), hands, elbows, knees, and ankles virtually clinches the diagnosis. Gottron papules are characteristic lesions resembling scaly erythematous papules on the extensor surfaces of the interphalangeal joints of the fingers, the elbows, and the knees. The weakness may advance to involve muscle groups used for swallowing, phonation, and respiration. Long-standing inflammation eventually results in calcium deposits in the skin and muscle, cutaneous striation, scarring, and significant muscle atrophy.

Diagnostic Evaluation

The most striking laboratory abnormality is marked elevation of **serum creatine kinase**, an enzyme released during muscle breakdown (as well as other muscle enzymes such as aldolase, aspartate aminotransferase, and lactic dehydrogenase). Specific electromyography and histologic results are characteristic of the disorder. Serum acute-phase reactant levels (erythrocyte sedimentation rate, C-reactive protein) correlate with disease severity. Half of these children have a positive ANA test. The most common myositis-specific antibody is Mi-2.

Treatment

Treatment consists of appropriate physical therapy and immunosuppressants. As long as muscle enzyme levels remain high, activity is limited, and the primary aim of therapy is to prevent contractures with positioning and splints. High-dose prednisone is prescribed in an attempt to control the inflammatory response. Once evidence of muscle destruction begins to abate, steroid doses are tapered and strengthening exercises are gradually added. Patients whose disease does not respond to oral steroids may require intravenous pulse steroids or second-line agents including methotrexate, intravenous immunoglobulin, cyclophosphamide, and cyclosporine.

Oropharyngeal, chest wall, and respiratory muscle weakness predisposes patients to aspiration. Respiratory failure necessitating mechanical ventilation is rare. Most children diagnosed with dermatomyositis recover with no permanent disability within a few years. Approximately 10% progress to wheelchair dependence. Gastrointestinal involvement with spontaneous perforation, although rare, is the leading cause of death.

11-8 KEY POINTS

1. Dermatomyositis is an inflammatory disease of the small vessels of the skin, striated muscle, and gastrointestinal tract.
2. The weakness begins in the proximal extremity muscle groups and is accompanied by a characteristic violaceous dermatitis.
3. Serum creatine kinase levels are markedly elevated.
4. The weakness may progress to involve the respiratory and oropharyngeal muscles.

VASCULITIDES

A number of other connective tissue diseases, including polyarteritis nodosa and Henoch-Schönlein purpura, present with vasculitis as the primary manifestation. **Kawasaki's disease**, a vasculitis postulated but not proven to be infectious in origin, is limited to the pediatric population.

Clinical Manifestations and Treatment

Polyarteritis Nodosa

Insidious in onset, variable in symptomatology, waxing and waning, polyarteritis nodosa often proves difficult to diagnose. Signs and symptoms may include any of the following: vague prolonged systemic complaints, painful erythematous skin nodules, purpura, hypertension, hematuria, abdominal pain, calf pain, encephalopathy, and neuropathy. The fingers and toes become gangrenous in extreme disease. The erythrocyte sedimentation rate is invariably elevated during active disease. Diagnosis rests on signature vascular lesions on biopsy. Corticosteroids and immune suppressants are the mainstays of therapy. Prognosis is fair; mortality is related to renal, CNS, or cardiac complications.

Henoch-Schönlein Purpura

Henoch-Schönlein purpura is an IgA mediated vasculitis involving the gastrointestinal tract, skin, joints, and kidneys. It occurs in young children, peaks in the winter months, and is preceded by a viral or group A streptococcal upper respiratory infection in 80%. Gastrointestinal involvement is usually significant, including spasmodic abdominal pain, vomiting, ileus, and upper and lower tract bleeding. Glomerulonephritis may rarely progress to renal failure. The characteristic nonthrombocytopenic palpable purpuric rash over dependent areas (typically the waist down, elbows down, and face) is almost always observed. Treatment is supportive; corticosteroids may be helpful if gastrointestinal symptoms and arthritis are present. The prognosis for full recovery within 4 to 6 weeks is excellent. Long-term complications parallel the severity of renal involvement. Initial proteinuria portends a worse prognosis than does hematuria.

Kawasaki's Disease

Kawasaki's disease is a systemic vasculitis characterized by high fever, lymphadenopathy, and mucocutaneous lesions. It occurs almost exclusively in infants and young children and is more common in boys. An infectious etiology has been suggested but never been confirmed. Table 11-5 notes the current criteria for diagnosis. Most symptoms arise during the first week (*acute phase*); coronary aneurysms may develop over the next few weeks (*subacute phase*), and the disease resolves over 2 to 3 months (*convalescent phase*).

The most serious complications are cardiac, including **coronary vasculitis** and concurrent or delayed **aneurysm formation**. Prognosis is tied to severity of cardiac involvement; cardiac instability can produce arrhythmias, infarction, or congestive heart failure within days of presentation. Aneurysms and coronary artery disease persist and may result in death months to years later.

Aspirin is prescribed until the end of the convalescent phase as an antiplatelet agent (provided there are no aneurysms). **IVIG therapy** results in rapid and profound improvement and significantly reduces the risk of coronary artery aneurysms.

■ **TABLE 11-5** Criteria for Diagnosis of Kawasaki Disease
Fever for 5 days or more, together with four of the following five signs on physical exam (or by history):
1. Bilateral conjunctivitis
2. Changes of lips and oral cavity (dry, red, fissured lips or strawberry tongue)
3. Changes of peripheral extremities (erythema or indurative edema of hands and feet)
4. Polymorphous rash (primarily on trunk)
5. Acute nonpurulent swelling of cervical lymph node to >1.5 cm in diameter

🔑 **11-9 KEY POINTS**
1. Henoch-Schönlein purpura is characterized by abdominal pain, vomiting, gastrointestinal bleeding, and palpable, nonthrombocytopenic purpura over dependent regions.
2. Kawasaki disease presents with high fever, lymphadenopathy, and mucocutaneous lesions.
3. High-dose IVIG reduces the risk of coronary artery aneurysms in Kawasaki disease.

Additional Suggested Reading

Boguniewicz M, Eichenfield LF, Hultsch T. Current management of atopic dermatitis and interruption of the atopic march. *J Allergy Clin Immunol.* 2003; 112:140–150.

Boxer LA. Neutrophil abnormalities. *Pediatr Rev.* 2003;24:52–62.

Goldman AS. Host responses to infection. *Pediatr Rev.* 2000;21:342–349.

Mahr TA, Sheth K. Update on allergic rhinitis. *Pediatr Rev.* 2005;26:278–283.

Chapter

12 Infectious Disease

Remarkable advances in the diagnosis, management, and prevention of infectious diseases have occurred during the past century. Newer techniques for diagnosis include fluorescent antibody testing, PCR, and imaging modalities such as MRI. Specific treatment of bacterial illnesses began with the introduction of sulfonamides in the 1930s and penicillin in the 1940s. Newer classes of antibacterial agents include semisynthetic penicillins, tetracyclines, macrolides, fluoroquinolones, aminoglycosides, carbapenems, and four generations of cephalosporins. Antifungal, antiviral, and antiparasitic agents have also been developed. Other anti-infectives include specific antibodies, intravenous immunoglobulin, phagocyte stimulating factors, and interferons. Vaccines have led to a dramatic decline in certain infectious diseases. Smallpox was eradicated worldwide in 1977, and indigenous poliomyelitis was eliminated from the United States in 1979. The annual incidence of measles, mumps, rubella, diphtheria, pertussis, tetanus, and *Haemophilus influenzae* type b meningitis has decreased by more than 98% because of vaccine use in the United States.

Unfortunately, new pathogens continue to emerge. Severe acute respiratory syndrome (SARS) appeared early in the new millennium, caused by a previously unknown coronavirus. Health organizations all over the world are concerned about the possibility of a bird flu mutation that would allow the disease to be spread among humans. Equally disconcerting is the rapid emergence of resistance to known antibiotics (e.g., methicillin- and vancomycin-resistant *Staphylococcus aureus* and penicillin-resistant *Streptococcus pneumoniae*). Thus, after 100 years of progress against infectious diseases, the current challenges are every bit as formidable as at the beginning of the last century.

VACCINATIONS

ROUTINE IMMUNIZATIONS

Active immunization involves stimulating an individual's immune system to develop a rapid protective response during future infectious exposures. A vaccine contains all or part of either a weakened or nonviable form of the organism. Table 12-1 contains a simplified version of the current vaccination guidelines recommended by the American Academy of Pediatrics (AAP). The AAP periodically releases additional vaccine recommendations. In particular, a policy statement released in July 2005 recommended that the new quadrivalent conjugate meningococcal vaccine (MCV4) be administered to all children at the 11- to 12-year-old well child care visit or to any adolescent entering high school or college (who plans to live in a dormitory) who has not yet been immunized against meningococcal disease.

Despite their long history of safe use and impressive cost-to-benefit ratio, vaccines should be held or delayed in certain circumstances. Table 12-2 lists absolute and relative contraindications to vaccine administration and some common misconceptions.

ADDITIONAL VACCINATIONS

Children with congenital, iatrogenic, or functional (e.g., sickle cell disease) asplenia should receive the polysaccharide meningococcal (MPSV4) and both pneumococcal (conjugate and polysaccharide) vaccines. A yearly influenza vaccine is recommended for children between 6 and 24 months of age and for patients 6 months of age or older who have chronic disease (including asthma, diabetes, HIV, cystic fibrosis,

■ TABLE 12-1 Childhood Immunization Schedule[d]

Age	Immunizations						
Birth–2 mo	HBV (1)[c]						
2 mo	HBV (2)	DTaP (1)	Hib (1)	IPV (1)	PCV (1)		
4 mo		DTaP (2)	Hib (2)	IPV (2)	PCV (2)		
6 mo[a]		DTaP (3)	Hib (3)		PCV (3)		
6–18 mo	HBV (3)			IPV (3)			
12–15 mo			Hib (4)		PCV (4)	MMR (1)	
>12 mo							Varicella
15–18 mo		DTaP (4)					
4–6 yr		DTaP (5)[b]		IPV (4)		MMR (2)	

NOTE: The numbers in parentheses indicate the number in the sequence of immunizations.
[a]Influenza vaccine also is recommended annually for all children 6 months to 24 months of age and for all children older than 6 months with chronic pulmonary, cardiovascular, metabolic, sickle cell, or HIV disease.
[b]Tetanus-diphtheria vaccine is given at 11 years of age and then every 10 years thereafter.
DTaP, diphtheria, tetanus, and acellular pertussis vaccine; HBV, hepatitis B virus vaccine; Hib, *Haemophilus influenzae* type b vaccine; IPV, inactivated polio virus vaccine; PCV, conjugated seven-valent pneumococcal vaccine.
[c] Adolescents who were not vaccinated against Hepatitis B in infancy should receive three doses of the vaccine.
[d] Adolescents entering middle school, high school or college should receive the conjugate meningococceal vaccine.

sickle cell disease, and cardiac conditions) or are receiving immunosuppressive therapy.

FEVER OF UNKNOWN ORIGIN

The phrase "fever of unknown origin" (FUO) implies fever of prolonged duration (≥14 days), documented temperature greater than 38.3°C (101°F) on multiple occasions, and uncertain etiology. FUO usually is caused by a common pediatric infection with an atypically prolonged time course.

DIFFERENTIAL DIAGNOSIS

FUO in the pediatric population is usually a common disorder presenting in an uncommon manner, rather

■ TABLE 12-2 Contraindications to and Precautions Regarding Vaccination

Absolute Contraindications	Precautions (Relative Contraindications)	Not Contraindications
Severe allergic reaction (e.g., anaphylaxis) after a previous vaccine dose	Shock/hyporesponsive episode ≤48 hr after previous dose of DTaP	Mild illness with or without low-grade fever
Known severe immune deficiency (MMR; varicella)	Fever >40.5°C (105°F) within 48 hr of previous dose of DTaP	Current antibiotic
Encephalopathy within 7 d of administration of the previous dose (DTaP)	Seizure ≤3 d after previous dose of DTaP	Positive PPD
Pregnancy (MMR; varicella)	Moderate-to-severe acute illness with or without fever	Prematurity[a]

[a]Premature infants should be vaccinated according to chronologic age. Hepatitis B vaccine should be delayed until the child weighs more than 2,000 g if the mother is HBsAg negative.
DTaP, diphtheria, tetanus, and acellular pertussis vaccine; HBsAg, hepatitis B surface antigen.

than a "zebra." Overall, infectious etiologies are more common than rheumatologic ones, which are more common than oncologic illnesses as a source for FUO. Diagnostic considerations include the following:

- **Infection**: Sinusitis, hepatitis, cytomegalovirus (CMV), EBV, parasites, cat-scratch disease, Rocky Mountain spotted fever, ehrlichiosis, Lyme's disease, brucellosis, leptospirosis, tularemia, endocarditis, septic arthritis, osteomyelitis, intra-abdominal abscess, enteric fever, tuberculosis, HIV, opportunistic infection
- **Connective tissue disease**: Systemic JRA, systemic lupus erythematosus
- **Malignancy**: Leukemia, lymphoma, neuroblastoma
- **Other**: Inflammatory bowel disease, Kawasaki's syndrome, drug fever, thyrotoxicosis, sarcoidosis, familial dysautonomia (Riley-Day's syndrome), and factitious fever

CLINICAL MANIFESTATIONS

History

The age and gender of the patient narrow the differential diagnosis. Inflammatory bowel disease and connective tissue disorders are uncommon in younger children. Autoimmune's disorders occur more frequently in girls. Sexual history, travel history, current medications, exposure to animals, tick bites, antecedent illness, trauma, associated symptoms, and family history are important areas of inquiry. Different fever patterns (constant, recurrent, cyclical) are more closely associated with particular diagnoses. A thorough history and physical exam (usually after repeated encounters) will reveal the diagnosis in more than half of the children in whom a cause of the fever is found.

Physical Examination

Conjunctivitis, the absence of tears, rashes, lymphadenopathy, joint tenderness, oral ulcers, thrush, heart murmurs, organomegaly, masses, abdominal tenderness, cutaneous manifestations (rash, hyperpigmentation, etc.), joint findings, and mental status changes may suggest a specific cause and guide further evaluation.

DIAGNOSTIC EVALUATION

The initial evaluation can be performed in the outpatient setting in older, well-appearing children. Neonates and ill-appearing children require hospitalization.

Screening laboratory tests include CBC and differential, serum electrolytes, BUN and creatinine levels, LFTs, alkaline phosphatase, and UA. Bacterial cultures should be obtained from specimens of blood, urine, stool, and possibly CSF. Stool may also be sent for viral antigen detection and parasite examination. Additional tests to consider include ESR, C-reactive protein, antinuclear antibodies, and specific serologic tests such as antibody studies for cat-scratch disease and EBV. A chest radiograph and skin testing for tuberculosis are typically performed. More expensive and invasive studies may be warranted based on screening results. In approximately 25% of cases, no etiology is determined and the children recover without sequelae.

12-1 KEY POINTS

1. The phrase "fever of unknown origin" implies fever of prolonged duration (≥14 days), documented temperature greater than 38.3°C (101°F) on multiple occasions, and uncertain etiology.
2. FUO is usually caused by a common pediatric infection with an atypically prolonged time course.
3. History, physical exam, and initial laboratory studies guide further evaluation.

BACTEREMIA AND SEPSIS

Bacteremia is the presence of bacteria in the blood. Bacteremia is further described as **occult** if it occurs in a well-appearing child without any obvious source of infection. The risk of occult bacteremia is highest (1.5% to 2.5%) in children between 2 and 24 months of age with a fever greater than 39.0°C and leukocytosis. The majority of episodes are caused by *Streptococcus pneumoniae* and resolve spontaneously. Rarely, localized infection (e.g., meningitis, pneumonia) occurs.

In contrast, **sepsis** implies bacteremia with evidence of a systemic response (tachypnea, tachycardia, etc.) and altered organ perfusion. Affected children appear quite ill and may develop shock. The cause of sepsis varies by age. In neonates, group B streptococci, enteric gram-negative bacilli, and *Listeria monocytogenes* are most prevalent. In older children, *S. pneumoniae* predominates, followed by *Neisseria meningitidis*. Less common causes include *Staphylococcus aureus*, *Salmonella* species, *Pseudomonas aeruginosa*, and viridans streptococci.

The evaluation of the child with suspected sepsis includes cultures from the blood, urine, and occasionally CSF. A chest radiograph is obtained if respiratory signs or symptoms are present. Empirical treatment with a third-generation cephalosporin and (occasionally) vancomycin is coupled with appropriate supportive measures.

ACUTE OTITIS MEDIA

PATHOGENESIS

Suspected or confirmed acute infection of the middle ear accounts for more physician visits (1 in 5) than any other pediatric illness. The middle ear is normally sterile; a patent but collapsible eustachian tube allows fluid drainage from the middle ear into the nasopharynx but normally prevents the retrograde entry of upper respiratory flora. In children, the angle of entry, short length, and decreased tone of the tube (*eustachian tube dysfunction*) increase susceptibility to infection. When the eustachian tube is further narrowed by edema from a concurrent viral URI, a relative vacuum is created, drawing secretions (and bacteria) from the nasopharynx into the middle ear, where they multiply.

EPIDEMIOLOGY

Acute otitis media (AOM) is most common in children 6 to 24 months of age. By 2 years of age, 90% of all children in the United States have had at least one episode of otitis media, and 50% have had at least three episodes. Approximately 20% of cases of acute OM are caused by viruses but may be complicated by bacterial superinfection. The other 80% represent bacterial infections, most commonly *S. pneumoniae* (50%), nontypeable *Haemophilus influenzae* (25%), and *Moraxella catarrhalis* (12%). Unfortunately, approximately 50% of *S. pneumoniae* isolates are resistant to penicillin, and many species of *H. influenzae* and *M. catarrhalis* have beta-lactamase activity.

RISK FACTORS

Caretaker smoking, bottle feeding, day-care attendance, allergic disease, craniofacial anomalies, immunodeficiency, genetic tendencies, and pacifier use all predispose children to AOM.

CLINICAL MANIFESTATIONS

History and Physical Examination

Children may have local or systemic complaints or both, including ear pain, fever, and fussiness. AOM is frequently preceded by symptoms of URI (cough, rhinorrhea, congestion). On physical examination, the affected tympanic membrane appears bulging, opaque, and erythematous or yellow with an aberrant light reflex. Pneumatic otoscopy reveals decreased tympanic membrane mobility. The diagnosis of AOM should only be made when there is an acute history of symptoms and a bulging, poorly or nonmobile tympanic membrane is noted in the presence of signs of local or systemic inflammation.

DIFFERENTIAL DIAGNOSIS

Otitis media with effusion is diagnosed when there is apparent fluid behind the tympanic membrane (reduced mobility on pneumatic otoscopy) but no evidence of inflammation (tympanic membrane translucent/gray, no fever, no evidence of ear pain). *Myringitis* is inflammation of the ear drum accompanied by normal mobility. This condition often accompanies a viral URI. *Otitis externa* (inflammation of the external ear canal) also causes ear pain; however, the tympanic membranes should appear normal on physical examination. The pain of otitis externa is exacerbated by manipulation of the external ear. A tympanic membrane that is erythematous without any other signs of disease may be caused by vigorous crying and should not be considered AOM.

TREATMENT

Because more antibiotics are prescribed for AOM than any other pediatric condition, and because antibiotic resistance is a growing concern, the Centers for Disease Control has issued consensus recommendations relating to the treatment of AOM. Patients younger than 24 months of age, patients thought to be at risk for poor follow-up, ill-appearing patients, and any patients with chronic illnesses (including immunodeficiencies) or recurrent, severe, or perforated AOM should be prescribed antibiotics. High-dose amoxicillin is the recommended first-line treatment. Patients who have been treated with antibiotics within the last month and those who have not improved within 48 hours are eligible for second-line therapy with amoxicillin/clavulanic acid, an oral second- or third-generation cephalosporin, or IM ceftriaxone. Children who are older than 24 months with less severe disease may be offered the choice of immediate antibiotic therapy versus pain control and watchful waiting. Those children who initially have antibiotics withheld should receive a prescription to fill 48 hours later if there has been no improvement. Patients with perforated tympanic membranes in addition to AOM should receive oral (and possibly topical) antibiotics at initial diagnosis. Most spontaneous perforations caused by AOM resolve within 24 to 72 hours.

The most common complication of AOM is otitis media with effusion, which follows virtually all cases of AOM and takes a variable amount of time to resolve. Children with otitis media with effusion that persists longer than 3 months should be referred for possible tympanostomy tube placement. Chronic otitis media with effusion increases the risk of delay of language acquisition and hearing loss. Tympanostomy tubes should also be considered for patients with at least 4 episodes of AOM within 6 months or 5 episodes within 12 months. Complications of frequent episodes of AOM include excessive scarring (tympanosclerosis), cholesteatoma formation, and chronic suppurative AOM.

Mastoiditis (infection of the mastoid bone of the skull) is a potentially severe but uncommon complication of AOM characterized clinically by high fever, tenderness of the mastoid bone, and anterior displacement of the external ear. Mastoiditis is treated with intravenous antibiotics; occasionally surgical drainage is required.

🔑 12-2 KEY POINTS

1. The three most common bacteria implicated in acute otitis media (AOM) are *S. pneumoniae*, nontypeable *H. influenzae*, and *Moraxella catarrhalis*.
2. In AOM, the tympanic membrane is bulging, opaque, and erythematous or yellow. Mobility is diminished as assessed by pneumatic otoscopy. Symptom onset is acute.
3. High-dose amoxicillin is the appropriate first-line treatment for most cases of AOM.
4. Tympanostomy tubes should be considered for children with recurrent episodes of AOM.
5. Chronic effusions and recurrent infection predisposes to permanent conductive hearing loss and language delay.

SINUSITIS

The maxillary and ethmoid sinuses are present at birth; the sphenoid and frontal sinuses develop later in childhood. The spectrum of pathogens responsible for sinusitis is virtually identical to that for otitis media (OM). Sinusitis is often difficult to diagnose in a young child because the classic symptoms of headache, facial pain, and sinus tenderness may be absent or difficult to articulate. Acute bacterial sinusitis has two common clinical presentations: (a) persistent respiratory symptoms (>10–14 days) without improvement, including either nasal discharge (clear or purulent) or a daytime cough, and (2) severe symptoms including high fever and purulent nasal discharge for at least 3 days. The differential diagnosis includes viral URIs, allergic rhinitis, and nasal foreign body. Sinusitis is primarily a clinical diagnosis. Plain films of the sinuses may be useful in older children when there is a poor response to therapy and the diagnosis is in doubt. CT is generally unnecessary. Sinus aspiration may be needed for recurrent or recalcitrant disease. Antibiotic coverage is similar to that for OM, although treatment should continue for 10 to 21 days. Complications are uncommon but include bony erosion, optic neuritis, orbital cellulitis, and intracranial extension. Children with recurrent or chronic sinusitis should be evaluated for cystic fibrosis, ciliary dyskinesia, or primary immune deficiency.

HERPANGINA

Herpangina is a symptom complex caused by enteroviruses (including groups A and B coxsackieviruses and other enterovirus serotypes). It is typically diagnosed during the summer and fall in younger children. Initially, the patient develops a high fever and very sore throat. On examination, characteristic vesicular lesions that progress to ulcers are scattered over the soft palate, tonsils, and pharynx. Primary herpetic gingivostomatitis (caused by herpes simplex virus [HSV]) presents in a similar manner, although the lesions are generally more widespread over the gums, lips, and mucosa. Herpangina is self-limited (5 to 7 days) and requires no specific therapy. When similar lesions are noted on the palms and soles (and occasionally on the buttocks), the more inclusive name **hand-foot-and-mouth disease** is used.

STREPTOCOCCAL PHARYNGITIS

PATHOGENESIS

Group A beta-hemolytic streptococci (group A *Streptococcus* [GAS]; *Streptococcus pyogenes*) are the most important cause of bacterial inflammation of the throat. Antimicrobial therapy for streptococcal disease is recommended because of the frequency of **suppurative** (peritonsillar abscess, retropharyngeal abscess) and **nonsuppurative** (rheumatic fever, post-streptococcal glomerulonephritis) complications.

EPIDEMIOLOGY

"Strep throat" afflicts older children and adolescents; it is uncommon before 3 years of age. The organism is spread person to person through infected oral secretions. At any one point in time, approximately 10% to 15% of well children carry GAS as part of their normal oral flora.

CLINICAL MANIFESTATIONS

History and Physical Examination

Classic symptoms include sore throat, fever, headache, malaise, nausea, and occasionally abdominal pain. Physical examination reveals enlarged, erythematous, exudative tonsils (approximately 50% of the time, patients with GAS pharyngitis do not have exudate on their tonsils) and tender anterior cervical lymphadenopathy. Petechiae may be present on the soft palate. Rhinorrhea, hoarseness, and coughing, the hallmarks of viral URIs, are notably absent. The diagnosis of scarlet fever is made when a characteristic erythematous, "sandpaperlike" rash accompanies the fever and pharyngitis. The rash appears on the neck or trunk, spreads to the extremities, and may desquamate 10 to 14 days later.

DIFFERENTIAL DIAGNOSIS

Differentiating viral pharyngitis and infectious mononucleosis from streptococcal pharyngitis may be impossible based on clinical symptoms; definitive diagnosis requires either throat culture or antigen detection test for GAS.

DIAGNOSTIC EVALUATION

Therapeutic decisions should be based on throat culture or rapid antigen detection test results. The specificity of most rapid antigen tests is greater than 95% (compared with throat culture), so false-positive test results are rare. The sensitivity of rapid antigen tests ranges from 80% to 90%, meaning false-negative results occasionally occur.

TREATMENT

Patients with documented group A streptococcal pharyngitis should receive a 10-day course of oral penicillin (or a single dose of IM benzathine penicillin G) to hasten symptom resolution, decrease transmissibility, and prevent acute rheumatic fever. Erythromycin, azithromycin, and clindamycin are acceptable alternatives for children allergic to penicillin. The treatment of scarlet fever is identical to that for streptococcal pharyngitis.

■ TABLE 12-3 Revised Jones Criteria for the Diagnosis of Acute Rheumatic Fever

Major manifestations

Carditis

Polyarthritis

Sydenham chorea

Erythema marginatum

Subcutaneous nodules

Minor manifestations

Clinical

  Fever

  Arthralgia

Laboratory

  Elevated C-reactive protein or ESR

  P-R interval prolongation on ECG

Additional criteria

Supporting evidence of preceding streptococcal infection

Positive throat culture for group A streptococci *or*

Positive rapid antigen test *or*

Increased streptococcal antibody titer[a]

NOTE: Diagnosis of acute rheumatic fever requires two major or one major and two minor criteria plus supporting evidence of antecedent group A streptococcal infection.
[a]Antibody tests include antistreptolysin-O (ASO), anti-DNase B, antihyaluronidase, or antistreptokinase.

Acute rheumatic fever (ARF) occurs 3 to 4 weeks after streptococcal pharyngitis in a small percentage of untreated patients. ARF is an inflammatory condition involving connective tissues of the heart (carditis, valvular destruction), joints (migratory polyarthritis), and CNS (transient chorea). Diagnosis rests on fulfilling the Jones criteria (Table 12-3). Initially, fever, dyspnea, chest pain, cardiac murmur, and arthritis predominate; long-term morbidity results from valvular destruction with consequent mitral or aortic valve insufficiency or stenosis. Acute episodes respond favorably to antibiotics, anti-inflammatory drugs, and cardiac management. ARF may recur after the initial episode. Therefore, individuals diagnosed with ARF should receive prophylactic penicillin therapy to prevent recurrent ARF.

Acute poststreptococcal glomerulonephritis may follow either group A streptococcal pharyngitis or skin infection (cellulitis) and is not prevented by timely antibiotic therapy. Clinical manifestations follow infection by approximately 10 days and include hematuria, edema, oliguria, and hypertension. Complement (C3) levels are low. Treatment consists of penicillin therapy and diuretics; steroids are rarely indicated. In contrast to affected adults, the majority of affected children recover without renal sequelae.

12-3 KEY POINTS

1. Children with pharyngitis should not be treated with antibiotics empirically because most episodes are caused by viruses. Therapeutic decisions should be based on throat culture or rapid antigen detection test results.
2. Penicillin is the antibiotic of choice for GAS pharyngitis.
3. Acute rheumatic fever (ARF) involves the heart, joints, and brain.
4. Acute poststreptococcal glomerulonephritis may follow either skin or pharyngeal infection and is not prevented by antibiotic therapy.

INFECTIOUS MONONUCLEOSIS

PATHOGENESIS

Infectious mononucleosis (IM) is a disease that occurs in older children and adolescents when they develop a primary EBV infection. Other pathogens,

notably cytomegalovirus and *Toxoplasma gondii*, can result in a similar clinical picture.

EPIDEMIOLOGY

Transmission occurs by mucosal contact with infected saliva (hence the term "kissing disease") or genital fluids. A majority of people are infected with EBV and seroconvert in early childhood. Such early infections are generally asymptomatic or mild in immunocompetent hosts, although the mononucleosis syndrome can occur in younger children as well.

CLINICAL MANIFESTATIONS

History and Physical Examination

The predominant symptom is usually a severe, exudative pharyngitis. Fever, generalized lymphadenopathy, and profound fatigue occur. Although the pharyngitis usually resolves within a week, the malaise may last 8 weeks or longer. Other manifestations include hepatosplenomegaly, palatal petechiae, jaundice, and rash. Patients infected with EBV who are misdiagnosed with a bacterial infection and receive amoxicillin or ampicillin are much more likely to manifest the rash, which involves the face and trunk and is generally maculopapular (but may be scarlatiniform, papulovesicular, or hemorrhagic as well).

DIFFERENTIAL DIAGNOSIS

Classic mononucleosis caused by EBV accounts for most cases. In CMV infection, typical signs of mononucleosis are present in only half the patients. Other infectious agents that cause similar symptoms include *Toxoplasma gondii*, human herpesvirus 6, and HIV. Pharyngitis caused by group A streptococci or adenovirus is difficult to distinguish from that of mononucleosis without laboratory studies. Pancytopenia in the presence of the clinical manifestations listed previously suggests malignancy.

DIAGNOSTIC EVALUATION

Leukocytosis or leukopenia may be present; lymphocytes account for more than 50% of leukocytes, and at least 10% are usually **atypical lymphocytes**. A heterophile antibody test allows rapid detection of EBV-associated mononucleosis in the outpatient setting; however, it has limited sensitivity in younger patients

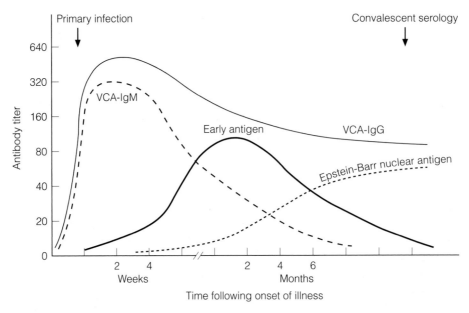

Figure 12-1 • Appearance of antibodies during EBV infection.

(<4 to 8 years of age) because they do not typically produce detectable heterophile antibodies. Specific serologic antibody testing is available for EBV (Fig. 12-1) and CMV. Other laboratory findings may include thrombocytopenia and elevated hepatic transaminase levels.

TREATMENT

The disorder is typically self-limited, requiring only supportive care. Activity restrictions (i.e., no contact sports) are advised until any associated splenomegaly resolves because of the possibility of splenic rupture.

Rare but serious complications include upper airway obstruction (treated with steroids), splenic rupture, and meningoencephalitis. Immunocompromised individuals are at risk for severe disseminated disease and lymphoproliferative disorders.

🔑 12-4 KEY POINTS

1. Classic mononucleosis is caused by EBV.
2. Clinical manifestations of mononucleosis include exudative pharyngitis, generalized lymphadenopathy, fever, and profound fatigue.
3. Helpful laboratory findings include lymphocytosis with a high percentage (10%) of atypical lymphocytes and a positive heterophile antibody test.

CROUP

The term **croup** refers to virus-induced inflammation of the laryngotracheal tissues, resulting in a syndrome of upper airway obstruction. Croup usually is caused by a parainfluenza virus but can also be caused by other viruses, such as influenza and RSV. It is most pronounced in young children because of the narrow caliber of the airway below the vocal cords (subglottic region); patients are typically between 3 months and 3 years of age. Incidence peaks during the late fall and winter. At its most severe, the disease progresses to partial or total airway obstruction.

CLINICAL MANIFESTATIONS

History and Physical Examination

Children typically experience the sudden onset of a hoarse voice, barky ("seal-like") cough, and inspiratory stridor, which may progress to respiratory distress. Patients may have a prodrome consisting of low-grade fever and rhinorrhea 12 to 24 hours prior to the onset of stridor. Respiratory compromise varies from minimal stridor with agitation to severe distress with tachypnea, hypoxia, nasal flaring, retractions, and impending airway obstruction.

DIAGNOSTIC EVALUATION

The diagnosis usually is made on the basis of clinical findings. If obtained, anteroposterior neck and chest

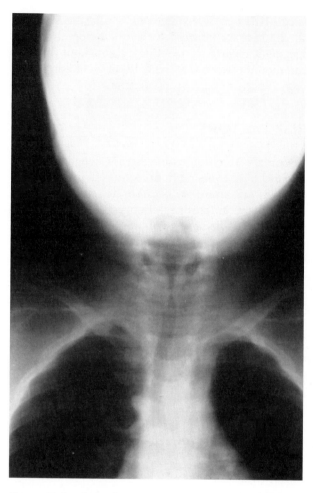

Figure 12-2 • Croup in a 3-year-old. Note the "steeple sign" indicative of subglottic narrowing.

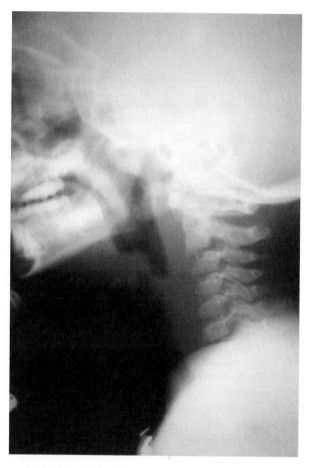

Figure 12-3 • Epiglottitis in a 4-year-old with massive edema of the epiglottis, thickened aryepiglottic folds, and effacement of the valleculae.

radiographs often reveal a tapered, narrow subglottic airway (steeple sign) (Fig. 12-2). This finding is present in 50% of cases and does not correlate with disease severity.

DIFFERENTIAL DIAGNOSIS

The differential diagnosis of upper airway obstruction (see Chapter 20) includes epiglottitis, bacterial tracheitis, foreign body aspiration, anaphylaxis, and angioneurotic edema. **Epiglottitis** consists of inflammation and edema of the epiglottis and aryepiglottic folds. It is considered a life-threatening emergency because of the propensity of the swollen tissues to result in sudden and irreversible airway occlusion. Most cases occur during the winter months in children 3 to 5 years of age. Fever, sore throat, hoarseness, and progressive stridor

develop over 1 to 2 days. On examination, the child appears toxic, drools, and leans forward with chin extended to maximize airway patency. Lateral neck radiographs show "thumb-printing" of the epiglottis (Fig. 12-3). Although radiographs may aid in diagnosis, they are not recommended because they delay appropriate care. The child with suspected epiglottitis requires timely transport to the operating room and emergent endotracheal intubation. Emergency cricothyroidotomy may be performed if an endotracheal airway cannot be secured in the face of rapidly progressive obstruction. Intravenous ampicillin-sulbactam provides appropriate empirical coverage until the organism is identified by culture and sensitivities are known. The incidence of epiglottitis has decreased markedly since the advent of routine administration of the **Hib** (*Haemophilus influenzae* type b) **vaccine** in the late 1980s (cases caused by *S. pneumoniae* and group A streptococci increasingly are reported); failure to maintain current Hib shots is the biggest risk factor for developing epiglottitis.

TREATMENT

Most children with croup never become symptomatic enough to prompt a visit to the pediatrician. They are usually treated at home; cough and stridor respond well to cool night air or humidity, and the disease resolves over 4 to 7 days. In the emergency department, stridulous infants receive cool mist, nebulized racemic epinephrine, and oral, intravenous, or IM steroids. Impending respiratory failure and airway obstruction constitute medical emergencies and are addressed accordingly (see Chapter 1).

🔑 12-5 KEY POINTS

1. Children with croup develop a hoarse voice, barky ("seal-like") cough, and stridor, which may progress to respiratory distress.
2. Infants with severe stridor caused by croup are treated with steroids and nebulized epinephrine.
3. Epiglottitis is a life-threatening emergency.
4. The typical patient with epiglottitis has a toxic appearance, with drooling and severe, progressive respiratory distress.
5. When epiglottitis is suspected, the child should be transported to the operating room for endotracheal intubation and direct visualization under general anesthesia.

BRONCHIOLITIS

PATHOGENESIS

Bronchiolitis is an acute viral lower respiratory tract infection that results in inflammatory obstruction of the peripheral airways. There is a predominantly lymphocytic infiltrate into the peribronchial and peribronchiolar epithelium that promotes submucosal edema. Intraluminal mucous plugs and cellular debris accumulate because of impaired mucociliary clearance.

EPIDEMIOLOGY

RSV causes 65% of cases; parainfluenza, influenza, human metapneumovirus, and adenovirus are responsible for the remaining 35%. Bronchiolitis typically occurs between November and April. At least half of all children are infected with RSV before 1 year of age, and recurrent infections throughout life are common. Between 0.5% and 1% of all children with bronchiolitis require hospitalization.

RISK FACTORS

Children with chronic lung disease, congenital heart disease, and congenital or acquired immunodeficiencies are more susceptible to severe disease. Hospitalization rates peak between 2 and 5 months of age. Predictors of severe illness include respiratory rate greater than 70 per minute, hypoxia, atelectasis on chest radiograph, and history of preterm birth.

CLINICAL MANIFESTATIONS

History

The acute illness lasts for 5 to 10 days, followed by gradual recovery over the next 1 to 2 weeks. Infected neonates may develop life-threatening **apnea**. Infants initially present with fever, cough, and rhinorrhea followed by progressive respiratory distress. Household contacts usually have upper respiratory symptoms.

Physical Examination

Findings on exam include fever, tachypnea, and mild to severe respiratory distress. Wheezing, rhonchi, crackles, and accessory muscle use during respiration (tugging) may be noted. Ill infants may be restless or lethargic. Hypoxia is common in severely affected patients.

DIFFERENTIAL DIAGNOSIS

The wheezing associated with bronchiolitis may be difficult to distinguish from asthma or airway foreign body in older infants. Causes of recurrent episodes of wheezing include vascular rings, cystic fibrosis, and ciliary dyskinesia.

DIAGNOSTIC EVALUATION

Rapid assays exist for RSV and influenza detection. Most respiratory viruses may be cultured from nasal secretions. Chest radiograph should be obtained for ill or hypoxic patients and for those with recurrent or unexplained wheezing. Findings consistent with bronchiolitis include lung hyperinflation, peribronchial thickening ("cuffing"), and increased interstitial markings.

TREATMENT

Hypoxic or ill-appearing children require hospitalization. Children with oxygen saturation greater than 94%, minimal respiratory distress, good fluid intake, reliable caretakers, and good follow-up may be treated as outpatients.

Most hospitalized infants require only supportive care (oxygen, fluid support) for their self-limited illness. The benefit of bronchodilators and corticosteroids is controversial. Although beta-agonists may transiently improve respiratory symptoms, they do not appear to shorten the duration of illness or hospitalization. α-Adrenergic agents such as epinephrine, given by inhalation, appear to be more beneficial. Corticosteroids have *not* been clearly shown to affect the course of the disease; however, administration early in the course of illness may benefit those infants with a familial predisposition to reactive airways disease. Nebulized ribavirin, an antiviral agent that suppresses viral RNA polymerase activity, improves respiratory status in hospitalized patients with RSV but is expensive and does not decrease the duration of hospitalization. Its use should be considered in patients with underlying chronic lung disease or immunosuppressive conditions.

RespiGam, an intravenous polyclonal immunoglobulin with high RSV antibody concentration, and **palivizumab**, an injectable RSV monoclonal antibody, provide passive prophylaxis and are recommended during the winter months for patients younger than 2 years of age who are at risk for severe disease (former premature infants and children with bronchopulmonary dysplasia who require oxygen). Palivizumab is currently preferred because it is easier to administer and not a blood product.

The mortality rate for hospitalized patients is approximately 1%. Children with congenital heart defects, chronic lung disease, and immunodeficiency fare particularly poorly. Patients with documented RSV bronchiolitis have more airway hyperresponsiveness later in life than the general population.

12-6 KEY POINTS

1. Bronchiolitis is a self-limited but potentially severe infection in infants, especially those with underlying conditions.
2. The classic presentation includes fever, wheezing, tachypnea, rhinorrhea, and respiratory distress.
3. Apnea is a frequent presentation in neonates.
4. Palivizumab is an injectable RSV monoclonal antibody. Prophylactic administration during the winter months should be considered in patients younger than 24 months who were premature infants or who have chronic lung disease (bronchopulmonary dysplasia) requiring oxygen.

PERTUSSIS

Infection with *Bordetella pertussis* causes a URI and persistent cough in adults but may result in life-threatening respiratory disease in neonates and infants. The organism is spread via aerosolized droplets expelled during intense coughing. The agent is highly infective among unimmunized hosts. The vaccine is 95% effective against severe disease, but immunity wanes significantly within several years.

CLINICAL MANIFESTATIONS

History and Physical Examination

Patients with pertussis are almost invariably afebrile. The classic presentation in young children is "whooping cough." The **catarrhal phase** follows a 7- to 10-day incubation period and consists of 1 to 2 weeks of low-grade fever, cough, and coryza. Then comes a 2- to 6-week **paroxysmal phase** characterized by intense spasms of coughing followed by sudden inhalation, which produces the characteristic whoop. Posttussive emesis is common. Facial petechiae and scleral hemorrhages often develop as a consequence of forceful coughing. Most symptoms remit during the **convalescent phase**, but the cough may last for 2 to 8 weeks. Infants with severe disease may present with apnea or the typical paroxysmal cough followed by choking and progressive cyanosis. The characteristic "whoop" is absent in very young infants because they cannot generate sufficient negative inspiratory force.

Adolescents and adults can also be infected with pertussis and usually present with nonspecific upper respiratory symptoms and a protracted cough.

DIAGNOSTIC EVALUATION

Laboratory evaluation usually reveals leukocytosis (>20,000 WBCs per µL) with a predominance of lymphocytes. Nasopharyngeal secretions contain the organism, which may be detected by fluorescent antibody staining, PCR, or culture. The chest radiograph usually is normal, but nonspecific infiltrates may be seen.

TREATMENT

Young infants with severe disease should be hospitalized to manage apnea, cyanosis, hypoxia, and feeding difficulties. Erythromycin estolate (and other macrolides) shorten the duration of illness *if given early in the catarrhal phase.* After the coughing paroxysms begin, antibiotics do not affect the course of illness but are recommended to decrease the period of infectivity. A 14-day course completely eradicates the organism from the nasopharynx and respiratory tract. Household and other close (daycare) contacts require chemoprophylaxis with erythromycin regardless of immunization status.

There is some discussion about whether adolescents and adults should receive the DTaP (acellular pertussis) vaccine rather than the Td vaccine every 10 years to protect against both tetanus and pertussis. The DTaP vaccine currently in use is not recommended for patients older than 7 years.

🔑 12-7 KEY POINTS

1. The "whoop" in pertussis is the long stridulous inspiration after the paroxysmal cough.
2. Neonates and young infants may present with apnea rather than the cough and whoop.
3. Leukocytosis with a predominance of lymphocytes is typical of pertussis.
4. The drug of choice is erythromycin estolate or another macrolide.

PNEUMONIA

PATHOGENESIS

Pneumonia refers to an acute inflammatory process occurring in the lungs. It may be infectious or noninfectious. Inflammation can occur in the alveolar space (lobar pneumonia), the alveolar walls (interstitial pneumonia), and/or the bronchi.

EPIDEMIOLOGY

The age of an immunocompetent child suggests an etiologic organism (Table 12-4). Viruses are the most common cause of pneumonia in young children. *Chlamydia trachomatis* pneumonia manifests at 2 to 3 months of age in infants born to women with untreated genital *C. trachomatis* infection. *S. pneumoniae* should be considered in any community-acquired lower respiratory tract infection. *Mycoplasma pneumoniae* pneumonia is uncommon in children younger than 5 years but, along with *Chlamydia pneumoniae* (Taiwan acute respiratory [agent] [TWAR]), becomes a more frequent and important pathogen in school-age children and adolescents. Less common bacterial causes include nontypeable *H. influenzae, M. catarrhalis, S. aureus, N. meningitidis,* and group A streptococci.

RISK FACTORS

Conditions associated with an increased risk of bacterial pneumonia include the following:

- Chronic lung disease, including cystic fibrosis and asthma
- Neurologic impairment (swallowing dysfunction or neuromuscular disease)
- Gastroesophageal reflux with aspiration of gastric contents
- Upper airway anatomic defects (tracheoesophageal fistula, cleft palate)
- Hemoglobinopathies (including sickle cell disease)
- Immunodeficiency or immunosuppressive therapy

CLINICAL MANIFESTATIONS

History

Viral pneumonia develops gradually over 2 to 4 days. It is usually preceded by upper respiratory symptoms such as cough, rhinorrhea, postnasal drip, coryza, and low-grade fever. Infants with pneumonia caused by *C. trachomatis* are afebrile and have conjunctivitis and a staccato cough. Infants and young children with bacterial pneumonia may present with nonspecific constitutional complaints, including fever, irritability, poor feeding, vomiting, abdominal pain, and lethargy. Abrupt onset of fever, chills, dyspnea, and chest pain

■ TABLE 12-4 Causes of Infectious Pneumonia by Age

1 Month	1 to 6 Months	6 Months to 5 Years	School Age/Adolescent
Group B streptococci	Streptococcus pneumoniae[a]	S. pneumoniae[a]	Mycoplasma pneumoniae
Escherichia coli/gram-negative enteric bacilli	Staphylococcus aureus	Moraxella catarrhalis	Chlamydia pneumoniae
Haemophilus influenzae	Moraxella catarrhalis	Haemophilus influenzae	S. pneumoniae[a]
Streptococcus pneumoniae	H. influenzae	Staphylococcus aureus	H. influenzae
Group D streptococci	Bordetella pertussis	Neisseria meningitidis	S. aureus
Listeria monocytogenes	Chlamydia trachomatis[b]	M. pneumoniae	Mycobacterium tuberculosis
Anaerobes	Ureaplasma urealyticum[b]	Group A streptococci	Viruses[c]
Cytomegalovirus	Cytomegalovirus[b]	M. tuberculosis	
Herpes simplex virus	Viruses[c]	Viruses[c]	
Ureaplasma urealyticum			
Staphylococcus aureus			

[a]Most common cause of bacterial pneumonia in this age group.
[b]Although acquired perinatally, these infections often do not present as pneumonia until after 1 month of age.
[c]Including RSV, influenza, parainfluenza, and adenovirus.

is typical. Productive cough is more common in older patients. *M. pneumoniae* and *C. pneumoniae* pneumonia present initially with fever, headache, and myalgia. These symptoms gradually subside over 5 to 7 days, whereas coughing increases and persists for 2 weeks or more.

Physical Examination

Any indication of respiratory distress can signal pneumonia, although tachypnea and dyspnea are most common. Tachypnea out of proportion to fever is an important clue to pneumonia in the young child. Diffuse wheezing and crackles suggest involvement of multiple areas of the lung, characteristic of viral or atypical (*M. pneumoniae, C. pneumoniae, C. trachomatis*) pneumonia. Focal findings such as focal crackles or decreased breath sounds, dullness to percussion, egophony, and bronchophony suggest pneumonia of bacterial origin. Pneumonia can also present with only fever and tachypnea in the absence of chest findings.

Cyanosis is uncommon except in severe disease. Approximately 10% of patients with *M. pneumoniae* infection develop a rash, usually macular and erythematous or urticarial; erythema multiforme has also been reported.

DIFFERENTIAL DIAGNOSIS

Pneumonia is much more common in the pediatric population than are other conditions with similar presentations, including CHF, chemical pneumonitis, pulmonary embolism, sarcoidosis, and primary or metastatic malignancy.

DIAGNOSTIC EVALUATION

A thorough history and physical examination usually suggest the diagnosis. Sputum culture is not likely to be helpful because pediatric patients generally do not produce adequate sputum samples. Chest radiograph remains an excellent test for defining the extent and pattern of involvement and assessing related complications (i.e., pleural effusion, pneumatocele). Bacterial pneumonia causes lobar consolidation. Diffuse interstitial infiltrates suggest viral or atypical pneumonia, although children with *Mycoplasma* pneumonia may have lobar consolidation. Aspiration pneumonia is typically located in the right middle or right upper lobe. *C. trachomatis* pneumonia is diagnosed by direct fluorescent antibody testing of conjunctival or nasopharyngeal specimens. *M. pneumoniae* can be noted by PCR of specimens obtained by nasopharyngeal swab or by specific antimycoplasmal IgM antibody determination. Cold-agglutinin titters are elevated not only in *M. pneumoniae* infections but also in many cases of viral pneumonia and in some cases of bacterial pneumonia.

TREATMENT

Therapy depends on the most likely pathogen. In the outpatient setting, amoxicillin/clavulanic acid is appropriate for most cases of bacterial pneumonia when antibiotics are thought to be necessary. Erythromycin, clarithromycin, or azithromycin is recommended for so-called walking pneumonia caused by *M. pneumoniae* or *C. pneumoniae*. Erythromycin is used to treat infants with infection caused by *C. trachomatis*.

Any child with persistent hypoxia (which necessitates oxygen therapy), moderate to severe respiratory distress, and/or hemodynamic instability requires hospitalization. Intravenous ampicillin/sulbactam is appropriate initial therapy for hospitalized children with suspected bacterial pneumonia. (Neonates with suspected bacterial pneumonia receive additional workup [LP] and are started on ampicillin and cefotaxime [or gentamicin if the CSF is sterile].) Cefuroxime and ceftriaxone are reasonable alternatives. Additional antibiotics (macrolides, vancomycin) may be appropriate depending on the suspected pathogen and community susceptibility patterns. Most viral infections are self-limited. Patients with severe disease (bacterial or viral) may require supportive therapy and intubation.

The most frequent complication is development of a pleural effusion large enough to compromise respiratory effort. Although virtually any infectious agent can cause an effusion, large effusions are much more likely to result from *S. aureus*. Pleurocentesis (with possible chest tube placement) provides rapid relief. Empyema results when purulent fluid from an adjacent lung infection drains into the pleural space. Lung abscesses may complicate anaerobic infections.

🔑 12-8 KEY POINTS

1. *S. pneumoniae* is the most common cause of bacterial pneumonia in most age groups. Amoxicillin/clavulanic acid is the outpatient oral antibiotic of choice.
2. *M. pneumoniae* and *C. pneumoniae* (TWAR) should be considered in older children and adolescents. Macrolide antibiotics are the treatment of choice for these pathogens.
3. The pattern of infiltrate on chest radiograph may suggest the etiologic agent.
4. The majority of large pleural effusions are caused by *S. aureus* pneumonia.

MENINGITIS

PATHOGENESIS

Almost any pathogen can infect the leptomeninges and CSF. Viral meningitis is typically an acute, self-limited illness; bacterial meningitis is a life-threatening condition associated with substantial morbidity and mortality. The term **aseptic meningitis** refers to meningeal inflammation caused by an antigenic stimulus other than pyogenic bacteria (e.g., enterovirus or *Borrelia*).

EPIDEMIOLOGY

The likely etiology of meningitis depends on age (Table 12-5). Beyond the neonatal period, viral meningitis is much more common than bacterial meningitis. Both infants and older children are at risk for meningitis caused by enteroviruses (the most common cause of viral meningitis). Enteroviruses primarily circulate in the late summer and early fall. Overall, *S. pneumoniae* and *N. meningitidis* are the most common bacterial pathogens. Neonates and children younger than 3 years are at highest risk for bacterial meningitis. Hib vaccine has nearly eliminated *H. influenzae* type b meningitis in the United States. Lyme meningitis, caused by *Borrelia burgdorferi*, usually affects school-age children and adolescents. Rare causes of meningitis and meningoencephalitis include EBV,

TABLE 12-5 Causes of Meningitis by Age

1 Month	1 to 2 Months	2 Months to 6 Years	School Age/Adolescent
Group B streptococci	Escherichia coli	Streptococcus pneumoniae	S. pneumoniae
Escherichia coli	S. pneumoniae	Neisseria meningitidis	N. meningitidis
Other gram-negative bacilli	Enteroviruses	Enteroviruses	Enteroviruses
Herpes simplex virus	Haemophilus influenzae type b[a]	Borrelia burgdorferi	B. burgdorferi
Listeria monocytogenes	Group B streptococci	H. influenzae type b[a]	
Streptococcus pneumoniae			

[a]Rare in immunized populations.

Bartonella henselae (cat-scratch disease), *M. pneumoniae*, *M. tuberculosis*, and *Cryptococcus neoformans*.

RISK FACTORS

Risk factors for bacterial meningitis are the same as those for sepsis because most cases result from hematogenous seeding. Direct invasion (nonhematogenous) occurs as a result of trauma, mastoiditis, sinusitis, and anatomic defects in the scalp or skull. In the neonate, low birth weight, prolonged rupture of membranes, and chorioamnionitis predispose to septicemia and meningitis; myelomeningocele also increases the risk.

CLINICAL MANIFESTATIONS

History

Classic symptoms of meningitis include nausea, vomiting, photophobia, irritability, lethargy, headache, and stiff neck. Viral meningitis is preceded by a nonspecific prodrome including fever, malaise, sore throat, and myalgias. Unless complicated by encephalitis, symptoms of most viral CNS infections generally resolve over 2 to 4 days and may improve after LP. In bacterial meningitis, the prodromal phase is absent and the fever is generally quite high. Mental status changes, focal neurologic signs, ataxia, seizures, and shock are not uncommon. Lyme meningitis is characterized by low-grade fever, headache, stiff neck, and photophobia developing over the course of 1 to 2 weeks. Cranial nerve palsies may occur.

Physical Examination

Patients with bacterial meningitis often appear toxic and may be hypertensive, bradycardic, and even apneic. Mental status changes and seizures can also occur. In older children, signs of increased intracranial pressure include cranial nerve palsies and papilledema. Nuchal rigidity and positive **Kernig** (flexion of the leg at the hip with subsequent pain on knee extension) and **Brudzinski** (involuntary leg flexion on passive neck flexion) **signs** are markers for meningeal irritation. These findings are rarely present in children younger than 1 year. Infants may present with a bulging fontanelle. A rash is often present in instances of *N. meningitidis* (petechial or purpuric) and Lyme (erythema migrans) CNS infections.

DIFFERENTIAL DIAGNOSIS

The differential diagnosis includes encephalitis, which may develop concurrently or subsequently (see Chapter 15). Other conditions that may present with a similar clinical picture include drug intoxication or side effects, recent anoxia or hypoxia, primary or metastatic CNS malignancy, bacterial endocarditis with septic embolism, intracranial hemorrhage/hematoma, malignant hypertension, and demyelination disorders.

DIAGNOSTIC EVALUATION

CSF analysis is diagnostic. Tests include cell counts and differential, Gram stain, glucose and protein levels, and culture. Bacteria are detected on Gram stain in 80%

■ TABLE 12-6 Cerebrospinal Fluid Findings Suggesting a Specific Etiology for Meningitis in Childhood

CSF Parameter	Bacterial	Viral	Lyme
WBCs/mm³	>1200	<500	<100
Neutrophils	>75%	<50%ᵃ	<30%
Protein	↑↑	Normal or ↑	Normal or ↑
Glucose	↓ or ↓↓	Normal	Normal

ᵃNeutrophils may predominate early in the course of viral meningitis; mononuclear cells usually predominate in Lyme meningitis.
↑, mild increase; ↑↑, moderate or severe increase; ↓, mild decrease; ↓↓, moderate or severe decrease.

of cases of bacterial meningitis. PCR assays for CSF HSV, enteroviruses, and Lyme's disease are available and are highly sensitive and specific. Table 12-6 describes CSF findings that suggest a specific etiology. Because of the potential for brainstem herniation, LP should not be attempted in a child with focal neurologic deficits and/or increased intracranial pressure until an expanding mass lesion is excluded by CT or MRI. Other contraindications include cardiopulmonary instability and skin infection overlying the LP site.

TREATMENT

When the diagnosis of uncomplicated viral meningitis is unequivocal, hospitalization is generally not necessary. If bacterial meningitis cannot be excluded, the patient should be hospitalized for intravenous antibiotic therapy.

Vancomycin plus a third-generation cephalosporin (cefotaxime or ceftriaxone) achieve therapeutic levels in the CSF and provide broad-spectrum coverage of the most likely pathogens in infants and older children. Neonates should be treated with ampicillin to treat group B streptococci and *L. monocytogenes*; cefotaxime is added to treat gram-negative pathogens. Once an organism and its susceptibility pattern are known, antibiotic coverage may be adjusted. The course of therapy for bacterial meningitis is usually 10 to 14 days. Exceptions include meningococcal meningitis (5 to 7 days), Lyme meningitis (14 to 28 days), and neonatal meningitis (14 to 21 days). Corticosteroids are often added during the first 2 days of therapy for bacterial meningitis to decrease the inflammatory response and limit CNS tissue damage.

The current mortality rate for bacterial meningitis is 30% for neonates and less than 5% for infants and older children. However, 10% to 20% of patients experience some persistent neurologic deficit, most commonly hearing loss, developmental delay, motor incoordination, seizures, and hydrocephalus.

🔑 12-9 KEY POINTS

1. Meningitis may be septic (bacterial) or aseptic.
2. Immunization with Hib vaccine has dramatically decreased the incidence of childhood meningitis. The conjugate pneumococcal vaccine appears to be associated with a decreased frequency of pneumococcal meningitis among infants and young children.
3. LP is invaluable in the diagnosis and development of a treatment strategy of meningitis.
4. New PCR-based assays facilitate the diagnosis of HSV, enteroviral, and Lyme CNS infections.
5. Appropriate empirical antibiotic choices for presumed bacterial meningitis are ampicillin and cefotaxime (in the neonate) and vancomycin and a second- or third-generation cephalosporin (in the child).

GASTROENTERITIS

Pathogens cause diarrhea by a variety of mechanisms. For example, some bacteria invade intestinal tissue directly, whereas others secrete injurious toxins before or after ingestion. Viruses, parasites, and protozoa also are capable of inflicting disease. Excessive stooling causes dehydration, inadequate nutrition, and electrolyte abnormalities, all of which are poorly tolerated in infants and small children.

CLINICAL MANIFESTATIONS

History

The history should include information about symptoms in other family members, recent travel, medication use, immune status, day-care attendance, source of drinking water, contact with animals, duration of symptoms, fever, and number, color, and character of stools.

The most common **bacterial** causes of gastroenteritis include *Salmonella* species, *Shigella* species, *Escherichia coli*, *Yersinia enterocolitica*, and *Campylobacter jejuni*; *Vibrio cholerae* may be acquired during travel to developing nations and from eating undercooked Gulf Coast shellfish. Patients with bacterial diarrhea present with fever, significant abdominal cramping, malaise, and tenesmus; vomiting is less common. The stools contain mucous and may be guaiac positive or streaked with blood. Occasionally, children with shigellosis present with **neurologic** manifestations (lethargy, seizures, mental status changes), possibly caused by a neurotoxin elaborated by the organism. *Salmonella* species are capable of invading the bloodstream and causing extraintestinal disease, including meningitis and osteomyelitis (particularly in children with sickle cell disease). *Shigella dysenteriae* and *E. coli* O157:H7 produce an enterotoxin (Shiga or Shigalike toxin) associated with **hemolytic uremic syndrome**, a serious complication consisting of microangiopathic hemolytic anemia, nephropathy, and thrombocytopenia. Almost 25% of individuals infected with *Y. enterocolitica* develop subsequent **erythema nodosum**. In some patients, particularly those with *Yersinia*, severe pain localizes to the right lower quadrant, creating a "pseudoappendicitis" picture.

In cholera, the stools quickly become colorless and flecked with mucus, termed "rice-water" stools. Severe diarrhea leading to hypovolemic shock may develop in hours to a few days.

Rotavirus is the major cause of nonbacterial gastroenteritis in infants and toddlers in the Western world. Infections peak between January and April. Complaints include profuse diarrhea, vomiting, and low-grade fever. Severe diarrhea may lead to significant dehydration, acidosis, and electrolyte disturbances.

Giardiasis is the most commonly reported parasitic disease in the United States. More water-related outbreaks of diarrhea are caused by *Giardia lamblia* than any other organism. The illness presents with frequent, foul-smelling, watery stools that rarely contain blood or mucus; abdominal pain, nausea, vomiting, anorexia, and flatulence often accompany the diarrhea. Symptoms generally resolve within 5 to 7 days, although some cases linger for more than a month. Patients with chronic giardiasis are at risk for failure to thrive resulting from ongoing malabsorption.

Physical Examination

The main goals of the physical examination are estimating the degree of dehydration (see Chapter 7), judging the stability of the patient's condition, identifying findings that may point to a specific infectious or noninfectious etiology, and ruling out a surgical condition.

DIFFERENTIAL DIAGNOSIS

Acute diarrhea in childhood is usually caused by infection. Other conditions associated with diarrhea include malabsorption, celiac disease, antibiotic use, cystic fibrosis, and inflammatory bowel disease.

DIAGNOSTIC EVALUATION

Electrolyte and renal function studies (Na^+, K^+, Cl^-, CO_3^-, BUN, creatinine) guide replacement therapy in significantly dehydrated children (see Chapter 7). Abdominal radiographs, if obtained, are generally normal or nonspecific. Blood, mucus, and fecal leukocytes suggest a bacterial origin for the illness. Blood culture should be performed at the time of initial evaluation if bacterial disease is suspected. Bacterial stool culture results take several days but are helpful in determining the need for antibiotics. If there is a history of antibiotic use, stool should be tested for *Clostridium difficile* toxins A and B. Rapid antigen testing is available for rotavirus. If *G. lamblia* infection is suspected, multiple stool samples from different times should be examined for cysts. Immunofluorescent antibody detection in stool can also be used to diagnose *G. lamblia* infection. Endoscopic biopsy may be indicated if the diarrhea becomes chronic and no etiology has been identified.

TREATMENT

Treatment incorporates oral rehydration whenever possible; aggressive parenteral therapy may be required in severe cases. Antidiarrheal agents are to be avoided in children.

Unless the patient is a febrile infant younger than 12 months or appears toxic, antibiotics should generally be withheld pending culture results. Antibiotic therapy prolongs *Salmonella* shedding and should be reserved for systemic infections. Antibiotics may enhance the likelihood of development of hemolytic uremic syndrome among patients with diarrhea caused by *E. coli* O157:H7. If symptoms persist once culture results are known, antibiotic therapy should be considered. Trimethoprim-sulfamethoxazole is usually effective in treating shigellosis. Erythromycin is the treatment of choice for *C. jejuni*. Patients with *C. difficile* enterocolitis usually improve with suspension of antibiotic therapy, but if treatment is warranted, metronidazole is the treatment of choice. Patients with giardiasis may also be treated with oral metronidazole.

As long as the patient does not develop hypovolemic shock, prognosis for full recovery is excellent. Even in life-threatening cases, appropriate management may prevent permanent sequelae.

🔑 12-10 KEY POINTS

1. Infectious diarrhea may be bacterial, viral, parasitic, or toxin mediated.
2. Careful fluid and electrolyte management is the most important treatment in infectious diarrhea.
3. Children with shigellosis may present with mental status changes.
4. *S. dysenteriae* and *E. coli* O157:H7 are associated with hemolytic uremic syndrome.

HEPATITIS

PATHOGENESIS

Acute hepatic inflammation in children can be caused by a large number of infectious and noninfectious causes. Viruses that are primarily hepatropic include hepatitis A virus (HAV), hepatitis B virus (HBV), hepatitis C virus (HCV), hepatitis D virus (HDV, formerly delta hepatitis), and hepatitis E virus (HEV). Table 12-7 compares features of HAV, HBV, and HCV.

EPIDEMIOLOGY

HAV and HEV are acquired via fecal–oral transmission. Hepatitis A is the most common infectious cause of jaundice in children. HBV, HCV, and HDV are transmitted by percutaneous or mucosal exposure to infectious body fluids and by vertical transmission from an infected mother to her infant. HDV, or delta antigen, consists of single-stranded RNA. It is a "defective" virus in that it requires the presence of an active HBV infection to replicate. HBV and HCV can persist for many years following acute infection. This "carrier state" is associated with development of hepatocellular carcinoma. The incidence of hepatitis B infection is decreasing in the pediatric population because of routine vaccination against hepatitis B in infancy.

RISK FACTORS

Intravenous drug users, those who have unprotected sex with multiple partners, and those who receive

TABLE 12-7 Viruses Responsible for Hepatitis: Comparison and Summary

Feature	Hepatitis A	Hepatitis B	Hepatitis C
Virus type	RNA	DNA	RNA
Incubation (days)	15–45	45–180	7–180
Period of infectivity	Late incubation to early symptomatic state	When HBsAg seropositive	Unknown
Fulminant hepatitis	<1%	1%–3%	1%
Chronic hepatitis	No	5%–10% of adults; 25% 50% of infants; 90% of neonates whose mothers are HBeAg⁺	50%
Diagnostic evaluation	Anti-HAV IgM	HBsAg, HBeAg, anti-HBs, anti-HBc, anti-HBe	Anti-HCV antibody, HCV PCR

anti-HBc, total antibody to hepatitis B core antigen; anti-HBe, total antibody to hepatitis B e antigen; anti-HBs, total antibody to hepatitis B surface antigen; HAV, hepatitis A virus; HBeAg, hepatitis B e antigen; HBsAg, hepatitis B surface antigen; HCV, hepatitis C virus.

blood transfusions are at increased risk of contracting HBV, HCV, and HDV. Risk factors for HAV and HEV include foreign travel, poor sanitation, and contact with other children in day care.

CLINICAL MANIFESTATIONS

History

Perinatally infected infants are usually asymptomatic. Clinical signs of acute hepatitis include anorexia, nausea, malaise, vomiting, jaundice, dark urine, abdominal pain, and low-grade fever. Children with HAV and HEV may also have diarrhea. However, a wide range of severity exists, and as many as 30% to 50% of infected children are asymptomatic. HBV and HCV infection are usually silent, in that the patient complains of no symptoms unless chronic infection has caused significant hepatic damage.

Physical Examination

Scleral icterus and jaundice are noted in some older children with HAV, 50% of children with HBV, and 20% to 30% of children with HCV. Hepatomegaly and right upper-quadrant tenderness may be present. A benign-appearing rash may appear early in the course.

DIFFERENTIAL DIAGNOSIS

EBV, CMV, enterovirus, and other viral infections can also cause hepatitis, but other organ systems are usually involved. Jaundice may also result from autoimmune hepatitis, metabolic liver disease, biliary tract disorders, and drug ingestions.

DIAGNOSTIC EVALUATION

Liver enzymes are uniformly elevated in hepatitis. Because the clinical manifestations are so similar, specific serologic tests are indispensable for securing an accurate diagnosis. The presence of anti-HAV IgM antibody confirms HAV infection (Fig. 12-4). Tests are also available to detect antibodies to the delta antigen.

Three different particles may be found in the serum of patients infected with HBV. The Dane particle is the largest, made up of a core antigen (HBcAg) and envelope antigen (HBeAg) surrounded by a spherical shell of HBsAg ("surface") particles. Figure 12-5 and Table 12-8 present the clinical course and serologic

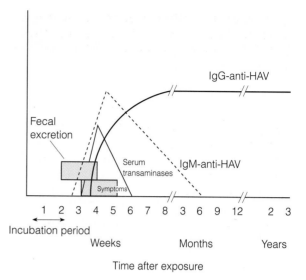

Figure 12-4 • The course of acute hepatitis A.

markers important in diagnosing HBV disease stage. Anti-HBs heralds resolution of the illness and confers lifelong immunity.

HCV antibody is present in both acute and chronic infection. HCV RNA can be detected by PCR within 1 week of infection, whereas the "window period" from infection to antibody response for HCV may be as long as 12 weeks. Therefore, the presence of HCV RNA in the absence of antibody response indicates acute infection. Recovery is characterized by disappearance of HCV RNA from the blood.

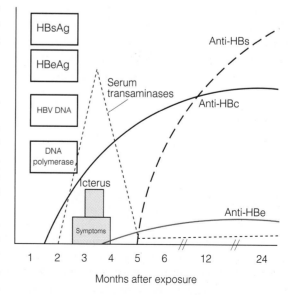

Figure 12-5 • The course of acute hepatitis B.

TABLE 12-8 Comparison of Disease States in Hepatitis B Virus

Test	Acute HBV	Resolved HBV	Chronic HBV
HBsAg	+	–	+
Anti-HBs	–	+	–
Anti-HBc	+	+	+
HBeAg	±	–	±
Anti-HBe	–	+	±

anti-HBc, total antibody to hepatitis B core antigen; anti-HBe, total antibody to hepatitis B e antigen; anti-HBs, total antibody to hepatitis B surface antigen; HBeAg, hepatitis B e antigen; HBsAg, hepatitis B surface antigen; HBV, hepatitis B virus.

TREATMENT

Both active and passive forms of immunization are available, depending on the source of infection. HAV immunization is recommended for all children in some parts of the United States where infection rates are relatively high. HAV immunoglobulin prevents clinical disease when administered within 14 days of exposure. The HBV vaccine series is recommended for all infants in the United States. Infants of infected mothers should receive both the vaccine and the HBV immunoglobulin at delivery to prevent the disease and development of the carrier state. Interferon alpha and lamivudine (a nucleoside analogue) are used to treat pediatric patients with chronic HBV hepatitis. There is no specific treatment for HDV. Interferon alpha may be effective in preventing conversion from acute to chronic HCV hepatitis in certain subsets of patients. No specific therapy is known for HEV.

The prognosis for patients with hepatitis depends on the virus responsible.

- *HAV*: Very few patients develop fulminant hepatitis, but the mortality rate among those who do is almost 50%.
- *HBV*: HBV may persist as chronic hepatitis, and the course may be relatively benign or more severe. Chronic persistent hepatitis B is characterized by little cellular inflammation and usually resolves within a year. Chronic active hepatitis is more aggressive, progressing to cirrhosis and increasing the risk of hepatocellular carcinoma.

Chronic infection is more likely among infected children than adults.
- *HDV*: When HDV and HBV are acquired simultaneously, the recipient is at greater risk for more severe chronic hepatitis B and fulminant hepatitis associated with a higher mortality rate. When an individual is infected with HDV on top of pre-existing HBV, acute exacerbation and an accelerated course result. The risk of progressing to cirrhotic liver disease is also increased when HDV is present.
- *HCV*: Half of those infected with HCV develop chronic hepatitis with an increased risk for cirrhosis.
- *HEV*: HEV does not appear to result in chronic hepatitis.

🔑 12-11 KEY POINTS

1. HAV and HEV are spread via fecal-oral transmission. HBV, HCV, and HDV are transmitted through infected bodily fluids.
2. Clinical signs of acute hepatitis include anorexia, nausea, malaise, vomiting, jaundice, dark urine, abdominal pain, and low-grade fever. However, a wide range of severity exists, and as many as 30% to 50% of infected children are asymptomatic.
3. Liver enzymes are uniformly elevated in hepatitis. Because the clinical manifestations are so similar, specific serologic tests are indispensable for securing an accurate diagnosis.

SYPHILIS

PATHOGENESIS

Syphilis is primarily a sexually transmitted disease (STD) resulting from infection with the spirochete *Treponema pallidum*.

EPIDEMIOLOGY

Syphilis in the pediatric population may be acquired transplacentally (congenital syphilis) or through sexual contact. The incidence of syphilis has increased sharply over the last several years. Coinfection with other STDs is common.

RISK FACTORS

Neonates born to a mother with untreated infection are at risk for congenital syphilis. Adolescents and adults who have unprotected sex with an infected partner or multiple partners are at risk for primary syphilis.

CLINICAL MANIFESTATIONS

History and Physical Examination

Approximately half of infants with congenital syphilis die shortly before or after birth. Those who survive are often asymptomatic at birth but develop symptoms within 1 month if untreated. Infants with congenital syphilis may have hepatomegaly, splenomegaly, mucocutaneous lesions, jaundice, lymphadenopathy, and the characteristic **snuffles**, a bloody, mucopurulent nasal discharge. Other findings include deafness and retardation.

Syphilis acquired through sexual contact progresses through three stages. After a 2- to 4-week incubation period, infected individuals enter the **primary** stage of syphilis, characterized by the classic chancre at the inoculation site: a well-demarcated, firm, strangely painless genital ulcer with an indurated base. Because the lesion heals spontaneously within 3 to 6 weeks, patients with primary syphilis often do not seek medical attention.

Thirty percent of untreated patients develop **secondary** syphilis, manifested by widespread dermatologic involvement coinciding with dissemination of the spirochete throughout the body. Onset follows the primary stage directly, often while the chancre is still present. The typical rash consists of generalized (including the soles and palms) erythematous macules (3–10 mm) that progress to papules. Some patients also develop systemic symptoms including fever, malaise, pharyngitis, mucosal ulcerations, and generalized lymphadenopathy; patchy alopecia and thinning of the lateral third of the eyebrow are also associated with secondary syphilis. Symptoms of secondary syphilis resolve in 1 to 3 months.

Tertiary syphilis develops years after primary exposure and is rare in the pediatric population. Granulomatous lesions called **gummas** destroy surrounding tissues, especially in the skin, bone, heart, and CNS. Unfortunately, tertiary syphilis may occur without any previous primary or secondary manifestations.

DIFFERENTIAL DIAGNOSIS

Syphilis is one of the great masqueraders, a disease with a wide spectrum of presentation. The presence of the rash, if characteristic, greatly aids in diagnosis.

DIAGNOSTIC EVALUATION

Chancre scrapings (and mucosal secretions in infected neonates) demonstrate rapidly mobile organisms moving in a corkscrewlike motion under dark-field microscopy. Aspiration of enlarged lymph nodes may also yield the organism. Both the VDRL (developed by the Venereal Disease Research Laboratory of the U.S. Public Health Service) and the RPR are excellent blood screening tests for high-risk populations, providing rapid, inexpensive, quantitative results. Both are nontreponemal tests for antibodies to a lipoidal molecule rather than the organism itself. Both are considered highly sensitive when titers are high or when the test is complemented by historical or physical evidence of the disease. However, infectious mononucleosis, connective tissue disease, endocarditis, and tuberculosis may all result in false-positive VDRL and RPR results. By contrast, treponemal tests, such as the fluorescent treponemal antibody absorption (FTA-ABS) and microhemagglutination assay for *T. pallidum* (MHA-TP), are much less likely to produce false positives, unless Lyme's disease is present. A positive screening VDRL or RPR coupled with a positive FTA-ABS in a newborn or sexually active adolescent is virtually diagnostic of untreated syphilis. Nontreponemal tests may become negative after treatment, whereas treponemal studies remain positive for life.

Neonates with suspected congenital syphilis require LP. CSF pleocytosis and elevated protein suggest neurosyphilis, but a positive CSF VDRL is diagnostic. Infants may develop radiographic abnormalities of the long bones. Anemia and thrombocytopenia may also develop in untreated infants.

TREATMENT

Parenteral penicillin G (IM or intravenous) remains the treatment of choice for any stage of infection and fully eradicates the organism from the body. Doxycycline may be used for those who are allergic to penicillin.

GENITAL HERPES SIMPLEX VIRUS INFECTION

Genital herpes usually results from infection with herpes simplex virus type 2 (in 90% of cases). Small mucosal tears or skin cracks are inoculated with the virus, usually during sexual activity. Genital herpes is one of the most common sexually acquired diseases; 10% to 25% of adults have a history suggestive of prior genital herpes infection. Transmission of HSV from mother to infant at the time of birth may result in devastating infection in the newborn.

CLINICAL MANIFESTATIONS

History and Physical Examination

After a variable incubation period (5 to 14 days), genital burning and itching progress to vesicular, often pustular, lesions. These burst to form painful shallow ulcers that heal without scarring. Fever, pharyngitis, headache, and malaise may accompany the primary episode. After acquisition, the virus ascends peripheral nerves to dorsal root ganglia, where it may lie latent or recur periodically. Recurrences have fewer symptoms than the primary episode, and asymptomatic shedding does occur.

DIAGNOSTIC EVALUATION

Giant multinucleated cells with intranuclear inclusions are found in scrapings from the ulcerous base (Tzanck testing). HSV may be cultured from the active lesions in 1 to 4 days; rapid antigen and PCR testing are also available.

TREATMENT

Oral antiviral agents (including acyclovir) diminish the length of both symptoms and shedding but do not eradicate the organism. They has limited efficacy in recurrent episodes. Continued prophylactic use of oral acyclovir prevents or reduces the frequency of recurrences.

PELVIC INFLAMMATORY DISEASE

PATHOGENESIS

Pelvic inflammatory disease (PID) is a constellation of signs and symptoms related to the ascending spread of pathogenic organisms from the lower female genital tract (vagina, cervix) to the endometrium, fallopian tubes, and contiguous structures.

EPIDEMIOLOGY

PID is generally polymicrobial, with *Chlamydia trachomatis* and *Neisseria gonorrhoeae* by far the most commonly isolated organisms. Other potential causes of PID include some anaerobes and other gram-negative organisms. Barrier contraceptive methods are protective. *N. gonorrhoeae* or genital *C. trachomatis* infection in a prepubertal child strongly suggests sexual abuse.

RISK FACTORS

Adolescence is a period of increased risk for development of PID because of the presence of cervical ectopy and the increased incidence of high-risk behavior in the teenage years. Risk factors also include sexual intercourse with multiple partners, unprotected intercourse, and a preexisting mucosal STD.

CLINICAL MANIFESTATIONS

The clinical diagnosis of PID is based on the presence of one of three **required** *and* one of several **supporting** symptoms:

- *Required*: Lower abdominal (uterine) pain and tenderness, cervical motion tenderness, or adnexal tenderness
- *Supporting*: Temperature greater than 38.3°C (101°F), elevated ESR or C-reactive protein, presence of WBCs on culdocentesis, intracellular

gram-negative diplococci found on endocervical smear, WBCs found on culdocentesis, laboratory evidence of *N. gonorrhoeae* or *C. trachomatis* at the cervix, abnormal cervical or vaginal mucopurulent discharge

History and Physical Examination

Other symptoms may include cramping, vaginal discharge or bleeding, nausea/vomiting, and malaise. The physical exam may be positive for peritoneal signs if the disease is severe.

DIAGNOSTIC EVALUATION

Nucleic acid amplification tests are sensitive and specific for both gonorrhea and chlamydia. If a patient is suspected of having PID, she should be tested for syphilis, HIV, typical vaginosis organisms, and other STDs. It is not uncommon not to identify a specific pathogen responsible for PID because PID is an upper genital tract disease, whereas samples are routinely taken from the lower tract.

DIFFERENTIAL DIAGNOSIS

Other gynecologic conditions and intra-abdominal pathology are included in the differential diagnosis:

* *Gynecologic*: mucopurulent cervicitis, ectopic pregnancy, ruptured ovarian cyst, septic abortion, endometriosis
* *Nongynecologic*: Appendicitis, pyelonephritis, inflammatory bowel disease

Patients with suspected PID should always receive a pregnancy test, both because treatment may need to be altered and because ectopic pregnancy is a life-threatening condition that must be ruled out.

TREATMENT

Patients with clinical PID should be treated for both *N. gonorrhoeae* and *C. trachomatis*. Coverage against anaerobes and other gram-negative organisms (such as metronidazole or clindamycin) is also desirable. A single dose of a long-acting parenteral third-generation cephalosporin, such as ceftriaxone or cefotaxime, is sufficient to eradicate *N. gonorrhoeae*. A 14-day course of oral doxycycline eradicates *C. trachomatis*. An alternative treatment for both organisms consists of oral ofloxacin or levofloxacin for 14 days. Significant infections require more extensive courses of therapy. All patients who are released for outpatient treatment should return for a follow-up visit within 72 hours. Sexual contacts need to be treated to avoid reinfection.

Patients who are admitted to the hospital for severe illness, vomiting, pregnancy, blood pressure instability, or a possible surgical condition should receive therapy with intravenous antibiotics, including both cefotetan or cefoxitin and doxycycline. An alternative regimen consists of clindamycin and gentamicin.

Twenty percent of infected women become infertile after a single episode of PID. Other gynecologic complications include increased risks for ectopic pregnancy, dyspareunia, chronic pelvic pain, and adhesions.

N. gonorrhoeae is capable of invading the bloodstream and thus any organ system. Joint involvement is most common. The **arthritis** may affect only one joint or may be polyarticular and migratory with associated tenosynovitis and skin lesions. Although *C. trachomatis* seldom causes systemic illness, untreated individuals may go on to develop **Reiter's syndrome** (a constellation of urethritis, conjunctivitis, and arthritis). **Fitz-Hugh-Curtis's syndrome**, a form of perihepatitis, is a known complication of infection with either organism.

🔑 12-13 KEY POINTS

1. *C. trachomatis* and *N. gonorrhoeae* are the most commonly isolated organisms in pelvic inflammatory disease (PID).
2. The diagnosis of PID is clinical, based on history, physical examination, and supporting laboratory results.
3. A single does of a parenteral cephalosporin (for *N. gonorrhoeae*) and 14 days of oral doxycycline (for *C. trachomatis*) constitute appropriate outpatient therapy in mild infections. Ideally, metronidazole is added for anaerobe and gram-negative coverage.

VULVOVAGINAL INFECTIONS

Trichomoniasis, bacterial vaginosis, and *Candida* vaginitis are all bothersome but relatively benign vaginal infections collectively manifested by changes in the amount and character of vaginal secretions. All three are easily diagnosed during the office visit by examination of vaginal fluid samples.

CLINICAL MANIFESTATIONS AND TREATMENT

Trichomoniasis

Trichomoniasis results from sexually transmitted *Trichomonas vaginalis*, a mobile flagellated protozoan. Most infected individuals remain asymptomatic, although urethritis is not uncommon in men. Typical symptoms in women include a malodorous, frothy gray discharge and vaginal discomfort. Some patients also develop dysuria and vague lower abdominal pain. The cervix and vaginal mucosa may be either normal or visibly irritated and inflamed. A fresh wet preparation of the vaginal fluid reveals polymorphonuclear leukocytes and the characteristic motile trichomonads. Oral metronidazole twice daily for 7 days is the treatment of choice for patients and their partners. Metronidazole gel and clindamycin gel are alternatives.

Bacterial Vaginosis

Bacterial vaginosis, long thought to be harmless, is now known to increase the risks of PID, chorioamnionitis, and premature birth. Bacterial vaginosis is caused by *Gardnerella vaginalis*, *Mycoplasma hominis*, and various anaerobic organisms. The epidemiology of the disease suggests sexual transmission, although the data remain unclear. Infection is usually asymptomatic except for a thin, white, foul-smelling discharge that emits a "fishy" odor when mixed with potassium hydroxide. The clinical diagnosis is based on patient history (much more common in sexually active females), the appearance and odor of discharge, a vaginal pH greater than 4.5, and characteristic "clue" cells on the wet prep (squamous epithelial cells with "smudged" borders caused by adherent bacteria). A single oral dose of metronidazole effectively cures the infection. Concurrent antibiotic treatment of male partners seems to have no effect on recurrence rates.

Vaginal Candidiasis

Vulvovaginal candidiasis is not a STD. All women are colonized with *Candida*; however, factors such as antibiotic use, pregnancy, diabetes, immunosuppression, and oral contraceptive use predispose women to candidal overgrowth (moniliasis). Signs and symptoms include a thick white vaginal discharge with vaginal itching and burning. Yeast and pseudohyphae are evident on wet preparation treated with potassium hydroxide. Over-the-counter topical antifungal creams are safe and generally effective. A single dose of oral fluconazole is an alternative.

🔑 12-14 KEY POINTS

1. Trichomoniasis is diagnosed by demonstrating motile trichomonads on fresh wet preparation and is treated with oral metronidazole twice daily for 7 days.
2. Bacterial vaginosis, often caused by *Gardnerella vaginalis* or *M. hominis*, should be suspected when the vaginal pH is greater than 4.5 and clue cells are seen on wet preparation. A single dose of oral metronidazole is effective treatment.

URETHRITIS

Urethritis is inflammation of the urethra caused by infection with a STD. It occurs much more commonly in adolescent males than females. *N. gonorrhoeae* and *C. trachomatis* are the most important pathogens. Symptoms include urethral discharge, itching, dysuria, and urinary frequency. Asymptomatic infections are common. The disease is diagnosed by notation of at least one of the following: mucoid or purulent urethral discharge; positive leukocyte esterase test or WBCs on microscopic examination of a first-void urine; and gram-negative intracellular diplococci on Gram stain. Patients with suspected urethritis should receive testing for other STDS including syphilis, *T. vaginalis*, and HIV. If gonorrhea is ruled out, the patient may be treated with one dose of oral azithromycin or 7 days of oral doxycycline. If *N. gonorrhoeae* is a consideration, IM ceftriaxone should be given in the office. Complications are rare.

HUMAN IMMUNODEFICIENCY VIRUS AND ACQUIRED IMMUNODEFICIENCY SYNDROME

PATHOGENESIS

HIV is a retrovirus that infects CD4 T lymphocytes. It remains latent until the T cell is stimulated by an antigen. The viral genome then replicates, filling the cell with viral proteins until it ruptures and the proteins go on to infect other cells. HIV produces a wide range of clinical manifestations in children, the most severe of which is AIDS. A child is defined as having AIDS when an AIDS-defining illness occurs (see later) or when the CD4+ lymphocyte count is less than a defined number for age (e.g., <200 per mm^3 for children older than 12 years).

EPIDEMIOLOGY

The disease is more common in urban populations, lower socioeconomic classes, and racial minorities. Most infections in children are acquired in utero or perinatally (>90%). The risk of HIV transmission from a seropositive mother to her fetus is approximately 25%. Treatment of infected pregnant women with zidovudine (AZT; a reverse transcriptase inhibitor) alone or in combination with other anti-retrovirals during the second and third trimesters, followed by treatment of the infant for the first 6 weeks of life, reduces the vertical transmission rate to approximately 2%. Asymptomatic HIV-positive women may not realize they are infected, and therefore they often do not receive therapy.

As a group, the adolescent population has the most rapidly increasing rate of HIV infection in the United States.

RISK FACTORS

Risk factors include birth to an HIV-positive mother, birth to a woman who uses intravenous drugs and shares needles, and birth to a woman with multiple sexual partners who does not practice safe sex. Other groups at risk include patients who received multiple units of blood products (e.g., hemophiliacs) before March 1985, victims of sexual abuse, and adolescents who engage in high-risk behavior (intravenous drug use or unprotected sexual activity with multiple partners).

CLINICAL MANIFESTATIONS

History and Physical Examination

HIV may present in infants and children with any one or several of the following signs and symptoms: generalized lymphadenopathy, hepatomegaly, splenomegaly, failure to thrive, recurrent or chronic diarrhea, oral candidiasis, parotitis, and developmental delay. Respiratory manifestations include lymphoid interstitial pneumonia (LIP) and *Pneumocystis jiroveci* pneumonia (PCP). Regression in developmental milestones and progressive encephalopathy may occur. Cardiomyopathy and nephropathy also occur. Recurrent, often severe, bacterial and opportunistic (fungal, disseminated HSV or CMV, and *Mycobacterium avium*) infections are the hallmark of the acquired helper T-cell immunodeficiency.

A significant percentage of infected adolescents present with a mononucleosis-type syndrome within 6 weeks of HIV acquisition. Symptoms and signs include sore throat, fatigue, fever, rash, and cervical or diffuse lymphadenopathy.

PCP and LIP are two of several AIDS-defining illnesses in the pediatric population. When any of these conditions occurs, the child is considered to have AIDS regardless of the absolute CD4 count.

DIFFERENTIAL DIAGNOSIS

HIV has become known as a "great masquerader" because of its variable presentation; the virus can affect any organ system, and symptoms are often nonspecific. A high degree of suspicion is required to diagnose the disease at an asymptomatic or early stage when it is most easily contained.

DIAGNOSTIC EVALUATION

Infants born to HIV-positive mothers are always seropositive for maternally derived IgG antibodies to the virus (i.e., ELISA and Western blot testing are always positive); these tests are not helpful in children younger than 18 months. If the mother is HIV positive, HIV DNA PCR or HIV culture of the infant's blood should be performed at birth. If this test is positive on two separate occasions, the infant is considered HIV positive. Negative tests should be repeated at regular intervals (1, 3, and 6 months of age). The combination of HIV DNA PCR and HIV culture detects 98% of all positive infants by 1 month of age and more than 99% by 4 months of age.

TREATMENT

The standard of care consists of nucleoside analogue reverse transcriptase inhibitor drugs such as AZT (zidovudine) and ddI (didanosine), nonnucleoside analogue reverse transcriptase inhibitors (NNRTIs), and protease inhibitors. Trimethoprim-sulfamethoxazole provides prophylaxis against PCP, the most common opportunistic infection. Prophylaxis against CMV and *Mycobacterium avium-intracellulare* may also be recommended. New pharmacologic therapies have drastically improved the chances of converting HIV infection from disease of near-certain death to a chronic lifelong condition.

✎ 12-15 KEY POINTS

1. Most HIV infections in children are acquired in utero or perinatally (>90%); smaller numbers result from early blood product transfusions and sexual transmission.
2. Infants born to HIV-positive mothers are always seropositive for maternally derived IgG antibodies to the virus; thus, the enzyme immunoassays used for screening older populations are not helpful in children younger than 18 months. HIV culture or HIV DNA PCR should be used in this population.
3. The manifestations of pediatric HIV are varied. Children may be asymptomatic or present with any one or several of the following signs and symptoms: adenopathy, hepatomegaly, splenomegaly, failure to thrive, recurrent or chronic diarrhea, oral candidiasis, parotitis, and developmental delay.

VIRAL INFECTIONS OF CHILDHOOD

Viral infections are quite common in the infant and young child but decrease with age because of acquired immunity. Several viral illnesses that are frequently encountered in the pediatric population are not usually seen in adults. Many of these present with characteristic rashes that permit reliable clinical diagnosis. Live attenuated vaccines are routinely administered to prevent measles, mumps, rubella, and varicella (chickenpox).

Roseola and erythema infectiosum are generally benign in children. Table 12-9 describes the typical presentations and complications of these viral illnesses in children, which are discussed further in Chapter 5.

ROCKY MOUNTAIN SPOTTED FEVER

PATHOGENESIS

Rocky Mountain spotted fever (RMSF) is a tick-borne disease caused by *Rickettsia rickettsii*, a gram-negative intracellular bacterium. Rickettsiae are introduced into the skin by a tick bite and subsequently spread via the lymphatics and blood vessels. They invade and multiply within the endothelial and smooth muscle cells of blood vessels, causing thrombosis and increasing vascular permeability (vasculitis).

EPIDEMIOLOGY

RMSF occurs more often between April and September in tick-infested areas of the south Atlantic states (but have been reported year round). Despite the name, none of the top ten states reporting RMSF is near the Rocky Mountains. Tick vectors include the wood tick, dog tick, and Lone Star tick.

RISK FACTORS

The most significant risk factor is residence in or travel to an endemic area during times of the year when ticks are most active.

CLINICAL MANIFESTATIONS

History and Physical Examination

The classic presentation of RMSF includes fever, headache, and rash. Symptoms develop approximately 7 days after a tick bite. Initial symptoms often are nonspecific and include fever, chills, headache, malaise, nausea, vomiting, and myalgias. The rash begins on the third or fourth day and consists of

TABLE 12-9	Presentations and Complications of Childhood Viral Illnesses		
Virus	**Exanthem**	**Other Features**	**Complications**
Measles	Confluent, erythematous maculopapular rash that starts on head and progresses caudally	Coryza, cough, conjunctivitis, Koplik spots (on buccal mucosa early in disease)	Pneumonia, myocarditis, encephalitis; rare: subacute sclerosing panencephalitis
Mumps	None	Swollen salivary glands, especially parotid glands	Orchitis, pancreatitis; rare: meningitis, encephalitis
Rubella	Similar to measles but does not coalesce	Suboccipital and posterior auricular lymphadenopathy	Polyarticular arthritis or arthralgias; rare: encephalitis
Roseola (human herpesvirus 6)	Maculopapular	High fever resolves as rash appears	Febrile seizures; rare: meningoencephalitis
Erythema infectiosum (fifth disease; parvovirus B19)	Facial erythema giving "slapped cheeks" appearance followed by spread to extremities in reticular pattern	Transient aplastic crisis in child with hemoglobinopathy	Arthritis; rare: encephalitis
Chickenpox (varicella)	Pruritic, erythematous macules evolve to vesicles and then crust over; begins on face and spreads to extremities	As initial lesions resolve, new crops form so lesions in different stages are observed simultaneously	Secondary bacterial infection; rare: pneumonia, cerebellar ataxia, encephalitis, hepatitis

blanching, erythematous, macular lesions that progress to form petechiae or purpura. It characteristically appears initially on the wrists and ankles and spreads proximally to involve the trunk and head over several hours. Typically, the palms and soles are involved as well. The rash is absent in 5% to 10% of children. Approximately 30% of children have some impairment of mental status.

DIAGNOSTIC EVALUATION

Although immunofluorescent staining of skin biopsies taken from rash sites may demonstrate the organism, there is no reliable diagnostic test that becomes positive early enough in the course of the disease to guide therapy. Thus, the clinician must maintain a high suspicion for the disease. Antibodies to confirm the clinical diagnosis are detectable approximately 10 days after symptom onset. Key laboratory features include thrombocytopenia and hyponatremia; however, these are only present in a minority of patients.

DIFFERENTIAL DIAGNOSIS

RMSF is essentially indistinguishable from ehrlichiosis (another tick-borne illness) and meningococcemia. Because approximately half of patients with RMSF and ehrlichiosis do not remember being bitten by a tick, initial antibiotic therapy for patients with these suspected illnesses and no tick history should include coverage for *N. meningitidis* as well. Atypical measles may present in a similar fashion; knowledge of a local outbreak should clarify this diagnosis.

TREATMENT

Treatment with doxycycline is effective in all age groups. Cefotaxime or ceftriaxone should be added if meningococcemia is a possibility. If RMSF is suspected, antibiotics must not be withheld pending laboratory results. Mortality is higher when treatment is delayed.

🔑 12-16 KEY POINTS

1. Rocky Mountain spotted fever (RMSF) is a tick-borne illness caused by infection with *Rickettsia rickettsii*.
2. The classic presentation of RMSF includes fever, headache, and rash.
3. RMSF is clinically indistinguishable from ehrlichiosis and meningococcemia.
4. The disease is rapidly progressive, and there is no laboratory test that becomes abnormal soon enough in the disease to guide therapy. Treatment should be started based on clinical suspicion alone.
5. Doxycycline is the treatment of choice. Coverage against *N. meningitidis* should be considered when there is no history of a tick bite, especially in the presence of severe disease.

LYME'S DISEASE

PATHOGENESIS

Lyme's disease is a tick-borne illness resulting from infection with the spirochete bacterium *Borrelia burgdorferi*. The pathogen lives in deer ticks (eastern United States) and western black-legged ticks (Pacific states).

EPIDEMIOLOGY

Although cases have been reported across the country, most occur in southern New England, southeastern New York, New Jersey, eastern Pennsylvania, Maryland, Delaware, Minnesota, and Wisconsin. The incidence of Lyme's disease is highest among children 5 to 14 years of age. Cases are usually clustered around the late spring and early summer.

RISK FACTORS

Individuals with increased occupational or recreational exposure to tick-infested woodlands in endemic areas are at highest risk of Lyme's disease. An infected tick must feed for more than 48 hours to transmit *B. burgdorferi*.

CLINICAL MANIFESTATIONS

History

Most patients do not recall a tick bite. The clinical manifestations depend on the stage of the disease: early localized, early disseminated, or late. **Erythema migrans**, the manifestation of **early localized** disease, appears at the site of the tick bite 3 to 30 days after the bite. The rash begins as a red macule or papule and progressively enlarges to form a large, annular, erythematous lesion with central clearing (resembling a bull's-eye) that is up to 10 inches in diameter. The skin lesion often is accompanied by fever, malaise, headache, arthralgias, and myalgias. **Early disseminated** Lyme's disease (days to weeks after tick bite) may manifest as multiple erythema migrans lesions (anywhere on the body), lymphadenopathy, cranial nerve palsy, meningitis, and carditis (heart block). The most common manifestation of **late** Lyme's disease (>6 weeks after tick bite) is arthritis, usually involving the knee.

Physical Examination

The rash, described earlier, may be present. Children with early disseminated Lyme may have multiple erythema migrans lesions, facial nerve palsy, or signs of meningitis (meningismus). Children with Lyme arthritis may have a swollen and tender joint.

DIFFERENTIAL DIAGNOSIS

The differential diagnosis depends on the presentation. When the rash is atypical, it may be confused with erythema multiforme or erythema marginatum (seen in rheumatic fever). The differential diagnosis of arthritis also includes JRA, reactive arthritis, and Reiter's syndrome. The differential diagnosis of Lyme meningitis includes other causes of aseptic meningitis.

DIAGNOSTIC EVALUATION

Testing for Lyme's disease in the presence of vague or nonspecific complaints is not helpful; false-positive test results can occur, especially with ELISA or immunofluorescent antibody testing. For the most part, early localized Lyme's disease is a clinical diagnosis, based on suggestive history and the characteristic rash on physical examination. The organism cannot be reliably cultured from the skin lesions, blood, and other body fluids. Lyme IgM titer is elevated several weeks after the tick bite. Antibodies to *B. burgdorferi* cross-react with other infectious agents, particularly other spirochetes including syphilis, although VDRL and RPR remain negative in patients with Lyme's disease. The Western blot is designed to be specific for antibodies to *B. burgdorferi* but does not usually become positive early enough in the course of disease to guide therapy.

Lyme PCR of CSF (or joint fluid) reliably diagnoses Lyme meningitis (or arthritis). Cardiac involvement, in the form of conduction abnormalities, is rare but can be diagnosed by ECG in conjunction with supporting history and antibody studies.

TREATMENT

Treatment of early localized Lyme's disease prevents early disseminated and late disease, including meningitis and arthritis. Younger children can be treated with oral amoxicillin or cefuroxime. Penicillin-allergic children can be treated with erythromycin. Children older than 8 years should receive oral doxycycline for 14 to 30 days. Children with vomiting or severe arthritis, cardiac disease, or neurologic involvement warrant parenteral therapy with high-dose penicillin G or ceftriaxone. A small minority of patients continue to experience low-grade, chronic symptoms despite appropriate therapy; long-term antibiotic treatment is not helpful in this population.

🔑 12-17 KEY POINTS

1. The classic rash of Lyme disease is erythema migrans.
2. Lyme disease is treated with oral amoxicillin in children younger than 8 years and with oral doxycycline in older children. Lyme meningitis requires intravenous ceftriaxone.

Additional Suggested Reading

Burstein GR, Murray PJ. Diagnosis and management of sexually transmitted diseases among adolescents. *Pediatr Rev.* 2003;24:119–127.

Centers for Disease Control National Immunization Program (NIP) Web site. Available at: http://www.cdc.gov/nip/default.htm

Gaston B. Pneumonia. *Pediatr Rev.* 2002;23: 132–140.

Harrison CJ. How will the new guideline for managing otitis media work in your practice? *Contemp Pediatr.* 2004;21:24–40.

Junker AK. Epstein-Barr virus. *Pediatr Rev.* 2005;26: 79–85.

Malhotra A, Krilov LR. Viral croup. *Pediatr Rev.* 2001;22:5–12.

McCarthy CA, Hall CB. Respiratory syncytial virus: Concerns and control. *Pediatr Rev.* 2003;24: 301–308.

Nash D, Wald E. Sinusitis. *Pediatr Rev.* 2001;22: 111–117.

Razzaq S, Schutze GE. Rocky Mountain spotted fever: a physician's challenge. *Pediatr Rev.* 2005; 26:125–130.

Siegal RM, Bien JP. Acute otitis media in children: A continuing story. *Pediatr Rev.* 2004;25:187–193.

Waggoner-Fountain L, Hayden GF. What's all the "whoop-la?" *Consultant Pediatricians.* 2004;3:184–187.

13 Neonatology

BIRTH

NEONATAL MORTALITY

The late fetal and early neonatal period is the time of life exhibiting the highest mortality rate of any pediatric age interval. The **perinatal mortality rate** refers to fetal deaths occurring from the 20th week of gestation until the 7th day after birth. Intrauterine fetal death (i.e., stillbirth) represents 40% to 50% of the perinatal mortality rate.

The **neonatal mortality rate** includes infants who die between birth and 28 days of life. Modern neonatal intensive care has delayed the mortality of many newborn infants who have life-threatening diseases, so that they survive beyond the neonatal period only to die of their original diseases or of complications of therapy sometime after the 28th day of life. This delayed mortality occurs during the **postneonatal** period, which begins after 28 days of life and extends to the end of the first year of life.

The **infant mortality rate** includes both the neonatal and the postneonatal periods and is expressed as the number of deaths per 1,000 live births. The infant mortality rate in the United States declined in 2000 to 6.9 per 1,000 live births. The rate for African American infants in 2000 remained a distressing 14.0 per 1,000 live births. There were 27 countries with lower infant mortality rates than the United States.

🔑 13-1 KEY POINTS

1. The 2000 infant mortality rate in the United States was higher than 27 other countries, and African American infants were twice as likely to die during the first year of life.

APGAR SCORING

The Apgar examination, a rapid scoring system based on physiologic responses to the birth process, is an excellent method for assessing the need for neonatal resuscitation. It is not generally useful as a prognostic tool. Table 13-1 shows the Apgar scoring system. At 1 and 5 minutes after birth, each of five physiologic parameters is evaluated. Full-term infants with a normal cardiopulmonary transition have a total score of 8 to 9 at 1 and 5 minutes. An Apgar score of 0 to 3 indicates either cardiorespiratory arrest or a condition resulting from severe bradycardia, hypoventilation, and/or CNS depression. Most low Apgar scores are caused by difficulty in establishing adequate ventilation or severe perinatal depression.

BIRTH TRAUMA

CEPHALOHEMATOMA

A cephalohematoma is a traumatic subperiosteal hemorrhage (usually involving the parietal bone) that does not cross suture lines. The scalp hematoma is characteristically firm without discoloration of overlying skin and may not become apparent until hours to days after delivery. Predisposing factors include large head size, prolonged labor, vacuum extraction, and forceps delivery. Spontaneous resolution occurs over several weeks. Two percent of hematomas organize, calcify, and form a central depression in the calvarium. Cephalohematoma dissolution may result in an indirect hyperbilirubinemia requiring phototherapy, especially in a premature infant.

■ TABLE 13-1 Apgar Scoring System			
Physical Exam Evaluated at 1 and 5 Minutes	0 Points	1 Point	2 Points
Heart rate	No pulse	<100	>100
Respiratory effort	No respirations	Irregular, weak cry	Vigorous cry
Color	Pale, cyanotic	Cyanotic extremities	Pink throughout
Muscle tone	Absent	Weak, slightly flexed extremities	Active
Reflex irritability	Absent	Grimace	Active cry and avoidance

CAPUT SUCCEDANEUM

A caput succedaneum is a diffuse, edematous, and often dark swelling of the soft tissue of the scalp that extends across the midline and/or suture lines and is commonly found in infants who are delivered vaginally in the customary occiput-anterior position. Pressure induced from overriding parietal and frontal bones against their respective sutures causes the molding associated with the caput. The caput is commonly seen after prolonged labor in both full-term and premature infants.

FRACTURED CLAVICLE

A fractured clavicle is found in 2% to 3% of vaginal deliveries, and the right clavicle is two times more likely to fracture than the left. This predilection exists because the right shoulder must move beneath the pubic symphysis during normal delivery and may get entrapped. Predisposing factors include large size, shoulder dystocia, and traumatic delivery. On examination, there may be swelling and fullness over the fracture site, crepitus, and decreased arm movement. Of neonates with clavicular fracture, 80% have no symptoms and only minimal physical findings. The injury is often diagnosed when a callus is detected at 3 to 6 weeks of age. Radiograph is not indicated. No specific treatment is necessary. The parents should be advised to avoid tension on the affected arm.

ERB PALSY

Injury to nerves of the brachial plexus results from excessive traction on the neck, producing paresis.

Erb palsy results from stretching of the fifth and sixth cervical nerves. The infant's arm is held in the "waiter's tip" position, where the arm is extended and internally rotated, and the wrist is flexed. When there is an absent Moro reflex in the right arm and the right hand grasp is intact, Erb palsy should be suspected. Ninety percent of these lesions resolve spontaneously by 4 months of age, but if the nerve deficit persists, nerve grafting may be beneficial.

🔑 13-2 KEY POINTS

1. A cephalohematoma is a traumatic subperiosteal hemorrhage that does not cross suture lines.
2. A caput succedaneum is a diffuse, edematous, and often dark swelling of the soft tissue of the scalp that extends across the midline and/or suture lines.
3. Clavicle fractures heal without intervention and are most common in babies with macrosomia and/or shoulder dystocia.
4. Erb palsy results from stretching of the fifth and sixth cervical nerves and should be suspected when there is an absent Moro reflex in the right arm and an intact right hand grasp.

PREMATURITY

Low-birth-weight (LBW) infants, defined as those having birth weights less than 2,500 g, represent a disproportionately large percentage of neonatal and infant deaths. Although these infants make up only 7% of all births, they account for two thirds of all neonatal deaths. Very low-birth-weight (VLBW) infants, weighing less than 1,500 g at birth, represent only approximately 1% of all births but account for 50% of neonatal deaths. In comparison with infants weighing 2,500 g or more, LBW infants are 40 times more likely to die in the neonatal period, and VLBW infants have a 200-fold higher risk of neonatal death.

In contrast to the improvements in the overall infant mortality rate, there has not been improvement in the rate of LBW *births*. This is one reason that the infant mortality rate of the United States is the worst of the large, modern, industrialized countries. If birth-weight mortality rates are calculated, the United States has one of the highest survival rates, but because of the large number of LBW infants, the total infant mortality rate remains high.

LBW is caused by premature birth or intrauterine growth retardation. Maternal factors associated with having an LBW infant include previous LBW birth, low socioeconomic status, low level of educational achievement, lack of prenatal care, maternal age younger than 16 years or older than 35 years, a short time interval between pregnancies, unmarried status, low prepregnancy weight (less than 100 lb) and/or poor weight gain during pregnancy (less than 10 lb), and African American race. Maternal use of cigarettes, alcohol, and/or illicit drugs is also associated with having an LBW infant. Table 13-2 lists specific medical causes of preterm birth.

■ TABLE 13-2 Medical Causes of Preterm Birth
Fetal
Fetal distress
Multiple gestations
Erythroblastosis fetalis
Nonimmune hydrops fetalis
Congenital anomalies
Placental
Placenta previa
Abruptio placenta
Uterine
Bicornuate uterus
Incompetent cervix
Maternal
Pre-eclampsia
Chronic medical illness
Infection (chorioamnionitis)
Drug abuse (esp. cocaine)
Other
Premature rupture of membranes
Polyhydramnios
Trauma
Diethylstilbestrol exposure

🔑 13-3 KEY POINTS

1. Low-birth-weight infants make up 7% of all births but account for two thirds of all neonatal deaths.
2. Very low-birth-weight infants represent 1% of all births but account for 50% of neonatal deaths.
3. In comparison with infants weighing 2,500 g or more, LBW infants are 40 times more likely to die in the neonatal period, and VLBW infants have a 200-fold higher risk of neonatal death.
4. One reason that the infant mortality rate of the United States is so high is that the rate of LBW births is high. If birth-weight mortality rates are calculated, the United States has one of the highest survival rates, but because of the large number of LBW infants, the infant mortality rate remains high.
5. LBW is caused by premature birth or intrauterine growth retardation.

POSTMATURITY

Infants whose gestation exceeds 42 weeks are considered postmature and are at risk for the syndrome of postmaturity. The cause of prolonged pregnancy is not known in most cases.

CLINICAL MANIFESTATIONS

The syndrome of postmaturity is characterized by normal length and head circumference but decreased weight. Infants with this syndrome are distinct from small for gestational age infants in that they were doing well until they went beyond 42 weeks' gestation and became nutritionally deprived from placental insufficiency. Common symptoms include dry, cracked, peeling, loose, and wrinkled skin and a malnourished appearance with decreased amounts of subcutaneous tissues. Conditions that appear more commonly in postmature infants include meconium aspiration and depression at birth, persistent pulmonary hypertension of newborn (PPHN), hypoglycemia, hypocalcemia, and polycythemia.

TREATMENT

Fetal well-being should be monitored closely by US, biophysical profile, and nonstress tests. Intrapartum treatment involves preparation for perinatal depression and meconium aspiration. Early feeding to reduce the risk of hypoglycemia and evaluation for the conditions just noted encompass postpartum treatment.

🔑 13-4 KEY POINTS

1. Infants whose gestation exceeds 42 weeks are considered postmature and are at risk for the syndrome of postmaturity.
2. Conditions that occur more frequently in postmature infants include meconium aspiration and depression at birth, persistent pulmonary hypertension of the newborn, hypoglycemia, hypocalcemia, and polycythemia.

INTRAUTERINE PROBLEMS

SMALL FOR GESTATIONAL AGE

Pathogenesis and Clinical Manifestations

Infants who are small for gestational age have birth weights below the 10th percentile for gestational age. The term "small for gestational age" is merely descriptive and includes normal infants who followed a stable growth curve through fetal development and infants who suffered growth restriction at some point in utero. Two broad categories of intrauterine growth retardation are described: early onset and late onset. A third of LBW neonates—infants weighing less than 2,500 g—are small for gestational age.

Early-onset, or symmetrical, intrauterine growth retardation is thought to result from an insult that begins before 28 weeks' gestation. The early insult results in a neonate whose head circumference and height are proportionately sized and whose weight-for-height ratio is normal. This pattern is seen in infants whose mothers have severe vascular disease with hypertension and renal disease or in infants with congenital malformations or chromosomal abnormalities.

Late-onset, or asymmetric, intrauterine growth retardation starts after 28 weeks' gestation. These infants have a normal, or close to normal, head circumference with a reduced height and weight. The weight-for-height ratio is low, and the infant appears long and emaciated. In this type of intrauterine growth retardation, the neonate initially has a normal growth trajectory and follows a normal percentile line, then "falls off" the curve late in gestation.

Risk Factors

Growth retardation may result from fetal causes such as multiple gestation, congenital viral infections, chromosomal abnormalities (trisomies or Turner syndrome), and congenital (especially CNS) malformation syndromes. Placental causes include chorionic villitis, chronic abruptio placentae, twin–twin transfusion, placental tumor, and placental insufficiency secondary to maternal vascular disease. Maternal causes of intrauterine growth retardation include severe peripheral vascular diseases that reduce uterine blood flow, such as chronic hypertension, diabetic vasculopathy, preeclampsia, sickle cell anemia, and cardiac and renal disease. Other maternal causes include reduced nutritional intake, alcohol or drug abuse, cigarette smoking, and uterine anomalies or uterine constraint. Uterine constraint is noted in mothers of small stature and reduced weight gain during pregnancy.

Treatment

Infants who are small for gestational age have a high risk for intrauterine fetal death. Therefore, prenatal management includes identification, evaluation, and monitoring. The standard intrauterine growth retardation workup includes a review of obstetric causes, examination for identifiable syndromes, and laboratory evaluation for congenital infection. Antepartum fetal monitoring with serial US, biophysical profile, nonstress test, and oxytocin challenge test is often used. Doppler examination of placental flow is used to determine if uteroplacental insufficiency exists. If early delivery is being contemplated, appropriate pulmonary maturity must be assured. Early delivery is necessary when it is determined that the risk to the fetus of staying in utero is greater than the risk of premature delivery. Fetal lung maturity can be accelerated, if necessary, by steroid administration. If there is placental insufficiency, the fetus may not tolerate labor and may require cesarean delivery.

Delivery should take place at a center with a high-risk nursery because infants who are very small for gestational age are at risk for life-threatening problems at the time of delivery. The delivery team should be prepared for perinatal asphyxia and/or depression, meconium aspiration, and hypothermia. Examination of the placenta after delivery for pathology consistent with congenital infection or infarction may be helpful in determining the cause of the intrauterine growth retardation. The newborn that is small for gestational age should be monitored for hypothermia, hypoglycemia, hypocalcemia, hyponatremia, polycythemia, pulmonary hemorrhage, and persistent pulmonary hypertension. Leukopenia, neutropenia, and thrombocytopenia may be seen in infants born to hypertensive mothers. Commencing feedings as soon as possible minimizes hypoglycemia.

LARGE FOR GESTATIONAL AGE

Infants whose weight is greater than 2 standard deviations above the mean or above the 90th percentile are defined as large for gestational age. Neonates at risk for being large for gestational age are those of diabetic mothers (class A, B, or C); postmature infants; and neonates with transposition of the great vessels, erythroblastosis fetalis, or Beckwith-Wiedemann's syndrome. Most infants who are large for gestational age are constitutionally large, from large parents or a family with a predilection for large infants. After birth, the infant should be evaluated for the disorders just described, as well as birth trauma, which occurs often in large for gestational age neonates. The blood sugar of the large for gestational age infant should be monitored and the child fed early because large for gestational age infants who have diabetic mothers or who suffer from Beckwith-Wiedemann's syndrome or erythroblastosis fetalis are prone to hypoglycemia. Obtaining a hematocrit after birth is advisable because large for gestational age neonates have an increased incidence of polycythemia.

Macrosomic neonates have birth weights greater than 4,000 g. All macrosomic infants are large for gestational age, but not all large for gestational age neonates are macrosomic. Macrosomic infants have an increased risk of shoulder dystocia and other birth trauma. Conditions such as maternal diabetes mellitus, obesity, and postmaturity are associated with an increased incidence of macrosomia.

13-5 KEY POINTS

1. It is useful to divide infants who are small for gestational age into two categories: symmetric (early onset) and asymmetric (late onset or "head sparing").
2. Intrauterine growth retardation may result from fetal, placental, or maternal causes.
3. Infants who are small for gestational age have a high risk for intrauterine fetal death; therefore, prenatal management includes identification, evaluation, and monitoring.
4. Neonates at risk for being large for gestational age are those of diabetic mothers (class A, B, or C); postmature infants; and neonates with transposition of the great vessels, erythroblastosis fetalis, or Beckwith-Wiedemann's syndrome.
5. Most infants who are large for gestational age are constitutionally large, from large parents or a family with a predilection for large infants.
6. Macrosomic neonates are a subcategory of large for gestational age infants and have birth weights greater than 4,000 g. They are at significant risk for shoulder dystocia.

POLYHYDRAMNIOS

Polyhydramnios is defined as an amniotic fluid volume greater than 2 L; it occurs in 1 in 1,000 births. Acute polyhydramnios is associated with premature labor, maternal discomfort, and respiratory compromise. More often, polyhydramnios is chronic and seen with gestational diabetes, immune or nonimmune hydrops fetalis, abdominal wall defects (omphalocele and gastroschisis), multiple gestations, trisomy 18 or 21, neural tube defects, and certain congenital anomalies of the GI tract. Anencephaly and meningomyelocele are neural tube defects that impair fetal swallowing, whereas esophageal or duodenal atresia, diaphragmatic hernia, and cleft palate interfere with swallowing and GI fluid dynamics.

OLIGOHYDRAMNIOS

Oligohydramnios is associated with intrauterine growth retardation, amniotic fluid leak, postmaturity, and congenital anomalies of the fetal kidneys. Bilateral renal agenesis results in **Potter's syndrome**. The syndrome is characterized by clubbed feet, compressed facies, low-set ears, scaphoid abdomen, and diminished chest wall size accompanied by pulmonary hypoplasia and pneumothorax. Uterine compression in the absence of amniotic fluid retards lung growth, and patients with this condition expire of respiratory failure rather than of renal insufficiency. Oligohydramnios increases the risk of fetal distress during labor. This risk may be reduced by normal saline amnioinfusion during labor.

🔑 13-6 KEY POINTS

1. Chronic polyhydramnios is seen with gestational diabetes, immune or nonimmune hydrops fetalis, abdominal wall defects (omphalocele and gastroschisis), multiple gestations, trisomy 18 or 21, neural tube defects, and certain congenital anomalies of the GI tract.
2. Oligohydramnios is associated with intrauterine growth retardation, amniotic fluid leak, postmaturity, and congenital anomalies of the fetal kidneys.

CONGENITAL INFECTIONS

Infections of the fetus during the first, second, or early third trimester are referred to as **congenital infections**. Classically, they are referred to as **TORCH infections**, an acronym for toxoplasmosis and *Treponema pallidum* infections, other infections, rubella, cytomegalovirus infection, and herpes simplex and HIV. Although it is important to be familiar with this acronym, it has several shortcomings. Herpes simplex and HIV are much more commonly perinatal (rather than congenital) infections, and there is an ever-expanding list of viruses that could be included in the "other" group. The most important congenital infections and their syndromes are discussed in this section. There are many similarities in the congenital syndromes, so focusing on the differences can help refine the evaluation. Table 13-3 summarizes disease-specific clinical findings and laboratory evaluation.

TABLE 13-3 Differentiating and Evaluating Some Congenital Infections

Agent Evaluation	Specific Clinical Features	Laboratory
Toxoplasma gondii	Hydrocephalus with generalized calcifications; chorioretinitis	Toxoplasmosis IgG antibody followed by IgM, which is more specific.
Treponema pallidum	Osteochondritis and periostitis; eczematoid skin rash; snuffles	Nontreponemal test such as RPR or VDRL, supported by treponemal test such as IgM FTA-ABS.
Rubella	Eye: Cataracts, cloudy cornea, pigmented retina; Skin: "Blueberry muffin" syndrome; Bone: Vertical striation; Heart: Patent ductus, pulmonary stenosis	Maternal rubella immune status. If immune, send infant's IgG and the more specific IgM. If IgM is negative, but IgG is positive, viral cultures from urine, CSF, and throat swabs may isolate the virus.
Cytomegalovirus	Microcephaly with periventricular calcifications; hepatosplenomegaly; chorioretinitis; inguinal hernias in males; thrombocytopenia	Urine for cytomegalovirus culture or calcifications; rapid CMV early antigen test.
Herpes simplex	Skin vesicles or denuded skin; keratoconjunctivitis; acute CNS findings such as seizures	Viral cultures from CSF, skin lesions, conjunctivae, urine, blood, rectum, and nasopharynx should grow within 2–3 days. PCR of CSF. Direct fluorescent antibody staining of scraping from skin lesion is specific but not sensitive.

CMV, cytomegalovirus; FTA-ABS, fluorescent treponema antibody test; VDRL, Venereal's Disease Research Laboratory test.

TOXOPLASMOSIS

Toxoplasmosis is caused by *Toxoplasma gondii*, an intracellular protozoal parasite found in mammals and birds. Members of the cat family are the definitive host. Infected cats excrete toxoplasma oocytes in their stool, resulting in fecal–oral transmission to humans.

There are approximately 3,000 cases of congenital infection annually in the United States. Only primary infection of the mother, which is usually asymptomatic, results in congenital infection. Among the infants of women infected with toxoplasmosis during the first trimester, less than 20% will be infected, but their disease will likely be severe. If the mother's infection is acquired in the third trimester, as many as 65% will give birth to an infected neonate, but the infection will be mild or asymptomatic.

Clinical Manifestations

Infants infected early in pregnancy suffer from intrauterine meningoencephalitis and present with microcephaly, hydrocephalus, microphthalmia, chorioretinitis, intracranial calcifications, and seizures. These infants may also appear septic and have jaundice, hepatosplenomegaly, purpura, petechiae, a maculopapular rash, and generalized lymphadenopathy. Of infants who are asymptomatic at birth, 70% suffer long-term sequelae, which may include mental retardation, learning disabilities, and chorioretinitis. Ocular disease can become reactivated years after the initial infection, both in healthy and immunocompromised individuals, resulting in impaired vision or blindness.

Serologic tests are the primary means of definitive diagnosis. A fourfold rise in antibody titer or seroconversion from negative to positive indicates the presence of infection. In congenital infection, diagnosis may be complicated by the presence of maternally derived transplacental antibody. If the maternal antibody status is negative, the diagnosis of congenital toxoplasmosis is excluded. If maternal and neonate levels are positive, serial studies of antitoxoplasma IgG for several months are necessary to distinguish transplacental antibody from congenital infection. Levels of transplacental antibody fall over the first year of life, whereas antibody levels from congenital infection remain stable or rise. Alternatively, infant IgM represents true infection in the neonate. A CT scan of the head may reveal cerebral calcifications in the CNS. The parasite may be visualized in the CSF by cytocentrifuge preparations or by growth in inoculated infant mice. Typical histopathology or cysts may be identified in biopsy specimens of involved lung, brain, bone marrow, or lymph node.

Treatment

Treatment includes both pyrimethamine and sulfadiazine, which act synergistically against *Toxoplasma*. These antibiotics inhibit folic acid, so supplementation is necessary. Corticosteroids are reserved for infants with severe CNS or ocular infection.

Ingestion of well-cooked meat and the avoidance of cats and soil in areas where cats defecate reduce the risk of toxoplasmosis in pregnant or immunocompromised patients. Cat litter should be disposed of daily because toxoplasma oocytes are not infectious for the first 48 hours after passage.

🔑 13-7 KEY POINTS

1. Toxoplasmosis is caused by *Toxoplasma gondii*, an intracellular protozoal parasite whose definitive host is the cat family.
2. Only primary infection of the mother, who is usually asymptomatic, results in congenital infection.
3. Infants infected early in pregnancy suffer from intrauterine meningoencephalitis and present with microcephaly, hydrocephalus, microphthalmia, chorioretinitis, intracranial calcifications, and seizures.
4. Of infected infants who are asymptomatic at birth, 70% suffer from long-term sequelae, which may include mental retardation, learning disabilities, and chorioretinitis.

SYPHILIS

Syphilis results from transplacental transmission of *Treponema pallidum*. Syphilis in the untreated pregnant woman may be transmitted to the fetus at any time, but fetal transfer is most common during the first year of maternal infection.

Clinical Manifestations

Neonates symptomatic at birth may exhibit nonimmune hydrops with anemia, thrombocytopenia, leukopenia, pneumonitis, hepatitis, osteochondritis, and rash.

Common manifestations described in the first year of life include intermittent fever, osteitis and osteochondritis, hepatosplenomegaly, lymphadenopathy, mucocutaneous lesions (maculopapular rash on the trunk, palms, and soles), persistent rhinitis (snuffles), jaundice, and failure to thrive. Laboratory tests may reveal hyperbilirubinemia, a transaminitis, thrombocytopenia, leukocytosis, and a Coombs-negative hemolytic anemia.

The late sequelae of congenital syphilis appear many years after birth. They include multiple bone signs (frontal bossing, saber shins), Hutchinson teeth, mulberry molars, a saddle-nose deformity, rhagades, juvenile paresis, juvenile tabes, interstitial keratitis, eighth nerve deafness, and Clutton joints (painless joint effusions). These manifestations are rare in the modern era in which penicillin therapy is used to treat congenital syphilis.

Diagnostic Evaluation

Laboratory tests include nontreponemal tests such as the RPR and the Venereal Disease Research Laboratory test (VDRL), and treponemal tests such as the IgM fluorescent treponemal antibody absorption test (IgM FTA-ABS). If a mother has a positive RPR screening test, a treponemal test should be used to confirm infection. If infection is suspected in the mother, the infant needs to be similarly evaluated. The IgM FTA-ABS test is the most specific for fetal infection. Radiographs of the long bones may provide evidence of metaphyseal demineralization or periosteal new bone formation. Dark-field examination of nasal discharge may reveal treponemes. CSF should also be sent for RPR and FTA-ABS.

Treatment

Pregnant women with primary, secondary, or latent syphilis are treated with penicillin.

If the infant's serologic test results are negative and no symptoms are present, no treatment is necessary. If the serologic test results are positive and the infant is symptomatic, treat the infant.

The asymptomatic infant is treated when any of the following conditions exists:

- The infant's titer is three to four times higher than the mother's.
- The FTA is 3 to 4.
- The mother has been inadequately treated or untreated.
- The mother is unreliable and follow-up is doubtful.

- The mother's infection was treated with a drug other than penicillin.
- The mother has had a recent sexual exposure to an infected person.
- The mother was treated in the last month of pregnancy.
- The mother has HIV and has been treated for syphilis with less than a neurosyphilis regimen.

If the infant has a positive RPR, and the history and clinical findings make infection unlikely, it is safe to await the results of the IgM FTA-ABS and repeat the RPR. Any significant rise in titer or any clinical signs require treatment. The infant should be treated if the serology is not negative by 6 months of age. For infants with no evidence of CNS disease, penicillin G is given intravenously for 10 to 14 days. Infants with CNS infection are treated with penicillin for 3 weeks. For infants at low risk for infection for whom follow-up is doubtful, treatment with one IM dose of benzathine penicillin G can be administered.

🔑 13-8 KEY POINTS

1. Congenital syphilis results from transplacental transmission of *T. pallidum*.
2. Common manifestations described in the first year of life include intermittent fever, osteitis and osteochondritis, hepatosplenomegaly, lymphadenopathy, maculopapular rash on the trunk, palms, and soles, persistent rhinitis (snuffles), jaundice, and failure to thrive.
3. Because the treatment of syphilis is so benign, an infant should be treated if the diagnosis is considered.

RUBELLA

Rubella virus is an RNA togavirus. Congenital rubella syndrome has become rare, reflecting the success of the rubella vaccine.

Clinical Manifestations

Anomalies occur primarily as a result of infection in the first trimester and include heart defects (patent ductus arteriosus, peripheral pulmonic stenosis, ventricular septal defect, atrial septal defects); ophthalmologic defects (cataracts, microphthalmia, glaucoma, and chorioretinitis); auditory deficits (sensorineural deafness); and neurologic malformations (microcephaly, meningoencephalitis, and mental retardation). Sequelae of chronic in utero infection are growth retardation, radiolucent bone disease, hepatosplenomegaly, thrombocytopenia, jaundice, and purple skin lesions ("blueberry muffin spots"). Mild forms of the disease can be associated with few or no obvious clinical manifestations at birth.

Rubella virus is most consistently isolated from nasopharyngeal secretions and urine. Infants with congenital rubella may excrete virus for months to years. Specific rubella IgM antibody or persistence of rubella IgG in the infant is diagnostic.

Treatment

There is no specific antiviral chemotherapy. Appropriate treatment of specific defects is recommended. Infants with congenital rubella are considered contagious until they are 1 year of age, unless they have negative nasopharyngeal and urine cultures after 3 months of age. Rubella vaccination should not be given during pregnancy, but inadvertent administration carries a very low risk of fetal disease.

13-9 KEY POINTS

1. Congenital rubella syndrome has become rare, reflecting the success of rubella vaccine. Anomalies occur primarily as a result of infection in the first trimester and include heart defects, ophthalmologic defects, auditory deficits, and neurologic malformations.
2. Sequelae of chronic infection include growth retardation, radiolucent bone disease, hepatosplenomegaly, thrombocytopenia, jaundice, and purple skin lesions ("blueberry muffin spots").
3. Rubella vaccination should not be given during pregnancy, but inadvertent administration carries a very low risk of fetal disease.

CYTOMEGALOVIRUS

Neonatal cytomegalovirus (CMV) infection is common, occurring in 1% of newborns in the United States. Higher rates are found in lower socioeconomic populations. Among fetuses of mothers who develop primary CMV infection during pregnancy, approximately 40% become infected, and of those infected, only 5% have residual neurologic deficits. Infection occurs in approximately 10% of pregnancies with recurrent or reactivated maternal infection. Neurologic sequelae in offspring are more severe after primary maternal infection; infection following reactivation during pregnancy may result in hearing loss and milder developmental problems for the infant. CMV infection acquired during the birth process, via breast-feeding, or from blood or platelet transfusions has not been associated with neurologic deficits.

Clinical Manifestations

Most cases are clinically inapparent. Late sequelae such as nerve deafness and learning disabilities may develop in 10% of clinically inapparent infections. The syndrome of congenital CMV (cytomegalic inclusion disease) is uncommon, occurring in 5% of infants with CMV infection, and includes intrauterine growth retardation, purpura, jaundice, hepatosplenomegaly, microcephaly, intracerebral calcifications, and chorioretinitis. The calcifications tend to be periventricular. A more common symptomatic presentation is intrauterine growth retardation, hepatosplenomegaly, and persistent jaundice. Severe interstitial pneumonia in premature infants can be fatal.

Infants with congenital infection excrete CMV in high titers in urine and saliva, and the virus may be grown in viral culture or identified by early antigen detection in the urine. Additional diagnostic studies to determine extent of infection include a CT scan of the head for detection of intracranial calcifications, liver function tests, long bone films, and chest radiograph to detect pneumonitis.

Treatment

Ganciclovir has been demonstrated to reduce the incidence or slow the progression of hearing loss in infants with documented CNS involvement. As a result, infected neonates with calcifications, retinitis, or positive CSF findings should be treated for several weeks with ganciclovir. Newborn hearing screening by brainstem auditory evoked responses is important. Repeated evaluations are imperative because postnatal development of deafness can occur. Neonates with congenital CMV shed the virus for some time, and pregnant health care workers should not take care of infected infants.

13-10 KEY POINTS

1. Cytomegalovirus infection is common in the newborn, occurring in 1% of all neonates.
2. Approximately 40% of fetuses whose mothers experience primary CMV infection during pregnancy experience congenital infection; of those infected, only 5% have residual neurologic deficits.
3. Infection occurs in approximately 10% of pregnancies with recurrent or reactivated maternal infection.
4. Most cases are clinically inapparent. Late sequelae such as nerve deafness and learning disabilities may develop in 10% of clinically inapparent infections.
5. Cytomegalic inclusion disease occurs in 5% of infants with CMV infection and includes intrauterine growth retardation, purpura, jaundice, hepatosplenomegaly, microcephaly, intracerebral calcifications, and chorioretinitis.

HERPES SIMPLEX VIRUS

There are two serotypes of herpes simplex virus (HSV): HSV-1 and HSV-2. They can both cause severe disease and mortality in the neonate, although HSV-1 in this setting generally produces milder disease. The incidence of neonatal infection is estimated to be approximately 1 in 3,500 live births. Most neonatal HSV infection is caused by HSV-2 because it accounts for the majority of genital herpes. The child is infected as he or she moves through the vaginal canal. The majority of neonatal herpes is therefore a result of perinatal infection, and true congenital herpes is rare.

Clinical Manifestations

Asymptomatic infection is rare. HSV manifests itself in three discrete constellations of symptoms. Infants may have disseminated infection involving the liver and other organs (occasionally including the CNS); localized CNS disease; or localized infection of the skin, eye, and mouth (SEM disease). Ocular manifestations include conjunctivitis, keratitis, and chorioretinitis. In approximately a third of the patients, SEM involvement is the first indication of the infection. Disseminated disease may present with findings described for sepsis. Localized CNS disease may present with fever, lethargy, poor feeding, hypoglycemia, DIC, and irritability, followed by intractable focal or generalized seizures. Vesicular lesions, when present, are an important clue to the diagnosis. Symptoms can occur shortly after birth or as late as 4 weeks after birth. Disseminated disease usually occurs during the first 2 weeks of life, whereas localized CNS disease and SEM disease typically occur during the second or third week.

Neonatal herpetic infections are frequently severe, with a high mortality rate and significant neurologic and/or ocular impairment of survivors, particularly in those not treated with antiviral therapy.

HSV is cultured easily; viral detection generally takes 1 to 3 days. Cultures are obtained from skin vesicles, the mouth or nasopharynx, conjunctiva, urine, blood, rectum, and CSF. Tzanck smear of vesicle scrapings may reveal multinucleated giant cells. Direct fluorescent antibody staining of vesicle fluid or scrapings from lesions is very specific but not very sensitive. HSV PCR of CSF is both sensitive and specific if there is CNS involvement. The diagnosis should be considered in any infant with vesicular lesions or denuded skin, infants with signs of sepsis, or in the setting of acute CNS disease.

Treatment

Antiviral therapy with acyclovir is indicated for all forms of neonatal herpes infection because even initially localized disease may disseminate with devastating effects.

13-11 KEY POINTS

1. Most neonatal herpes simplex virus infections are caused by HSV-2.
2. Asymptomatic infection is rare. HSV manifests itself in three discrete constellations of symptoms. Infants may have disseminated infection involving the liver and other organs (often including the CNS), localized CNS disease, or SEM disease.
3. Antiviral therapy with acyclovir is indicated for all forms of neonatal herpes infection because even initially localized disease may disseminate with devastating effects.

VARICELLA-ZOSTER VIRUS

Ninety percent of women of childbearing age are immune to varicella-zoster virus (VZV), so congenital and neonatal varicellas are rare. Only 25% of the infants of infected nonimmune mothers develop congenital or neonatal chickenpox.

Clinical Manifestations

Maternal VZV infection in the first and second trimesters has been associated with cutaneous scars, abnormalities of digits or limbs, defects of the eye, CNS anomalies, and low birth weight in newborns. Newborns who acquire VZV infection during the perinatal period have a clinical illness varying from mild to fatal. The acquisition of transplacental antibody determines the outcome in infants.

Diagnosis of congenital varicella is made by specific IgM VZV antibody or the persistence of significant titers of VZV IgG. Maternal history will reveal characteristic chickenpox illness during pregnancy. Neonatal varicella is characterized by diffusely disseminated skin lesions in varying states, from macules, papules, vesicles, and pustules to crusts. Recovery of VZV by culture, immunofluorescent staining of scrapings, or Tzanck smear of vesicle base scrapings is diagnostic. Direct immunofluorescence of cells differentiates VZV infection from HSV.

Treatment

Infants with congenital varicella do not require isolation because they are no longer shedding virus. Infants with neonatal varicella should be placed in strict isolation for at least 7 days after the onset of rash. Infants born to mothers with onset of varicella 5 or more days before delivery require no specific treatment other than isolation, if kept in the hospital. Infants whose mothers have onset of varicella within 5 days before delivery, or within 2 days after delivery, should receive varicella-zoster immune globulin (VZIG), preferably at birth or within 96 hours. Infants with acute varicella in the first week of life should receive acyclovir for 10 days. Infants who are exposed to VZV infection as a result of contact with nursery personnel should have their immune status verified and, if susceptible, they should receive VZIG within 96 hours of exposure.

13-12 KEY POINTS

1. Ninety percent of women of childbearing age are immune to varicella-zoster virus, and only 25% of infants of infected nonimmune mothers develop congenital or neonatal chickenpox.

HUMAN IMMUNODEFICIENCY VIRUS

HIV, an RNA retrovirus, causes AIDS. HIV is particularly tropic for CD4-containing cells, which include helper T cells, monocytes, and macrophages. It is the invasion and destruction of these cells that causes immunodeficiency. Eighty percent of pediatric AIDS cases result from maternal transmission. Most remaining cases are transfusion related or occur because of sexual transmission. Predisposing factors include mothers with HIV secondary to drug abuse or sexual contact with a male with HIV. Because of the relatively high prevalence of intravenous drug abuse in inner-city areas, minority children are disproportionately affected. Fifty percent of pediatric AIDS cases caused by maternal transmission occur in African American infants, and 25% in Hispanics. Transmission rates of HIV from the mother to the neonate are estimated at 15% to 30%. Postnatal transmission of HIV from infected mothers to infants by means of breast milk is documented.

Clinical Manifestations

Infected infants are generally asymptomatic at birth. Within the first month, they may develop persistent thrush, lymphadenopathy, and hepatosplenomegaly. During the first year of life, without appropriate antiretroviral therapy, common symptoms include recurrent refractory infections, severe intractable diarrhea, and failure to thrive. It is estimated that 20% of untreated infants with congenital/perinatal HIV infection die within the first year of life, and 60% of HIV-infected children have severe symptomatic disease by 18 months of age.

Diagnosis of HIV at birth is difficult because of maternal antibodies. If HIV is suspected and the mother is seronegative for HIV, the risk in the child is minimal. The diagnosis of HIV infection in children born to mothers who are HIV seropositive can be established before the onset of symptoms through detection of HIV in peripheral blood by HIV DNA detection (see Chapter 12).

Treatment

Studies have shown that maternal antiretroviral therapy in the last two trimesters can dramatically reduce transmission of HIV to the fetus to less than 10%, and multidrug regimens reduce the risk of transmission even further. Risk of transmission appears to correlate with viral load. Neonates who have HIV-positive mothers or mothers in whom HIV is suspected are also treated with antiretrovirals. At-risk infants are also treated prophylactically with trimethoprim-sulfamethoxazole to prevent *Pneumocystis jiroveci* pneumonia (PCP).

⚿ 13-13 KEY POINTS

1. Eighty percent of pediatric AIDS cases result from maternal vertical transmission. Most remaining cases are transfusion related.

2. Transmission rates of HIV from the mother to the neonate are estimated at 15% to 30% if neither mother nor infant is treated with antiretrovirals.

3. Maternal treatment dramatically reduces the risk of transmission to the infant.

4. Within the first month, infected infants may develop persistent thrush, lymphadenopathy, and hepatosplenomegaly. During the first year of life, common symptoms among untreated infants include recurrent refractory infections, severe intractable diarrhea, and failure to thrive.

5. Treatment involves nutritional support, PCP prophylaxis, antiviral therapy, and anti-infective agents for specific infections.

NEONATAL INFECTION

NEONATAL SEPSIS

Neonatal sepsis is generally divided into early onset, late onset, and nosocomial sepsis. Early-onset sepsis, occurring from birth to 3 days, can be an overwhelming multiorgan systemic disease manifested by respiratory failure, shock, meningitis (30%), DIC, and acute tubular necrosis. Early-onset sepsis is caused by infection by the bacteria in the mother's genitourinary tract. These organisms include group B streptococci, *Escherichia coli*, *Klebsiella*, and *Listeria monocytogenes*. Predisposing factors for early-onset sepsis include vaginal colonization with group B streptococci, prolonged rupture of the membranes (>24 hours), chorioamnionitis, maternal fever or leukocytosis, fetal tachycardia, and preterm birth. African American race and male sex are unexplained additional risk factors for neonatal sepsis.

Late-onset sepsis, occurring between days 3 and 28, usually occurs in the healthy full-term infant who was discharged in good health from the normal newborn nursery. Bacteremia leads to hematogenous seeding that results in focal infections such as meningitis (75%, usually caused by group B streptococci or *E. coli*); osteomyelitis (group B streptococci and *Staphylococcus aureus*); arthritis (*Neisseria gonorrhoeae*,

S. aureus, *Candida albicans*, gram-negative bacteremia); and urinary tract infection (gram-negative bacteremia).

Nosocomially acquired sepsis (occurring between day 3 and discharge) occurs predominantly among premature infants in the newborn intensive care unit (NICU) because many of these infants have been colonized with the multidrug-resistant bacteria indigenous to the NICU. Frequent treatment with broad-spectrum antibiotics for sepsis and the presence of central venous indwelling catheters, endotracheal tubes, umbilical vessel catheters, and electronic monitoring devices increase the risk for such serious bacterial or fungal infections. The most common pathogens are *S. aureus*, *Staphylococcus epidermidis*, gram-negative bacteria, and *Candida albicans*.

The incidence of group B streptococcal disease has dramatically decreased since the institution of maternal screening protocols and prenatal antibiotic regimens in culture-positive mothers. Group B streptococci are recovered from the vaginal cultures of approximately 25% of American women at the time of delivery.

Clinical Manifestations

Most infants with early-onset sepsis present with nonspecific cardiorespiratory signs such as grunting, tachypnea, and cyanosis at birth. As a result, it is often hard to differentiate early-onset sepsis from respiratory distress syndrome (RDS) in the preterm neonate. Because of this difficulty, most premature infants with RDS receive broad-spectrum antibiotics. Common signs and symptoms of early sepsis include poor feeding, emesis, lethargy, apnea, ileus, and abdominal distention. Petechiae and purpura are noted when DIC is present. Meningitis (with possible seizures) is present in 25% of neonates with early-onset sepsis.

Infants with suspected early-onset sepsis should have blood and CSF sent for culture. CSF should also be tested for Gram stain, cell count and differential, and protein and glucose levels. Serial CBCs are performed to identify signs of infection. A WBC less than 5,000 or greater than 40,000, a total neutrophil count under 1,000, and a ratio of bands to neutrophils of greater than 20% all correlate with an increased risk of bacterial infection. Thrombocytopenia may also be seen. The chest radiograph is used to determine the presence of pneumonia. ABGs should be monitored to detect hypoxemia and metabolic acidosis that may be caused by hypoxia and/or shock. Blood pressure, urine output, central venous pressure, and peripheral perfusion are monitored to determine the need to treat septic shock with fluids and vasopressor agents.

The clinical manifestations of late-onset sepsis include lethargy, poor feeding, hypotonia, apathy, seizures, bulging fontanelle, fever, and direct hyperbilirubinemia. The evaluation for late-onset sepsis is similar to that for early-onset sepsis, with special attention given to examination of the bones, the laboratory values, and urine culture obtained by sterile suprapubic aspiration or urethral catheterization. Late-onset sepsis may be caused by the same pathogens as early-onset sepsis *or* those usually found in the older infant (*Streptococcus pneumoniae*, *Neisseria meningitides*).

The initial clinical manifestations of nosocomial infection in the premature neonate may be subtle and include apnea and bradycardia, temperature instability, abdominal distention, and poor feeding. In the later stages, there may be severe metabolic acidosis, shock, DIC, and respiratory failure.

Treatment

A combination of ampicillin and gentamicin for 10 to 14 days is effective treatment against most organisms responsible for early sepsis. Once an organism is identified and antibiotic sensitivities are determined, antibiotic therapy may be tailored to treat the infecting organism. If meningitis is present, the treatment is extended, and a third-generation cephalosporin is recommended for improved penetration across the blood–brain barrier. Cefotaxime and amikacin (for synergy) are used to treat *E. coli* or *Klebsiella* meningitis. Sepsis resulting from group B streptococcal meningitis and *Listeria* are treated with ampicillin and gentamicin (for synergy). The treatment of late-onset neonatal sepsis and meningitis is the same as that for early-onset sepsis.

The treatment of nosocomially acquired sepsis depends on the indigenous microbiologic flora of the particular hospital and their antibiotic sensitivities. Because *S. aureus* (sometimes methicillin resistant), *S. epidermidis* (usually methicillin resistant), and gram-negative pathogens are the most common bacterial nosocomial infections, a combination of vancomycin and gentamicin is often used. Persistent signs of infection despite antibacterial treatment suggest candidal (fungal) sepsis, which is treated with amphotericin B.

13-14 KEY POINTS

1. Neonatal sepsis is generally divided into early-onset, late-onset, and nosocomial sepsis.
2. Early-onset sepsis (birth to 3 days of life) is caused by infection by the bacteria in the mother's genitourinary tract, which includes group B streptococci, *E. coli*, *Klebsiella*, and *Listeria monocytogenes*.
3. Late-onset sepsis (3 to 28 days of life) may be caused by the same pathogens as early-onset sepsis, but those infants presenting late in the neonatal period also may have infections caused by pathogens usually found in the older infant (e.g., *S. pneumoniae*, *N. meningitidis*).
4. Nosocomially acquired sepsis (3 days of life to discharge) occurs predominantly among premature infants in the newborn intensive care unit (NICU) and is most commonly caused by *S. aureus*, *S. epidermidis*, gram-negative bacteria, and *C. albicans*.

CHLAMYDIA INFECTION

Chlamydia trachomatis is transmitted from the genital tract of infected mothers to their newborn infants. Acquisition occurs in approximately 50% of infants born vaginally to infected mothers. Of the infants who acquire *C. trachomatis*, the risk of conjunctivitis is 25% to 50%, and the risk of pneumonia is 5% to 20%. The nasopharynx is the most commonly infected anatomic site. A symptomatic infection of the conjunctiva, pharynx, rectum, or vagina of the infant can persist for more than 2 years. Prevalence among pregnant women varies between 6% and 12% in most populations.

Clinical Manifestations

In neonatal chlamydial conjunctivitis, ocular congestion, edema, and discharge develop a few days to several weeks after birth and last for 1 to 2 weeks.

Pneumonia in young infants caused by *C. trachomatis* is usually an afebrile illness that presents between 3 and 19 weeks after birth. A repetitive, staccato cough and tachypnea are characteristic but not always present. Crackles can be present, whereas wheezing is less likely. Hyperinflation on chest radiograph is prominent. Untreated disease can linger or recur.

Treatment

Topical erythromycin may be instilled into the eye at birth to prevent gonococcal ophthalmia, but this treatment will not reliably prevent neonatal chlamydial pneumonia. Chlamydial conjunctivitis and pneumonia in young infants are treated with oral erythromycin for 14 days. Topical treatment of conjunctivitis is ineffective and unnecessary. The efficacy of erythromycin therapy is only 80%, so a second course is sometimes required. A specific diagnosis of C. trachomatis infection in the infant should prompt treatment of the mother and evaluation of her sexual partner.

13-15 KEY POINTS

1. Acquisition occurs in approximately 50% of infants born vaginally to infected mothers. Of the infants who acquire C. trachomatis, the risk of conjunctivitis is 25% to 50% and the risk of pneumonia is 5% to 20%.
2. In neonatal chlamydial conjunctivitis, congestion, edema, and discharge develop a few days to several weeks after birth and last for 1 to 2 weeks.
3. Pneumonia in young infants caused by C. trachomatis is usually an afebrile illness that presents between 3 and 19 weeks after birth. A repetitive, staccato cough and tachypnea are characteristic but not always present.

NEONATAL RESPIRATORY DISEASE

RESPIRATORY DISTRESS SYNDROME

Pathogenesis

RDS, or hyaline membrane disease, is the most common cause of respiratory failure in newborn infants. It occurs predominantly in premature infants who are born with immature lungs. In the average child, lung maturity occurs at 32 to 43 weeks' gestation, when surfactant, a phospholipid that lines the alveoli, is produced by the type II pneumocytes. RDS is caused by a deficiency of surfactant. The major function of surfactant is to decrease alveolar surface tension and increase lung compliance. Surfactant prevents alveolar collapse at the end of expiration and allows for opening of the alveoli at low intrathoracic pressures.

Because of the lack of surfactant, the lungs have poor compliance, which results in progressive atelectasis, intrapulmonary shunting, hypoxemia, and cyanosis. The forces generated by mechanical ventilation, oxygen exposure, and alveolar capillary leak result in formation of a hyaline membrane. This membrane lines the alveoli and is composed of protein and sloughed alveolar epithelium. The incidence of RDS increases with decreasing gestational age. A measure of amniotic fluid lecithin-to-sphingomyelin ratio can be used to predict lung maturity.

The production of surfactant is accelerated by maternal steroid administration, prolonged rupture of fetal membranes, maternal narcotic addiction, preeclampsia, chronic fetal stress caused by placental insufficiency, maternal hyperthyroidism, and theophylline. The production of surfactant is delayed by combined fetal hyperglycemia and hyperinsulinemia, as occurs in maternal diabetes.

Clinical Manifestations

Affected premature infants characteristically present with tachypnea, grunting, nasal flaring, chest wall retractions, and cyanosis in the first 3 hours of life. There is poor air entry on auscultation. The amniotic fluid lecithin-to-sphingomyelin ratio is less than 2.0, and phosphatidylglycerol is absent in the amniotic fluid. Diagnosis is confirmed by chest radiograph that reveals a uniform **reticulonodular or ground-glass** pattern and air bronchograms that are consistent with diffuse atelectasis.

The natural course is a progressive worsening over the first 24 to 48 hours of life. After the initial insult to the airway lining, the epithelium is repopulated with type II alveolar cells, which produce surfactant. Subsequently, there is increased production and release of surfactant, so there is a sufficient quantity in the air spaces by 72 hours of life. This results in improved lung compliance and resolution of respiratory distress, which is frequently preceded by an increase in urine output.

Acute complications associated with RDS include pulmonary interstitial emphysema, pneumothorax, pneumomediastinum, and pneumopericardium. Rupture of the alveolar epithelial lining produces pulmonary interstitial emphysema as air dissects along the interstitial spaces and the peribronchial lymphatics. Extravasation of gas into the lung parenchyma reduces lung compliance and worsens respiratory failure.

Treatment

The goal of therapy is to provide respiratory support to the infant until spontaneous resolution occurs. All attempts should be made to minimize barotrauma and damage from high FiO_2.

Conventional therapy for the affected infant includes respiratory support with oxygen, continuous positive airway pressure (CPAP), and/or mechanical ventilation. Therapy with artificial surfactant improves this condition dramatically and significantly decreases the rate of neonatal mortality in premature infants. After surfactant administration, the FiO_2 of oxygen should be titrated to keep the PaO_2 greater than 50 mm Hg. If the FiO_2 exceeds 60%, CPAP can be used to decrease the time spent in high oxygen concentrations and to lessen the need for mechanical ventilation. CPAP is also useful in treating apnea that is unresponsive to nasal cannula stimulation and during the weaning process after extubation. Intubation and intermittent positive pressure ventilation are used when CPAP has been optimized and the FiO_2 required to keep the PaO_2 greater than 50 mm Hg exceeds 60%. Other indicators that mechanical ventilation is needed include apnea that is unresponsive to CPAP and/or persistent respiratory acidosis ($PaCO_2$ greater than 60 and pH less than 7.25) on maximum CPAP. In general, CPAP is not sufficient for neonates with birth weights less than 1,000 g. As RDS resolves and surfactant therapy takes effect, the compliance of the lungs increases dramatically and ventilator parameters must be weaned quickly to avoid severe barotrauma. When amniotic fluid assessment of the premature infant reveals fetal lung immaturity and preterm delivery cannot be prevented, administration of corticosteroids to the mother 48 hours before delivery can induce or accelerate the production of fetal surfactant and minimize the incidence of RDS.

Very premature neonates who require mechanical ventilation for long periods of time are at risk for alveolar rupture and the development of pulmonary interstitial emphysema, pneumothorax, pneumomediastinum, and/or pneumopericardium. The risk of barotrauma increases as the duration of mechanical ventilation increases, mean airway pressure escalates, and the intermittent mandatory ventilation rate increases. When RDS is very severe, pulmonary hypertension may occur, causing a right-to-left shunt at the patent foramen ovale and the ductus arteriosus. Infants with respiratory distress deserve evaluation for sepsis and pneumonia because group B streptococcal infection may mimic RDS clinically and on chest radiograph. Until blood culture results are known, antibiotics are recommended. Intraventricular hemorrhage and necrotizing enterocolitis (NEC) are more likely to occur in the neonate with RDS.

Chronic lung disease, also referred to as **bronchopulmonary dysplasia** (BPD), is the long-term complication of RDS and is caused by prolonged mechanical ventilation of the premature infant with high airway pressures and high oxygen tensions. The incidence varies greatly among NICUs but may affect as many as 50% of premature infants whose birth weight is less than 1,000 g. Before surfactant and modern ventilation strategies, BPD was characterized by cystic areas of lung, squamous cell metaplasia, and hypertrophy of small airways with subsequent alveolar collapse or air trapping. Although this pathology is still seen in the sickest premature infants, BPD is now more commonly a disease of **arrested alveolar development**. Alveoli are large and mature appearing but are decreased in number. Complications include chronic respiratory insufficiency, requiring home use of continuous oxygen therapy, diuretics and bronchodilators; right-sided congestive heart failure secondary to pulmonary hypertension; and pneumothorax. Weaning the infant off oxygen to room air can take several months. Reactive airway disease is common and can be severe. SIDS is more common in infants with BPD. Lower respiratory infections caused by usually benign viral agents, most notably RSV, may cause severe respiratory distress. Some infants recover fully, but the healing process takes years.

13-16 KEY POINTS

1. Respiratory distress syndrome, or hyaline membrane disease, is the most common cause of respiratory failure in newborn infants. It occurs in premature infants who are born at 37 weeks' gestation or less and results from deficiency of surfactant.
2. Conventional therapy for the affected infant includes respiratory support with oxygen, continuous positive airway pressure, and/or mechanical ventilation.
3. Therapy with artificial surfactant improves RDS dramatically and has significantly decreased the rate of neonatal mortality in premature infants.
4. Chronic lung disease is a long-term complication of RDS and is caused by prolonged mechanical ventilation of the premature infant with high airway pressures and high oxygen tensions.
5. Modern-day bronchopulmonary dysplasia is characterized by arrested alveolar development.

MECONIUM ASPIRATION

Pathogenesis

The fetal lung produces fluid that flows out of the lung and contributes to amniotic fluid. Fetal respiratory movements are not of sufficient strength to draw amniotic fluid into the respiratory tree. Fetal hypoxia, however, may trigger the passage of meconium from the lower GI tract into the amniotic fluid; with severe fetal asphyxia and acidosis, a gasp reflex may generate adequate force to draw the meconium into the lung. Aspiration of meconium interferes with gas exchange and obstructs airways by a ball-valve mechanism, resulting in ventilation-perfusion mismatch and pneumothoraces. The resulting hypoxia and acidosis increase pulmonary vascular resistance and cause right-to-left shunting of blood across the patent foramen ovale or the ductus arteriosus or both. This shunting further worsens the hypoxia and acidosis created by aspiration, resulting in a vicious cycle of increasingly severe pulmonary arteriolar hypertension, respiratory distress, and cyanosis. This sequence of events can occur without meconium aspiration as a primary result of chronic fetal hypoxia and is referred to as **persistent pulmonary hypertension**.

Risk Factors

The risk of meconium aspiration is markedly increased in postmature infants and neonates who suffer from intrauterine growth retardation. Both have placental insufficiency as a common pathway for fetal hypoxia. Infants born in the breech position also have an increased risk of meconium in the amniotic fluid.

Clinical Manifestations

Meconium aspiration pneumonitis is characterized by tachypnea, hypoxia, and hypercapnia. Diagnosis is established by the presence of meconium in the tracheal or amniotic fluid, combined with symptoms of respiratory distress and a chest radiograph that reveals a pattern of diffuse infiltrates with hyperinflation. Of infants with meconium aspiration syndrome, 10% develop pneumothoraces.

Treatment

In pregnancies in which uteroplacental insufficiency is either documented or suspected, tests of fetal well-being, such as the nonstress test, biophysical profile, fetal monitoring, and scalp pH sampling, help identify those infants at high risk for meconium aspiration.

When meconium is noted, the obstetrician suctions the oropharynx before delivery of the thorax (and the first intake of breath). After delivery, if the infant appears depressed, the vocal cords are visualized by direct laryngoscopy and an endotracheal tube inserted. Suction is applied to the endotracheal tube as it is slowly removed. The procedure is repeated if significant meconium is recovered. If the infant exhibits poor respiratory effort, support by bag-valve mask is then initiated. An infant who appears vigorous immediately upon delivery does not require intubation but should have routine suctioning of the oropharynx.

If aspiration has occurred and the infant is in distress, therapy consists of administration of oxygen and/or mechanical ventilation. Because meconium inactivates endogenous surfactant, surfactant administration may be beneficial. The severity of disease is related to the amount of meconium the infant has aspirated and the severity of the pulmonary hypertension present caused by the prenatal asphyxia. For persistent hypoxia ($Pao_2 < 50$ mm Hg) or severe hypercapnia ($PCO_2 > 60$ mm Hg), intubation and mechanical ventilation are indicated. If severe hypoxia persists with conventional ventilation, it is likely that PPHN is present and high-frequency ventilation and/or ECMO may be beneficial.

🔑 13-17 KEY POINTS

1. Meconium aspiration syndrome is a disorder caused by perinatal asphyxia. Fetal hypoxia triggers passage of meconium into the amniotic fluid, which is likely aspirated in utero and immediately after birth.
2. Aspiration of the meconium interferes with gas exchange and obstructs airways by a ball-valve mechanism, resulting in ventilation-perfusion mismatch and pneumothoraces. The resulting hypoxia and acidosis increase pulmonary vascular resistance and causes right-to-left shunting of blood across the patent foramen ovale or the ductus arteriosus or both.
3. The risk of meconium aspiration is markedly increased in postmature infants (gestational age >42 weeks) and neonates who suffer from intrauterine growth retardation.

PERSISTENT PULMONARY HYPERTENSION OF THE NEWBORN

Pathogenesis

PPHN, or persistent fetal circulation, is a disorder of term or post-term infants who have experienced acute or chronic hypoxia in utero. The primary abnormality is the failure of the pulmonary vasculature resistance to fall with postnatal lung expansion and oxygenation. At birth, the systemic vascular resistance normally rises as a result of cessation of blood flow through the placenta, and pulmonary vascular resistance decreases after the first few breaths. With persistence of the fetal circulation, the pulmonary vascular resistance continues to be high and may in fact be higher than the systemic resistance. This results in shunting of the deoxygenated blood, which is returning to the right atrium, away from the lungs. The right-to-left shunt can occur at the foramen ovale, the ductus arteriosus, or both. Because the lungs are bypassed, the blood is not oxygenated and hypoxemia ensues. The hypoxemia and acidosis caused by the right-to-left shunt only worsens the baseline pulmonary arteriolar hypertension, resulting in a vicious cycle of increasingly severe pulmonary arteriolar hypertension and cyanosis culminating in cardiopulmonary failure.

Risk Factors

PPHN is associated with meconium aspiration, severe RDS, diaphragmatic hernia, pulmonary hypoplasia, and neonatal pneumonia.

Clinical Manifestations

The diagnosis is suggested by a history of perinatal hypoxia and rapidly progressive cyanosis associated with mild to severe respiratory distress. Often the clinical severity of pulmonary insufficiency is greater than the findings on chest radiograph; the chest radiograph may be normal or abnormal depending on the specific cause of the PPHN. Echocardiography reveals absence of structural heart disease, evidence of increased pulmonary vascular resistance, and the presence of right-to-left shunting at the foramen ovale, ductus arteriosus, or both. The severity varies from mild disease with spontaneous resolution to death from intractable hypoxemia. Pulmonary hypertension usually resolves within 5 to 10 days of birth.

Treatment

Treatment focuses on maximizing oxygen delivery and decreasing pulmonary arteriolar hypertension.

Conditions that potentiate PPHN include hypoxia, acidosis, hypoglycemia, hyperviscosity, anemia, and systemic hypotension. Hypoxia and acidosis promote increased pulmonary arteriolar hypertension, whereas systemic hypotension increases right-to-left shunting and tissue hypoxemia. Hypoglycemia results in ketosis, which exacerbates acidosis. Anemia reduces oxygen delivery to the tissues. Sludging caused by hyperviscosity increases pulmonary hypertension. The therapies used to treat PPHN combat the conditions that worsen pulmonary hypertension and include supplemental oxygen, hyperventilation, administration of sodium bicarbonate, pulmonary vasodilators, and support of systemic blood pressure.

Mild hyperventilation to a $PaCO_2$ less than 40 mm Hg prevents the pulmonary vasoconstrictive effects of a respiratory acidosis and results in improvement in PaO_2. Nitric oxide relaxes pulmonary arteriolar smooth muscle cells and is effective in PPHN. Sedation facilitates relaxation of the infant and pulmonary vasodilation, whereas muscle paralysis may be needed to assist with hyperventilation. The overall mortality rate associated with PPHN is 25% in term infants. Infants who require very high ventilator settings, marked by an alveolar-to-arterial gradient of greater than 600 mm Hg on room air, have a high mortality rate and may benefit from ECMO. ECMO improves outcomes in the group of most severely ill patients.

> ### ⚲ 13-18 KEY POINTS
>
> 1. PPHN is seen when there is failure of the pulmonary vasculature resistance to fall with postnatal lung expansion and oxygenation. It occurs in term and postterm infants who have experienced acute or chronic hypoxia in utero.
> 2. Hypoxemia and acidosis caused by right-to-left shunting worsen baseline pulmonary arteriolar hypertension, resulting in a vicious cycle of increasingly severe pulmonary arteriolar hypertension and cyanosis that culminates in cardiopulmonary failure.
> 3. The therapies used to treat PPHN include supplemental oxygen, hyperventilation, administration of sodium bicarbonate, pulmonary vasodilators, and support of systemic blood pressure.

NEONATAL GASTROINTESTINAL DISEASE

HYPERBILIRUBINEMIA

Hyperbilirubinemia manifests as jaundice—a yellowing of the skin, mucous membranes, and sclera. It occurs when serum bilirubin levels are greater than 5 mg per dL in neonates and greater than 2 mg per dL in children and adolescents. The two types of hyperbilirubinemia are unconjugated (indirect), which can be physiologic or pathologic in origin, and conjugated (direct), which is always pathologic. Conjugated hyperbilirubinemia is defined as the direct fraction of bilirubin in the blood exceeding 2 mg per dL or 15% of the total bilirubin. Bilirubin is a bile pigment formed from the degradation of heme that is derived from RBC destruction and ineffective erythropoiesis. Figure 13-1 illustrates normal bilirubin metabolism.

Abnormalities in any step in the process may result in unconjugated or conjugated hyperbilirubinemia.

Neonatal hyperbilirubinemia is monitored with great care because elevated levels of unconjugated bilirubin cause kernicterus. Unconjugated bilirubin is normally bound tightly to albumin in the blood, but at high levels the unconjugated bilirubin exceeds the binding capacity of albumin and free bilirubin crosses the blood–brain barrier and damages the cells of the brain. In premature infants, much lower levels of hyperbilirubinemia may result in kernicterus because the more immature the neonate, the more immature the blood–brain barrier. Kernicterus is characterized by a yellow staining of the basal ganglia and hippocampus, which results in widespread cerebral dysfunction. Clinical features include lethargy and irritability, hypotonia, opisthotonos, seizures, mental retardation, cerebral palsy, and hearing loss.

Most full-term and preterm neonates develop a transient, unconjugated hyperbilirubinemia during

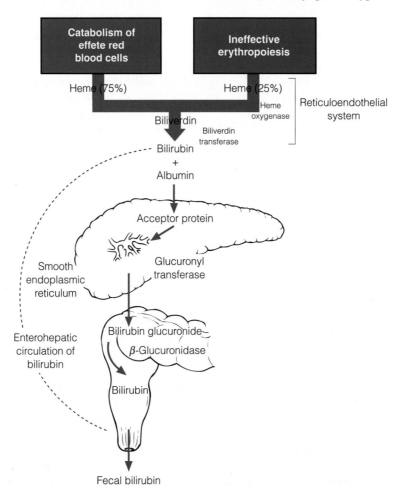

Figure 13-1 • Bilirubin metabolism in the neonate.

the first week of life. This episode of "physiologic jaundice" is caused by an elevated bilirubin load (secondary to an increased RBC volume, decreased RBC survival time, and increased enterohepatic circulation), defective hepatic uptake of bilirubin, inadequate bilirubin conjugation caused by decreased UDP-glucuronyl-transferase activity, and defective bilirubin excretion. Physiologic jaundice begins after 24 hours of life, is associated with a peak of 12 to 15 mg per dL at 3 to 5 days of life, and returns to normal levels by the end of the first week of life. Risk factors for developing more severe physiologic jaundice include prematurity, maternal diabetes, and Asian or Native American ancestry.

The mechanism of breast milk jaundice, which is also quite common, is not known. Some researchers have theorized that it is caused by an increase in enterohepatic circulation from an unknown maternal factor in the breast milk. The infant's peak bilirubin level tends to be higher and lasts longer than that found with physiologic jaundice.

Any infant who develops hyperbilirubinemia in the first 24 hours of life, has an increase in serum bilirubin greater than 5 mg/dL/day, is jaundiced, and has the risk factors noted earlier has prolonged jaundice (more than 1 week in the full-term infant or more than 2 weeks in the premature neonate) or has conjugated hyperbilirubinemia that needs to be evaluated.

Differential Diagnosis

Unconjugated Hyperbilirubinemia
- Physiologic jaundice
- Hemolytic process

  Immune etiology: ABO/Rh incompatibility, erythroblastosis fetalis, drug reaction (penicillin, sulfonamides, oxytocin)
  Red cell defects: Structural (spherocytosis, elliptocytosis); hemoglobinopathy (sickle cell, α-thalassemia); enzyme deficiency (G6PD or pyruvate kinase deficiency)
  DIC

- Polycythemia
- Extravascular blood loss: Bruising from birth trauma (petechiae, cephalohematoma), hemorrhage (pulmonary, cerebral)
- Increased enterohepatic circulation: Intestinal obstruction (pyloric stenosis, duodenal stenosis or atresia, annular pancreas), Hirschsprung's disease, meconium ileus and/or meconium plug syndrome, drug-induced paralytic ileus (magnesium)

- Breast milk jaundice
- Disorders of bilirubin metabolism: Gilbert's syndrome, Crigler-Najjar syndrome, and Lucey-Driscoll syndrome
- Endocrine's disorders: Hypothyroidism, infants of diabetic mothers, hypopituitarism
- Bacterial sepsis

Conjugated Hyperbilirubinemia
- Extrahepatic obstruction: Biliary atresia, choledocholithiasis, choledochal cyst, common duct stenosis, inspissated bile syndrome from cystic fibrosis, extrinsic bile duct compression, pancreatitis
- Persistent intrahepatic cholestasis: Paucity of intrahepatic ducts, benign recurrent intrahepatic cholestasis, arteriohepatic dysplasia
- Acquired intrahepatic cholestasis: Neonatal hepatitis (bacterial sepsis; congenital infections; hepatitis A, B, and C; varicella; Epstein-Barr virus; echovirus; coxsackie virus; tuberculosis; leptospirosis; amoebiasis; idiopathic), drug-induced cholestasis, total parenteral nutrition cholestasis, cirrhosis, drug or metal toxicity, neoplasms (hepatoblastoma, secondary liver metastases)
- Genetic and metabolic disorders: Disorders of bilirubin metabolism (Dubin-Johnson's syndrome, Rotor's syndrome), disorders of carbohydrate metabolism (galactosemia, fructosemia), disorders of amino acid metabolism (tyrosinemia, hypermethioninemia), disorders of lipid metabolism (Niemann-Pick's disease, Gaucher's disease), chromosomal disorders (trisomy 18 and 21), metabolic liver disease (Wilson's disease, α_1-antitrypsin deficiency)

Clinical Manifestations

History

An important fact on history is whether the child is bottle or breast fed. Other important clues include a history of red cell structural defects, hemoglobinopathies, or enzyme deficiencies in the family or whether a previous child had an ABO incompatibility. There may be a family history of genetic or chromosomal disorders. Prenatal screens should be reviewed for possible indications of congenital infection. The length of time the jaundice has been present, whether it is worsening or improving, and associated GI or constitutional symptoms should be explored. Also, it is important to ask whether the stool color has changed (to a gray color) or the urine has darkened.

Physical Examination

In neonates, the examination should focus on the level of jaundice because progression is reliably cephalopedal. When jaundice has reached the umbilicus, the serum level is approximately 10. If the palms and soles are involved, the level is likely greater than 15.

Diagnostic Evaluation

Because the most common causes of unconjugated hyperbilirubinemia are physiologic (including breast milk jaundice) and hemolytic, the initial evaluation should include a CBC with peripheral blood smear and reticulocyte count, a determination of maternal and infant blood types, a Coombs test (direct and indirect), and a determination of the conjugated and unconjugated fractions of the hyperbilirubinemia. Figure 13-2 shows an algorithm for the evaluation of hyperbilirubinemia.

Treatment

The goal in treating unconjugated hyperbilirubinemia is to avoid kernicterus or sublethal bilirubin encephalopathy. The two modalities used to decrease unconjugated bilirubin are phototherapy and exchange transfusion. When to use these treatments depends on the birth weight of the neonate. Given a specific LBW, Table 13-4 provides a general guide for

TABLE 13-4 Hyperbilirubinemia in Low-Birth-Weight Neonates		
	Bilirubin Level (mg/dL)	
Weight (g)	Consider Phototherapy	Consider Exchange Transfusion
<1,000	5–7	12–15
1,000–1,500	7–10	15–18
1,500–2,500	10–15	8–20
>2500	>15	>20

treatment at different levels of unconjugated hyperbilirubinemia. When to use phototherapy in the full-term neonate is quite controversial. No studies show evidence of encephalopathic damage from unconjugated hyperbilirubinemia peak levels less than 25 mg per dL in the full-term healthy neonate with uncomplicated physiologic jaundice. As a result, there is much debate among pediatricians as to when to begin phototherapy. However, because kernicterus continues to be a problem in the United States, the American Academy of Pediatrics released a policy statement in 2004 recommending that every infant have a bilirubin level checked before discharge. The statement includes elaborate treatment recommendations differentiating among infants of low, moderate, and high risk. Phototherapy converts the unconjugated bilirubin into several water-soluble photoisomers that can be excreted without conjugation, so it is important to optimize the infant's hydration status. Exchange transfusion directly removes the bilirubin from the intravascular space and removes maternal immunoglobulin that may be contributing to a hemolytic process. Exchange transfusion is usually reserved for the bilirubin levels above 25 in the setting of hemolytic disease.

Treatment of conjugated hyperbilirubinemia is directed at the underlying cause of the hyperbilirubinemia. Phototherapy of conjugated bilirubin "bronzes" the skin and takes months to resolve.

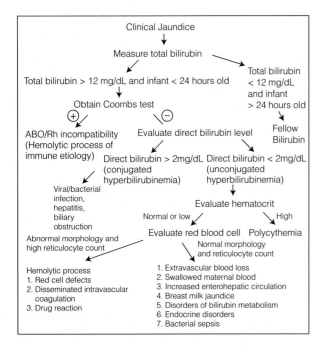

Figure 13-2 • Algorithm for the evaluation of hyperbilirubinemia in the neonate.

☙ 13-19 KEY POINTS

1. Hyperbilirubinemia may be conjugated or unconjugated. Conjugated hyperbilirubinemia is always pathologic, whereas unconjugated hyperbilirubinemia may or may not be pathologic.
2. The two most common causes of unconjugated hyperbilirubinemia are physiologic (including breast milk) jaundice and hemolytic disease.
3. Most neonatal unconjugated hyperbilirubinemia is physiologic.

NECROTIZING ENTEROCOLITIS

Pathogenesis

NEC refers to a process of transluminal and mucosal necrosis that is seen in premature infants. The cause is unknown but likely involves a component of ischemia or reperfusion injury, followed by translocation of bacteria into the wall of the intestine. Occasional epidemics in NICUs implicate a primary role for infection in some instances. **Pneumatosis intestinalis** results from gas production in the bowel wall. It can be detected on abdominal radiography and is pathognomonic for NEC.

NEC occurs primarily in premature infants and is ultimately diagnosed in almost 25% of very low-birth-weight infants (<1,500 g). Prenatal factors associated with NEC include maternal age greater than 35, maternal infection requiring antibiotics, premature rupture of membranes (PROM), and cocaine exposure. Perinatal factors include maternal anesthesia, depressed Apgar score at 5 minutes, birth asphyxia, RDS, and hypotension. Postnatal factors include patent ductus arteriosus, congestive heart failure, umbilical vessel catheterization, polycythemia, and exchange transfusion. The osmotic load of formula is also implicated.

Clinical Manifestations

The presentation may be mild to fulminant and occurs in the first 6 weeks of life. The earliest signs are feeding intolerance with bilious aspirates and abdominal distention. The patient may develop occult blood in the stool, which can become grossly bloody. Extreme abdominal tenderness with discoloration, hyperglycemia, severe metabolic acidosis, sepsis, shock, DIC, temperature instability, and ineffective respiratory effort (caused by severe abdominal distention) requiring mechanical ventilation are seen in the more severe cases.

Long-term complications include intestinal strictures, which may be demonstrated by contrast study. Laboratory findings include leukocytosis, neutropenia, thrombocytopenia, and metabolic acidosis.

Treatment

If NEC is suspected, feeds should be discontinued immediately and a NG tube should be placed for gastric and intestinal decompression. Systemic antibiotics should be started and blood cultures sent. Abdominal radiographs are obtained at least every 6 hours to monitor for pneumatosis intestinalis, portal air, and free peritoneal air. Intravenous fluids are administered to prevent shock. If free air is seen in the peritoneal cavity or intestinal necrosis is suspected, surgical intervention is indicated. If there is no free air, a 10- to 14-day course of bowel rest and broad antibiotic treatment generally leads to full recovery, although mortality rates remain high for this disease.

🔑 13-20 KEY POINTS

1. Necrotizing enterocolitis refers to a process of acute intestinal necrosis seen in premature infants.
2. Infants with medical NEC present with feeding intolerance, abdominal distention, occult blood in the stool, and dilated bowel loops on abdominal radiograph.
3. Pneumatosis intestinalis is the diagnostic radiographic finding. Free peritoneal air is evidence of perforation and an indication for surgical intervention.

NEONATAL HEMATOLOGIC DISORDERS

POLYCYTHEMIA

Pathogenesis

Polycythemia is defined as a greater than normal number of RBCs. Neonatal polycythemia (defined as a venous hematocrit >65%) is almost always a consequence of fetal hypertransfusion. Delayed clamping of the cord after delivery with consequent transfer of placental blood to the infant is the most common cause in term infants. A significantly elevated hematocrit leads to hyperviscosity of the blood, resulting in vascular stasis, microthrombi, hypoperfusion, and tissue ischemia. Neonatal erythrocytes are less filterable and deformable than adult erythrocytes, further contributing to hyperviscosity. Although a central venous hematocrit of greater than 65% occurs in 3% to 5% of infants, not all infants have symptoms of hyperviscosity syndrome.

Risk Factors

Infants at risk for polycythemia are postterm and small for gestational age neonates; infants of diabetic mothers; infants with delayed cord clamping (maternal–fetal transfusion); and infants suffering from neonatal hyperthyroidism, adrenogenital syndrome, the trisomies (13, 18, and 21), twin–twin transfusion (recipient), or

Beckwith-Wiedemann's syndrome. In some infants, polycythemia reflects a compensation for prolonged periods of fetal hypoxia from placental insufficiency; these infants have increased erythropoietin levels at birth.

Clinical Manifestations

Polycythemic infants appear ruddy and plethoric. Irritability, lethargy, poor feeding, emesis, tremulousness, and seizures all reflect abnormalities of the microcirculation of the brain. Acute renal failure results from inadequate renal perfusion. Hepatomegaly and hyperbilirubinemia are caused by poor hepatic circulation and to the increased amount of hemoglobin that is metabolized into bilirubin. Because of stasis in the pulmonary vessels, pulmonary vascular resistance increases, and PPHN may result. Other complications include NEC and hypoglycemia. Vascular impairment in the penis can cause priapism, and the formation of microthrombi may result in thrombocytopenia. If ischemia is severe enough, both the EEG and the ECG may be abnormal. Chest radiograph often reveals cardiomegaly, increased vascular markings, pleural effusions, and interstitial edema.

Long-term complications from neonatal polycythemia are more likely in the symptomatic child, particularly if hypoglycemia is present. Neurodevelopmental abnormalities include mild deficits in speech, hearing, and coordination. If cerebral infarction occurs, cerebral palsy and mental retardation are likely.

Treatment

Long-term complications may be prevented by treatment of symptomatic infants with partial exchange transfusion after birth. A partial exchange transfusion removes whole blood and replaces it with normal saline or albumin.

13-21 KEY POINTS

1. Hyperviscosity syndrome, which occurs when the hematocrit exceeds 65%, results in vascular stasis, microthrombi, hypoperfusion, and tissue ischemia.
2. Polycythemic infants appear ruddy and plethoric.
3. Long-term complications from neonatal polycythemia are more likely in the symptomatic child, particularly if hypoglycemia is also present, and include mild deficits in speech, hearing, and coordination.
4. Treatment of polycythemia is primarily by partial exchange transfusion.

ANEMIA

Anemia in the neonate can result from blood loss, hemolysis, decreased RBC production, or (physiologic) decreased erythropoiesis. Blood loss may result from obstetric causes, occult blood loss, or iatrogenic causes and may occur during the prenatal, perinatal, or neonatal period.

Obstetric causes of blood loss include abruptio placenta, placenta previa, incision of the placenta during cesarean delivery, rupture of anomalous vessels (vasa previa, velamentous insertion of the cord, or rupture of communicating vessels in a multilobed placenta), hematoma of the cord caused by varices or aneurysm, or rupture of the cord.

Occult blood loss may result from fetomaternal bleeding, fetoplacental bleeding, or twin-to-twin transfusion. Fetomaternal bleeding may be chronic or acute. It occurs in 8% of all pregnancies. The diagnosis of this problem is by Kleihauer-Betke stain of maternal smear for fetal cells.

Bleeding in the neonatal period may be caused by intracranial bleeding, massive cephalohematoma, retroperitoneal bleeding, ruptured liver or spleen, adrenal or renal hemorrhage, GI bleeding, or bleeding from the umbilicus. Excessive blood loss may result from blood sampling with inadequate replacement. With acute blood loss, the hematocrit is often normal, as is the reticulocyte count.

Hemolysis is manifested by a decreased hematocrit, increased reticulocyte count, and an increased bilirubin level. Hemolysis may result from immune mechanisms, hereditary red cell disorders, or acquired hemolysis. Immune-mediated hemolysis results from Rh incompatibility, ABO incompatibility, minor blood group incompatibility (c, E, Kell, Duffy), and maternal hemolytic anemia from systemic lupus erythematosus. Hereditary red cell disorders that result in hemolysis include RBC membrane defects (spherocytosis), enzymopathies (G6PD deficiency, pyruvate kinase deficiency), and hemoglobinopathies (sickle cell disease, α- and β-thalassemias). Causes of acquired hemolysis include bacterial or viral infection, DIC, vitamin E deficiency, or microangiopathic hemolytic anemia.

Diminished RBC production is manifested by a decreased hematocrit, decreased reticulocyte count, and normal bilirubin level. Etiologies include Diamond-Blackfan's syndrome, Fanconi anemia, congenital leukemia, infections (especially rubella and parvovirus), osteopetrosis leading to inadequate erythropoiesis, drug-induced RBC suppression, physiologic anemia, or anemia of prematurity.

Physiologic anemia of the full-term or premature neonate is caused by physiologically decreased erythropoiesis. Full-term infants have a nadir of the hemoglobin level at 6 to 12 weeks, premature infants (1,200 to 2,400 g) have a nadir at 5 to 10 weeks, and very LBW neonates (birth weight < 1,200 g) have a nadir at 4 to 8 weeks. The laboratory manifestations of physiologic anemia are a decreased hematocrit and a low reticulocyte count. When the infant's oxygen demand increases, erythropoietin will increase; if iron stores are adequate, the reticulocyte count will increase and the hemoglobin level will rise.

Clinical Manifestations

A complete family history, including questions about anemia, jaundice, cholestatic disease, and splenectomy, may give important clues to newborn disease. The obstetric history may identify blood loss as the cause of the anemia. The physical examination can usually differentiate acute blood loss, chronic blood loss, and chronic hemolytic disease. Manifestations of acute blood loss include shock, tachypnea, tachycardia, low venous pressure, weak pulses, and pallor. Chronic blood loss is manifested by extreme pallor and a low hematocrit. These infants are typically normovolemic and may have congestive heart failure or hydrops fetalis. Chronic hemolysis is associated with pallor, jaundice, and hepatosplenomegaly.

Neonatal anemia may be classified by evaluation of the reticulocyte count, bilirubin level, Coombs test, and RBC morphology (Table 13-5). The **Apt test** helps identify maternal blood that has been swallowed by the neonate, and the **Kleihauer-Betke preparation** determines if fetomaternal transfusion has occurred. US of the head is used to define an intracranial bleed. Laboratory tests on the parents help determine the likelihood of a hemolytic process. If a congenital infection is suspected as the cause of the anemia, appropriate diagnostic tests may be done. Bone marrow aspiration is performed in rare cases in which bone marrow failure is suggested.

Treatment

Healthy, term, asymptomatic newborns self-correct a mild anemia, provided that iron intake is adequate. Although non-breast-feeding infants are sent home

TABLE 13-5 Classification of Anemia in the Newborn

Reticulocytes	Bilirubin	Coombs Test	RBC Morphology	Diagnostic Possibilities
Normal or decreased	Normal	Negative	Normal	Physiologic anemia of infancy or prematurity; congenital hypoplastic anemia; other causes of decreased production
Normal or increased	Normal	Negative	Normal	Acute hemorrhage (fetomaternal, placental, umbilical cord, or internal hemorrhage)
			Hypochromic microcytes	Chronic fetomaternal hemorrhage
Increased	increased	Positive	Spherocytes	Immune hemolysis (blood group incompatibility or maternal autoantibody)
Normal or increased	increased	Negative	Spherocytes	Hereditary spherocytosis
			Elliptocytes	Hereditary elliptocytosis
			Hypochromic microcytes	α- or γ-thalassemia syndrome
			Spiculated RBCs	Pyruvate kinase deficiency
			Schistocytes and RBC fragments	DIC; other microangiopathic processes
			Bite cells (Heinz bodies with supravital stain)	Glucose-6-phosphate dehydrogenase deficiency
			Normal	Infections; enclosed hemorrhage (cephalohematoma)

on iron-fortified formulas, iron supplementation is not required until 2 months of age when reticulocytosis resumes.

If the neonate has acute blood loss at birth, immediate access should be obtained, and blood must be sent for typing and crossmatching. If hypovolemic shock is present (decreased venous pressure, pallor, tachycardia), 20 mL per kg of volume expander is recommended. Unmatched type O blood should be available for transfusion if needed. Albumin and normal saline are also useful to replete the intravascular volume temporarily. Chronic blood loss and the anemia from hemolysis are generally well tolerated. Only if the neonate is symptomatic with congestive heart failure should he or she be transfused. It is recommended that the hematocrit in the child with cardiac or respiratory diseases be kept above 35 to 40.

Anemia of prematurity is tempered by vitamin E and iron administration in premature formulas. Premature infants tolerate hemoglobins of 6.5 to 8.0 g per dL. The level itself is not an indication for transfusion. Transfusion should occur if another condition exists that requires increased oxygen-carrying capacity, such as sepsis, NEC, pneumonia, chronic lung disease, and apnea.

🔑 13-22 KEY POINTS

1. Anemia in the neonate can result from blood loss, hemolysis, decreased RBC production, or physiologically decreased erythropoiesis.
2. Neonatal anemia may be classified by evaluation of the reticulocyte count, bilirubin level, Coombs test, and RBC morphology (Table 13-5).

NEONATAL CENTRAL NERVOUS SYSTEM DISORDERS

APNEA OF PREMATURITY

Pathogenesis

Apnea in the premature infant is defined as a cessation of breathing for longer than 20 seconds or a shorter pause associated with cyanosis, pallor, hypotonia, or a heart rate of less than 100 beats per minute (bpm). Apnea in the full-term neonate (apnea of infancy; see Chapter 20) is defined as absent breathing for longer than 16 seconds. In the premature infant, apneic episodes may be caused by central, obstructive, or mixed mechanisms. In central apnea, there is a complete cessation of air flow and respiratory effort with no chest wall movement, whereas in obstructive apnea, there is respiratory effort and chest wall movement but no air flow. Apnea of prematurity usually has a mixed central and obstructive picture. Periodic breathing, which must be differentiated from apnea, is defined as pauses of 5 to 10 seconds followed by a short period of rapid breathing. Periodic breathing is normal.

Epidemiology

Apnea occurs in most infants of less than 28 weeks' gestation, approximately 50% of infants 30 to 32 weeks' gestation, and in less than 7% of infants 34 to 35 weeks' gestation.

Clinical Manifestations

Apnea of prematurity is associated with bradycardia, which is a heart rate less than 80 bpm. Bradycardia and cyanosis are usually present after 20 seconds of apnea but may occur more rapidly in the small, premature infant. After 30 to 40 seconds, pallor and hypotonia are also seen, and the infant may be unresponsive to tactile stimulation. A neonate may rouse itself and stop the apneic spell, but more symptomatic apnea is apparent if a caregiver must touch the infant to discontinue the apnea. With hypotonia and pallor, bag-mask ventilation is required to return the child to a normal breathing pattern.

A diagnosis of apnea of prematurity is made after excluding other causes of apnea, which can be grouped into the following broad categories: hypoxemia, diaphragmatic fatigue, respiratory center depression, infection, vagal stimulation, airway obstruction, and inappropriate environmental temperature. Hypoxemia may result from anemia, hypovolemia, and congenital heart disease, whereas RDS and pneumonia can cause diaphragmatic fatigue. Respiratory center depression can occur with metabolic abnormalities (hypoglycemia, hypocalcemia, hyponatremia), drugs, seizures, or intraventricular hemorrhage (IVH). Infectious processes such as sepsis, NEC, and meningitis all can cause apnea, whereas gastroesophageal reflux, suctioning of the oropharynx, and NG tube passage can cause vagally mediated depression of the respiratory center. Excessive oral secretions, anatomic obstruction, or malposition may result in obstructive apnea.

Treatment

Treatment for apnea of prematurity includes maintenance of a skin-core temperature gradient in the incubator, supplemental oxygen, tactile stimulation, and administration of respiratory stimulants (caffeine or theophylline). Apnea of prematurity may also be managed by increasing the mean airway pressure through the use of CPAP or intermittent assisted ventilation. For the other causes of apnea, treatment of the underlying disorder usually leads to cessation of the apneic episodes.

When an infant reaches 34 to 35 weeks' postconceptional age, is tolerating feeds orally, and has not had an apneic or bradycardiac episode for 7 days, the infant is ready to be discharged home. The apnea monitor sent home with the patient can be discontinued when the infant has been apnea free for 2 months.

⚜ 13-23 KEY POINTS

1. Apnea in the premature infant is defined as a cessation of breathing for longer than 20 seconds or a shorter pause associated with cyanosis, pallor, hypotonia, or a heart rate of less than 100 bpm.
2. In the premature infant, apneic episodes may be caused by a central, obstructive, or mixed mechanism.
3. The treatment for apnea of prematurity includes maintenance of a skin-core temperature gradient in the incubator, supplemental oxygen, tactile stimulation, administration of respiratory stimulants, and, in the most severe cases, CPAP or intermittent assisted ventilation.

INTRAVENTRICULAR HEMORRHAGE

Pathogenesis

IVH is seen almost exclusively in preterm infants and results from bleeding of the germinal matrix, an area of immature vasculature that is the site of pluripotent cells that migrate to form neurons and glia. Changes in cerebral blood flow have been proposed as a contributing mechanism. Surges of cerebral arterial flow may occur with seizures, episodes of hypoxia, apnea, respiratory distress, rapid infusion of colloid, patent ductus arteriosus, and ECMO. Increased venous pressure may be associated with RDS, pneumothorax, congestive heart failure, ventilator parameters such as CPAP, and hyperviscosity. IVH is very common among VLBW infants, and the risk decreases as gestational age increases. Approximately 50% of infants under 1,500 g have evidence of intracranial bleeding. Small intraventricular hemorrhages that are confined to the germinal matrix (grade I) or are associated with a small amount of blood in the ventricle (grade II) often resolve without sequelae. Large IVHs that are associated with ventricular dilatation (grade III) or with extension into the brain parenchyma (grade IV) are associated with permanent functional impairment and hydrocephalus.

Posthemorrhagic hydrocephalus is a consequence of obstruction of the ventricular outlets (obstructive hydrocephalus) or of obliteration of the arachnoid villi that ultimately absorb the CSF (communicating hydrocephalus). Hydrocephalus may be static, in which case no intervention is made, or it may be progressive, requiring the surgical placement of a ventriculoperitoneal shunt.

Clinical Manifestations

Approximately 50% of hemorrhages occur in the first day of life, and approximately 90% occur within the first 3 days of life. Most hemorrhages are asymptomatic. If a severe hemorrhage occurs, the neonate may develop anemia, pallor, hypotension, focal neurologic signs, seizures, an acute increase in ventilatory assistance needs, apnea, and/or bradycardia.

US through the anterior fontanelle is the method of choice to screen for, grade, and follow IVH. All premature infants with birth weights less than 1,500 g should have a diagnostic US performed within the first week of life.

Treatment

The risk of IVH is minimized by preventing premature delivery, if possible, or through the use of appropriate neonatal resuscitation measures to minimize hypoxemia by stabilizing the arterial blood pressure, intravascular volume, hematocrit, and oxygenation. The goal in acute management of IVH is to maintain adequate cerebral perfusion and to control intracerebral pressure. Normal arterial blood pressure is preserved by volume replacement with packed RBCs and/or inotropic support. IVH is followed by serial US evaluations because ventriculomegaly occurs before there is an increase in head circumference. Progressive posthemorrhagic hydrocephalus is treated by placement of a ventriculoperitoneal shunt.

Outcome is dependent on the severity of the IVH. Grades I and II hemorrhages rarely result in long-term morbidity. Of infants with grade III IVH, 30% to 45% have motor and intellectual impairment. An estimated 60% to 80% of neonates with grade IV IVH develop motor and intellectual disabilities.

> ### 🔑 13-24 KEY POINTS
>
> 1. Intraventricular hemorrhage is seen almost exclusively in preterm infants and results from bleeding of the germinal matrix.
> 2. Approximately 50% of hemorrhages occur in the first day of life, and approximately 90% occur within the first 3 days of life.
> 3. The risk of IVH is minimized by preventing premature delivery, if possible, or through the use of appropriate neonatal resuscitation measures to minimize hypoxemia and rapid cerebral flow changes by stabilizing the arterial blood pressure, intravascular volume, hematocrit, and oxygenation.
> 4. Grades I and II hemorrhages result in no long-term morbidity. Of infants with grade III IVH, 30% to 45% have motor and intellectual impairment; of neonates with grade IV IVH, 60% to 80% develop motor and intellectual disabilities.

HYPOXIC ISCHEMIC ENCEPHALOPATHY

Pathogenesis

Hypoxic ischemic encephalopathy (HIE) occurs with an incidence of approximately 6 per 1,000 full-term infants. HIE is a significant cause of neonatal morbidity and mortality with long-term neurologic sequelae. It is a consequence of ischemia-reperfusion injury related to a number of prenatal or perinatal events. Maternal risk factors include hypotension, hypothyroidism, and infertility treatment. Intrapartum events commonly include cord prolapse, placental abruption, breech extraction, or difficult forceps delivery. Postnatal events such as sepsis, severe respiratory failure, or congenital heart disease are far less common causes.

Clinical Manifestations

Most commonly, an infant presents at birth with severe perinatal depression or asphyxia requiring full resuscitation in the delivery room. Significant metabolic and respiratory acidosis is often present, and the infant may have poor respiratory effort. However, if the insult occurred well before delivery, there may be few initial signs in the delivery room. In the case of perinatal injury, the infant has depressed mental status for several hours because of the depression of cortical activity. Up to 50% of these infants have seizures within the first 6 to 12 hours of birth. Normal infant reflexes such as the Moro or grasp are often absent, and severely affected newborns do not have a gag reflex. This period is often followed by a time of improved alertness; however, infants with significant brain injury frequently regress to a depressed level of consciousness with signs of brainstem dysfunction. Hypotonia, apnea, fixed and dilated pupils, poor suck and swallow, and proximal weakness are all signs of substantial injury. Metabolic disturbances including hypoglycemia, hypocalcemia, hyponatremia, and acidosis are common. A diffusion-weighted MRI obtained within 48 to 72 hours of the injury may demonstrate the extent of injury and in severe cases may help delineate a poor prognosis. EEG may document seizures or a burst suppression pattern indicative of global injury. However, the best predictor of outcome remains the neurologic exam at 1 week of life. If an infant has a normal exam and is able to take full oral feeds, the chance for a full recovery are excellent.

Treatment

Although no treatment is available for established brain injury, preliminary studies of head cooling after acute perinatal depression show promise in reducing the severity of neurologic sequelae. Further studies are needed before this approach is universally recommended.

NEONATAL SEIZURES

The causes of neonatal seizures are categorized in the following list:

- *Metabolic*: Hypoglycemia, electrolyte abnormalities (hypocalcemia, hypomagnesemia, hyponatremia), inborn errors of metabolism (organic acidemias, error of amino acid metabolism, pyridoxine deficiency)
- *Toxic*: Maternal drug ingestion, neonatal drug withdrawal, inadvertent local anesthetic poisoning, hyperbilirubinemia
- *Hemorrhagic*: Intraventricular, subdural, or subarachnoid hemorrhage

- *Infectious*: Bacterial meningitis, viral encephalitis
- *Asphyxia*: Hypoxic ischemic encephalopathy
- *Genetic/dysmorphic syndromes*: Cerebral dysgenesis, chromosomal abnormalities, phakomatoses (tuberous sclerosis)

Seizures are difficult to differentiate from benign jitters or clonus in neonates with hypoglycemia or hypocalcemia, in infants of diabetic mothers, in newborns with narcotic withdrawal syndrome, and in infants after an episode of asphyxia. In contrast to seizures, jitters and tremors are sensory dependent, elicited by stimuli, and may be interrupted by holding the extremity. Seizure activity is coarse, with fast and slow clonic activity, whereas jitters are characterized by fine, very rapid movement. It is often difficult to identify seizures in the newborn period because the infant, especially the LBW infant, usually does not demonstrate the tonic-clonic major motor activity typical of the older child.

Subtle seizures constitute 50% of seizures in newborns (both term and preterm). Subtle seizure activity may include rhythmic fluctuations in vital signs, apnea, eye deviation, nystagmus, tongue thrusting, eye blinking, staring, and "bicycling" or "swimming" movements. Continuous bedside EEG monitoring can help identify subtle seizures.

The movements in **focal clonic seizures** involve well-localized clonic jerking. These types of seizures are not associated with loss of consciousness and are most often provoked by metabolic disturbances. Subarachnoid hemorrhage and focal infarct may also promote this type of seizure. The EEG during seizure activity is unifocally abnormal, but the prognosis is generally good.

Multifocal clonic seizures are characterized by random clonic movements of the limbs. Multifocal anomalies are seen on the EEG, and the prognosis is poor.

Tonic seizures manifest as extensor posturing with tonic eye deviation and are most often seen in premature neonates with diffuse CNS disease or IVH. The EEG has multifocal abnormalities. The prognosis is generally poor.

Synchronized single or multiple slow jerks of the upper or lower limbs (or both) characterize **myoclonic seizures**. These seizures are noted when there is diffuse CNS pathology, and the prognosis is poor. The EEG shows a burst/suppression pattern.

Seizures noted in the delivery room may be caused by direct injection of local anesthetic into the fetal scalp, severe anoxia, or congenital brain malformation. Seizures because of hypoxic-ischemic encephalopathy (postasphyxial seizures), a common cause of seizures in the full-term neonate, usually occur 12 to 24 hours after a history of birth asphyxia and are often refractory to conventional doses of anticonvulsant medications. Postasphyxial seizures may also result from metabolic disorders such as hypoglycemia and hypocalcemia. IVH is a common cause of seizures in premature infants and often occurs from the first to third days of life. Seizures with IVH may be associated with a bulging fontanelle, hemorrhagic spinal fluid, anemia, lethargy, and coma. Seizures after the first 5 days of life may be caused by infection or drug withdrawal. Seizures associated with lethargy, acidosis, ketonuria, respiratory alkalosis, and a family history of infantile death may be caused by an inborn error of metabolism.

Clinical Manifestations

A careful prenatal and perinatal history may shed light on the seizure etiology. The diagnostic evaluation of infants with seizures should include a determination of blood levels of glucose, sodium, calcium, magnesium, and ammonia. In the jaundiced neonate, measurement of the bilirubin level is indicated. When infection is suspected, a blood culture and LP are performed. If an inborn error of metabolism is suspected, urine organic acids and serum amino acids may be examined. Further evaluation may include a US or a CT scan of the head. If physical examination or head imaging suggests a congenital infection, appropriate cultures, antibody determinations, and PCR should be done. Continuous bedside video and EEG monitoring provides the best information in defining the type of seizure present. Continuous EEG with pyridoxine infusion helps establish the presence or absence of pyridoxine deficiency. If seizures result from narcotic withdrawal syndrome, a controlled wean is indicated.

Treatment

If possible, the primary cause of the seizure should be identified and treated. Any metabolic disturbances must be corrected. If a toxin (hyperammonemia, hyperbilirubinemia) is isolated as the etiology of the seizure, exchange transfusion may be used to remove it. Meningitis is treated with the appropriate antibiotic agent. In the absence of an identifiable cause, anticonvulsant therapy is used. Agents include phenobarbital, phenytoin (Dilantin), lorazepam (Ativan), and diazepam (Valium). Phenobarbital is standard primary therapy. Phenytoin is used when seizures persist with a phenobarbital level greater than 50 mg per L. The long-term outcome of neonatal seizures is determined by the type and etiology of the seizure.

🔨 13-25 KEY POINTS

1. Seizures may result from metabolic disturbances, inborn errors of metabolism, toxic exposures, hemorrhagic brain insult, infectious etiologies, asphyxia, and genetic defects.
2. Neonatal seizures are divided into focal clonic, multifocal clonic, tonic, myoclonic, and tonic-clonic seizures.
3. Continuous bedside video EEG monitoring provides the best information in defining the type of seizure present.
4. Phenobarbital is the primary anticonvulsant used to manage neonatal seizures.

NEONATAL DISORDERS OF THE ENDOCRINE SYSTEM

HYPOTHYROIDISM

The physical stigmata of congenital hypothyroidism in the newborn are often too subtle for physical diagnosis, so clinicians rely heavily on diagnostic screening. All states currently require newborn screening for hypothyroidism. The sooner treatment is initiated, the better the prognosis for normal intellectual development in the child. In most cases the diagnosis can be made and treatment initiated within 4 weeks.

The etiology is usually sporadic athyreosis or thyroid ectopy. Less common is familial goitrous hypothyroidism. Children of mothers with Graves' disease who are receiving propylthiouracil have transient hypothyroidism.

Clinical Manifestations

Primary hypothyroidism is indicated by a low T_4 level and an elevated TSH. Serum levels should be drawn to confirm abnormal screening results.

A low T_4 level accompanied by a low TSH value may indicate a physiologically normal thyroid status caused by a low concentration of thyroid-binding globulin (TBG). This is frequently observed in premature infants or may be seen on a hereditary basis. Alternatively, a low T_4 and low TSH with a normal TBG level may indicate hypopituitarism or hypothalamic deficiency. Hypothalamic deficiency usually is accompanied by growth hormone or corticotropin deficiency, which may cause acute hypoglycemia. Figure 13-3 delineates an algorithm for the diagnosis of hypothyroidism.

Treatment

If the screening results indicate primary hypothyroidism, the T_4 and TSH studies should be repeated and therapy started. Serum T_4 is measured after 5 days of therapy, and the thyroxine dosage is adjusted to keep the T_4 level in the upper half of the normal range for age. The TSH concentration may remain elevated for months in some patients because of immaturity of the feedback mechanism. Levothyroxine is administered at an initial dose of 10 µg per kg. Tablets are crushed and given orally.

Before therapy commences, a bone age and a thyroid scan should be done. An iodinated ^{123}I or technetium scan of the thyroid gland evaluates the presence of a rudimentary or ectopic thyroid gland. Scans must be performed before therapy commences and the TSH decreases. Maternal antibodies can suppress the newborn thyroid gland function temporarily so there is no uptake by the thyroid gland on scan.

If therapy is started within the first month after birth, the prognosis is excellent. The thyroxine dose must be carefully adjusted because too little thyroxine results in persistent hypothyroidism, whereas too much thyroxine may result in advanced bone age and craniosynostosis.

🔨 13-26 KEY POINTS

1. All states currently require newborn screening for hypothyroidism.
2. If therapy is started within the first month after birth, the prognosis for normal intellectual development in the child is excellent.

NEONATAL HYPOGLYCEMIA

The definition of hypoglycemia in the neonate has been the subject of decades of debate. Full-term neonates frequently have a transient hypoglycemia with blood glucose measurements in the 30s (mg per dL)

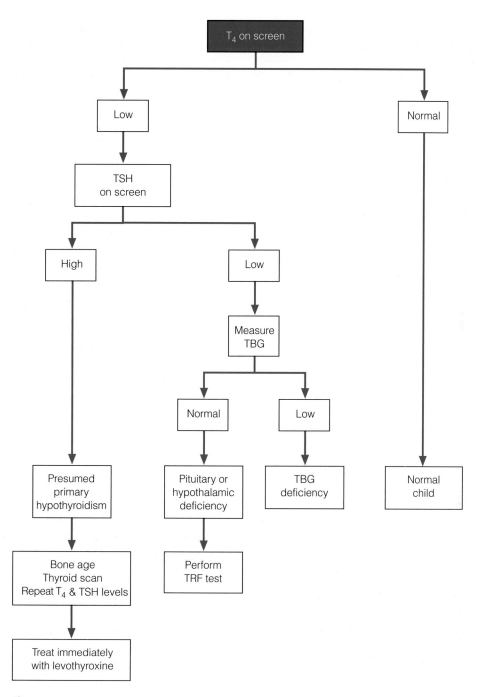

Figure 13-3 • Algorithm for the diagnosis of hypothyroidism.

and spontaneously recover. As a result, published statistical definitions of hypoglycemia generally use a level in the mid-30s. However, persistent levels of less than 60 should prompt consideration of and evaluation for pathologic processes.

Pathogenesis

Infants with hypoglycemia may be divided into those with hyperinsulinism and those without hyperinsulinism. Infants with transient hyperinsulinism include infants of diabetic mothers and infants with Rh hemolytic disease. Infants with protracted hyperinsulinism include those who have Beckwith-Wiedemann's syndrome, islet cell adenomas, and functional hyperinsulinism. Infants who do not have hyperinsulinism and have transient hypoglycemia include those with intrauterine growth retardation, birth asphyxia, polycythemia, cardiac disease, CNS disease, sepsis, maternal use of propranolol, oral hypoglycemic agents, or narcotic addiction. Infants who do not have hyperinsulinism but have protracted hypoglycemia include those with neonatal hypopituitarism or defects in carbohydrate and/or amino acid metabolism. Deficiencies of growth hormone or corticotropin or both cause hypoglycemia in neonatal hypopituitarism. Defects in carbohydrate metabolism that result in hypoglycemia include glycogen storage disease type I, glycogen synthetase deficiency, fructose-1,6-diphosphatase deficiency, fructose intolerance, galactosemia, and pyruvate carboxylase deficiency. Disorders of amino acid metabolism that result in hypoglycemia include methylmalonic acidemia, tyrosinosis, propionic acidemia, and maple syrup urine disease.

Clinical Manifestations

The onset of hypoglycemia may occur anywhere from a few hours after birth to several days of age. Subtle symptoms such as poor feeding, apathy, lethargy, and hypotonia are most common, but life-threatening manifestations such as seizures, apnea, and cyanosis may also occur.

Inborn errors of metabolism may cause persistent or recurrent hypoglycemia. When the infant is hypoglycemic, serum should be obtained for glucose, insulin, cortisol, growth hormone, lactate, and pyruvate levels. Serum amino acid screening is indicated if no definitive diagnosis is made; the infant need not be hypoglycemic at the time of the sample collection.

Treatment

In asymptomatic infants, oral feedings can be attempted. If oral feedings are not accepted, an intravenous infusion of maintenance dextrose at 5 to 7 mg/kg/minute is initiated.

In symptomatic infants, an intravenous push of 2 mL per kg 10% dextrose precedes infusion of intravenous dextrose at a rate of 5 to 7 mg/kg/minute. The rate is adjusted to keep the blood glucose level between 60 and 120 mg per dL. Rebound hypoglycemia may occur if the dextrose infusion is abruptly decreased. Dextrostix values are useful for screening blood sugar; abnormal values should be verified with a true blood sugar. When the infant is stabilized, the dextrose infusion rate is slowly decreased, with careful monitoring of blood glucose. After dextrose infusion is discontinued, the blood glucose level should be monitored for 24 hours.

Glucagon in doses of 300 µg per kg to 1 mg per kg can be used in conditions with adequate glycogen stores, such as hyperinsulinism. Glucocorticoids are used as replacement therapy in infants with hypoadrenalism. Growth hormone is helpful in those infants with growth hormone deficiency. Diazoxide can be administered in hyperinsulinemic states and may serve as a diagnostic technique because patients with insulinomas are far less likely to respond to diazoxide than are functional hyperinsulinemic patients. Pancreatectomy is reserved for intractable hypoglycemia caused by hyperinsulinism. If an isolated tumor is found, it must be removed.

🔑 13-27 KEY POINTS

1. Infants with hypoglycemia may be divided into those with hyperinsulinism and those without hyperinsulinism.
2. Infants who do not have hyperinsulinism and have transient hypoglycemia include those with intrauterine growth retardation, birth asphyxia, polycythemia, cardiac disease, CNS disease, and sepsis, and infants whose mothers have used propranolol, oral hypoglycemic agents, and narcotics.
3. Infants who do not have hyperinsulinism and have protracted hypoglycemia include those with neonatal hypopituitarism and defects in carbohydrate or amino acid metabolism.
4. In symptomatic infants, an intravenous push of 2 mL per kg 10% dextrose is followed by an infusion of intravenous dextrose at a rate of 5 to 7 mg/kg/minute.

CONGENITAL ANOMALIES

TRACHEOESOPHAGEAL FISTULA

The lower section of the esophagus develops as an elongation of the superior portion of the primitive foregut. When there is abnormal anastomosis of superior and inferior portions of the esophagus, esophageal atresia results. Of neonates with esophageal atresia, 85% have tracheoesophageal fistula (TEF). Figure 13-4 shows the four types of tracheoesophageal atresias. Esophageal atresia with distal TEF accounts for 85% of the cases of TEF. Forty percent of patients with TEF have other defects. Associated cardiovascular anomalies include patent ductus arteriosus, vascular ring, and coarctation of the aorta. The incidences of imperforate anus, malrotation, and duodenal anomalies also are increased. VACTERL syndrome describes the association of vertebral, anal, cardiac, tracheal, esophageal, renal, and limb anomalies.

Clinical Manifestations

Neonates with TEF have excessive oral secretions, inability to feed, gagging, and respiratory distress. Polyhydramnios often is noted on US while the child is in utero. Lateral and anteroposterior chest radiographs of the thoracocervical region and abdomen with a Replogle tube in the proximal esophagus reveal a blind pouch with air in the GI tract. In esophageal atresia without TEF, gas is absent from the GI tract, whereas in TEF without esophageal atresia (H type), infants may have nonspecific symptoms for several months, including chronic cough with feeding and recurrent pneumonia.

Treatment

Placing the infant in a 60-degree head-up prone position and minimizing disturbance of the infant are recommended to prevent reflux and aspiration of gastric contents. To remove swallowed oral secretions from the proximal esophageal pouch, a Replogle tube may be placed to suction. The usual corrective procedure is division and closure of the TEF and end-to-end anastomosis of the proximal and distal esophagus. If the distance between esophageal segments is too long for primary anastomosis, delayed anastomosis follows stretching of the upper segment. Strictures at the anastomosis site require periodic dilation.

🔑 13-28 KEY POINTS

1. When there is abnormal anastomosis of superior and inferior portions of the esophagus in utero, esophageal atresia results. Eighty-five percent of neonates with esophageal atresia have tracheoesophageal fistula.

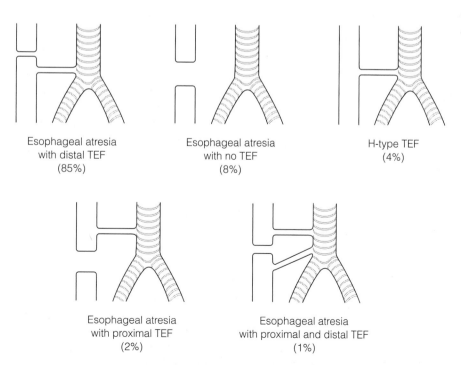

Esophageal atresia
with distal TEF
(85%)

Esophageal atresia
with no TEF
(8%)

H-type TEF
(4%)

Esophageal atresia
with proximal TEF
(2%)

Esophageal atresia
with proximal and distal TEF
(1%)

Figure 13-4 • Types of tracheoesophageal fistulas with relative frequencies.

DUODENAL ATRESIA

Duodenal obstruction may be complete (atresia) or partial (stenosis) because of a web, band, or annular pancreas. Duodenal atresia results from a failure of the lumen to recanalize during the eighth to tenth weeks of gestation. Seventy percent of the cases of duodenal atresia are associated with other malformations, including cardiac anomalies and GI defects such as annular pancreas, malrotation of the intestines, and imperforate anus. Twenty-five percent of infants with duodenal atresia are premature. Duodenal atresia is often associated with trisomy 21.

Clinical Manifestations

With complete obstruction, in utero polyhydramnios may be present. After birth, bilious emesis begins within a few hours after the first feeding. Abdominal radiographs usually show gastric and duodenal gaseous distention proximal to the atretic site. This finding is known as the "double bubble" sign. The presence of gas in the distal bowel suggests partial obstruction, and a contrast radiographic study of the abdomen should be performed.

Treatment

Treatment is surgical. Mortality is related to prematurity and other associated anomalies.

⚲ 13-29 KEY POINTS

1. Duodenal atresia results from a failure of the lumen to recanalize during the eighth to tenth weeks of gestation.
2. Seventy percent of the cases of duodenal atresia are associated with other malformations, including cardiac anomalies and GI defects such as annular pancreas, malrotation of the intestines, and imperforate anus.

CONGENITAL DIAPHRAGMATIC HERNIA

Congenital diaphragmatic hernia results from a defect in the posterolateral diaphragm that allows abdominal contents to enter the thorax and compromise lung development. This defect is commonly referred to as a **Boch-dalek hernia**. Ninety percent of congenital diaphragmatic hernias occur on the left side of the diaphragm. The combination of pulmonary hypoplasia and pulmonary arteriolar hypertension makes this congenital defect lethal in many cases.

Clinical Manifestations

Early symptoms include respiratory distress with decreased breath sounds on the affected side and shift of heart sounds to the opposite side with a scaphoid abdomen. Diagnosis is sometimes made via US while the fetus is in utero. If the diagnosis is not known at birth, a simple chest radiograph makes the diagnosis.

Treatment

Because of pulmonary hypoplasia and pulmonary hypertension, the child must be intubated and ventilated. Sometimes conventional ventilation is not sufficient to provide adequate oxygen delivery and carbon dioxide excretion; in such cases, high-frequency ventilation or ECMO may be needed to manage the child's pulmonary hypertension. A Replogle tube is placed to minimize GI distention that would further diminish effective lung volume. Operative repair with balanced chest drainage is needed to avoid excessive transalveolar pressure gradients.

⚲ 13-30 KEY POINTS

1. Congenital diaphragmatic hernia results from a defect in the left posterolateral diaphragm that allows abdominal contents to enter the thorax and compromise lung development.
2. The combination of pulmonary hypoplasia and pulmonary arteriolar hypertension makes this congenital defect lethal in many cases.

OMPHALOCELE

Omphalocele results when the abdominal viscera herniate through the umbilical and supraumbilical portions of the abdominal wall into a sac covered by peritoneum and amniotic membrane. The defect results from arrested folding of the embryonic disc. Large defects may contain the entire GI tract and the liver and spleen. The sac covering the defect is thin and may rupture in utero or during delivery. The incidence of omphalocele is 1 in 6,000 births.

Clinical Manifestations

Polyhydramnios is noted in utero, and 10% of infants with omphaloceles are born prematurely. Diagnosis is often made by prenatal US. Thirty-five percent of afflicted infants have other GI defects, and 20% have congenital heart defects. Ten percent of children with omphalocele have Beckwith-Wiedemann's syndrome (exophthalmos, macroglossia, gigantism, hyperinsulinemia, and hypoglycemia).

Treatment

Cesarean section may prevent rupture of the sac. Small defects are closed primarily, whereas larger defects often require a staged repair that involves covering the sac with prosthetic material.

Treatment of the intact omphalocele sac includes low-pressure intermittent NG tube suction to minimize GI distention, covering the sac with petrolatum-impregnated gauze, wrapping the infant in a dry sterile towel to minimize heat loss, and wrapping the sac on the abdomen with Kling gauze to support the viscera on the abdominal wall. There should be no attempt to reduce the sac because this may cause rupture of the sac, interfere with venous return from the sac, and cause respiratory distress. Broad-spectrum antibiotics should be given. Definitive surgery is delayed until the infant is thoroughly resuscitated. Definitive care can be postponed as long as the sac remains intact.

Treatment of the ruptured sac is similar to that of the intact sac, except that saline-soaked gauze is placed over the exposed intestine and emergent surgical intervention is needed to cover the intestine.

🗝 13-31 KEY POINTS

1. Omphalocele results when the abdominal viscera herniate through the umbilical and supraumbilical portions of the abdominal wall into a sac covered by peritoneum and amniotic membrane.
2. Omphalocele has a high association with other anomalies, including GI and cardiac abnormalities and Beckwith-Wiedemann's syndrome.

GASTROSCHISIS

Gastroschisis, by definition, contains no sac; the intestine is herniated through the abdominal wall lateral to the umbilicus. The eviscerated uncovered mass is adherent, edematous, dark in color, and covered by a gelatinous matrix of greenish material. The pathogenesis of this abdominal wall defect is not clear.

Clinical Manifestations

Polyhydramnios is noted in utero. Sixty percent of these infants are born prematurely, and 15% have associated jejunoileal stenoses or atresias.

Treatment

Treatment of gastroschisis involves placement of a NG tube to suction, covering the exposed intestine with saline-soaked gauze, wrapping the infant in a dry, sterile towel to minimize heat loss, and starting antibiotics to cover for infection caused by bowel flora. Gastroschisis is a surgical emergency; single-stage primary closure is possible in only 10% of infants.

🗝 13-32 KEY POINTS

1. Gastroschisis, by definition, contains no sac; the intestine is herniated through the abdominal wall lateral to the umbilicus.
2. Gastroschisis has a lower association with other anomalies compared to omphalocele.

CLEFT LIP AND CLEFT PALATE

Pathogenesis

Cleft lip with or without cleft palate occurs in 1 in 1,000 births and is more common in boys. Unilateral cleft lip is the result of failure of fusion of the ipsilateral maxillary prominence with the medial nasal prominence. This process produces a persistent labial groove. Failure of bilateral fusion produces bilateral cleft lip.

Cleft palate occurs in 1 in 2,500 births. Development of the palate proper, which includes the hard palate, soft palate, uvula, and maxillary teeth, is completed by the ninth week of gestation. This region develops from the maxillary bone plates that are initially separated by the tongue. As the tongue descends in the floor of the mouth and moves forward, the two plates fuse. Failure of the tongue to descend produces the midline palatal clefts.

Epidemiology

Multiple genetic and environmental factors play a role in the etiology of the cleft lip. The recurrence risk in siblings is 3% to 4%. The risk for a child with a mother with cleft lip is 14%. Genetic factors are also important in cleft palate, and the recurrence risk is the same as that for cleft lip. Cleft palates are common in patients with chromosomal abnormalities.

Clinical Manifestations

Malformations associated with cleft lip include hypertelorism, hand defects, and cardiac anomalies. In general, feeding difficulties are not seen in isolated cleft lip.

Treatment

Most cleft lips are repaired shortly after birth or once the infant demonstrates steady weight gain. Cleft palate repair is usually undertaken at 12 to 24 months of age. In the newborn period, respiratory and feeding problems may occur. Repositioning the tongue and feeding the infant on his or her side should resolve respiratory difficulties. Most patients do well with a long soft nipple with a hole that is longer than usual. Complications after cleft palate repair include speech difficulties, dental disturbances, and recurrent otitis media. Although two thirds of children demonstrate acceptable speech, it may have a nasal quality or a muffled tone.

🔑 13-33 KEY POINTS

1. Most cleft lips are repaired shortly after birth or once the infant demonstrates steady weight gain.
2. Cleft palate repair is usually undertaken at 12 to 24 months of age.
3. In the newborn period, respiratory and feeding problems may occur with cleft lip or cleft palate.

NEURAL TUBE DEFECTS

Neural tube defects are discussed in detail in Chapter 15.

NEONATAL DERMATOLOGIC PROBLEMS

ERYTHEMA TOXICUM NEONATORUM

The rash of erythema toxicum consists of evanescent papules, vesicles, and pustules on an erythematous base that usually occur on the trunk (but sometimes appear on the face and extremities). Rash onset usually occurs 24 to 72 hours after birth but may be seen earlier. Gram stain of vesicular contents reveals sheets of eosinophils. The lesions resolve over 3 to 5 days without therapy. Fifty percent of full-term babies have erythema toxicum. This figure decreases as the gestational age decreases. The cause of the rash is unknown.

MILIA

Milia are characterized by pearly white or pale yellow epidermal cysts found on the nose, chin, and forehead. The benign lesions exfoliate and disappear within the first few weeks of life. No treatment is necessary.

SEBORRHEIC DERMATITIS

Seborrhea is characterized by erythematous, dry, scaling, crusty lesions. It occurs in areas rich in sebaceous glands (face, scalp, perineum, and postauricular and intertriginous areas). Affected areas are sharply demarcated from uninvolved skin. Seborrhea appears between 2 and 10 weeks and is commonly called "cradle cap" when it appears on the scalp. For severe cradle cap, baby oil is applied to the scalp for 15 minutes, followed by washing with a dandruff shampoo. For seborrhea of the diaper area, 1% hydrocortisone cream can be used. If candidal superinfection occurs, nystatin ointment is recommended.

MONGOLIAN SPOTS

Mongolian spots are transient dark blue-black pigmented macules usually seen over the lower back and buttocks in 90% of African American, Indian, and Asian infants. The spots are never elevated or palpable and result from infiltration of melanocytes deep within the dermis. The hyperpigmented areas fade as the child ages. They present no known long-term problems but may occasionally be mistaken for bruises inflicted by abusive trauma.

1. Erythema toxicum neonatorum occurs 24 to 72 hours after birth and resolves 3 to 5 days later without therapy. Fifty percent of full-term babies have erythema toxicum.
2. Milia are epidermal cysts of the nose, chin, and forehead.
3. Seborrheic dermatitis appears between 2 and 10 weeks of life and is commonly called "cradle cap" when it appears on the scalp.
4. Mongolian spots are benign, transient, dark blue-black pigmented macules seen over the lower back and buttocks in 90% of African American, Indian, and Asian infants.

DRUGS OF ABUSE

FETAL ALCOHOL SYNDROME

Alcohol is the most common teratogen to which fetuses are exposed. Maternal alcohol ingestion results in a spectrum of effects in the neonate, ranging from mild reduction in cerebral function to classic fetal alcohol syndrome. The amount of alcohol consumed by the mother appears to correlate with the degree to which the fetus is affected. Fetal alcohol syndrome occurs in 1 in 1,000 newborns. The incidence is much higher in the Native American population because of a higher incidence of alcoholism. The syndrome affects 40% of the offspring of women who consume more than four to six drinks per day while pregnant.

Clinical Manifestations

Features of fetal alcohol syndrome include microcephaly and mental retardation, intrauterine growth retardation, facial dysmorphisms, and renal and cardiac defects. Facial anomalies include midfacial hypoplasia, micrognathia, a flattened philtrum, short palpebral fissures, and a thin vermillion border.

Treatment

Treatment is aimed at minimizing morbidity and mortality from renal and cardiac defects and assisting the child with mental retardation with activities of daily living.

1. Alcohol is the most common teratogen to which fetuses are exposed.
2. Fetal alcohol syndrome affects 40% of the offspring of women who consume more than four to six drinks per day while pregnant.
3. Features of fetal alcohol syndrome include microcephaly and mental retardation, intrauterine growth retardation, facial dysmorphisms, and renal and cardiac defects.

COCAINE

Cocaine causes maternal hypertension and placental vasoconstriction with diminished uterine blood flow and fetal hypoxia. These effects are associated with increased rates of spontaneous abortion, placental abruption, fetal distress, meconium staining, preterm birth, intrauterine growth retardation, and low Apgar scores at birth.

Clinical Manifestations

Maternal cocaine use is associated with congenital anomalies, intracranial hemorrhage, and NEC. Congenital anomalies include cardiac defects, skull abnormalities, and genitourinary malformations. Cocaine-exposed infants have demonstrated abnormalities in respiratory control and have an increased risk of SIDS. Long-term defects include attention and concentration deficits and an increased incidence of learning disabilities.

Infants may undergo withdrawal, characterized by irritability, increased tremulousness, lability, inability to be consoled, and poor feeding in the first few days of life.

Treatment

During the perinatal period, therapy is supportive. Sedative medications may be helpful, but frequently soothing nonpharmacologic interventions are adequate. At school age, many of these children have special learning needs.

⚷ 13-36 KEY POINTS

1. Cocaine causes placental insufficiency and fetal hypoxia, which is associated with increased rates of spontaneous abortion, placental abruption, fetal distress, meconium staining, preterm birth, intrauterine growth retardation, and low Apgar scores at birth.
2. Infants may undergo withdrawal, characterized by irritability, increased tremulousness, state lability, inability to be consoled, and poor feeding in the first few days of life.
3. Long-term defects include attention and concentration deficits and an increased incidence of learning disabilities.

HEROIN AND METHADONE

Heroin and methadone are the two narcotics to which fetuses are most commonly exposed. Approximately 10,000 heroin-dependent babies are born in the United States each year, and 5,000 narcotic-addicted pregnant women are in methadone treatment programs. Methadone maintenance is prescribed for pregnant women to decrease the stress that unreliable heroin dosing and uncontrolled withdrawal in utero place on the fetus.

Clinical Manifestations

Opiate abuse is not associated with congenital anomalies, but maternal use causes intrauterine growth retardation, an increased risk of SIDS, and infant narcotic withdrawal syndrome. It is unclear whether the abnormalities of fetal growth seen with narcotic abuse are caused by the direct effect of the drug or to other environmental factors, such as poor maternal nutrition.

Narcotic withdrawal syndrome, which generally occurs within the first 4 days of life, is characterized by irritability, poor sleeping, a high-pitched cry, diarrhea, sweating, sneezing, seizures, poor feeding, and poor weight gain. The risk of neonatal withdrawal is higher with methadone (75%) than with heroin (50%). Methadone withdrawal tends to be later in onset and more protracted, sometimes lasting as long as 1 month. Symptoms appear soon after birth, improve, and then may recur at 2 to 4 weeks.

Treatment

The treatment for narcotic withdrawal syndrome attempts to minimize irritability, emesis, and diarrhea and to maximize sleep between feedings. Symptomatic care includes holding, rocking, and swaddling the infant and providing the neonate with frequent small feedings of a hypercaloric formula.

Infants of narcotic-abusing mothers should never be given naloxone in the delivery room because it may precipitate seizures. Narcotic withdrawal symptoms unresponsive to nonmedicinal care can be mitigated by a controlled wean of morphine, phenobarbital, or benzodiazepines. Paregoric and tincture of opium also are used.

⚷ 13-37 KEY POINTS

1. Heroin and methadone are the two narcotics to which fetuses are most commonly exposed.
2. Heroin and methadone are not associated with congenital anomalies, but maternal use does cause intrauterine growth retardation and infant narcotic withdrawal syndrome.
3. Infants of narcotic-abusing mothers should never be given naloxone in the delivery room because it may precipitate seizures.
4. Narcotic withdrawal symptoms unresponsive to nonmedicinal care can be mitigated by the use of sedative medications.

Additional Suggested Reading

AAP Subcommittee on Neonatal Hyperbilirubinemia. Neonatal jaundice and kernicterus. *Pediatrics*. 2001; 108:763–765.

Aly H. Respiratory disorders in the newborn: identification and diagnosis. *Pediatr Rev*. 2004; 25:201–208.

Armentrout DC, Husby V. Neonatal polycythemia. *J Pediatr Health Care*. 2002;16:40–42.

Farrell PA, Weiner GM, Lemons JA. SIDS, ALTE, apnea, and the use of home monitors. *Pediatr Rev*. 2002;23:3–9.

Gotoff SP. Group B Streptococcal Infections. *Pediatr Rev*. 2002;23:381–386.

Suchy FJ. Neonatal Cholestasis. *Pediatr Rev*. 2004; 25:388–396.

Vaucher YE. Bronchopulmonary dysplasia: an enduring challenge. *Pediatr Rev*. 2002;23:349–358.

Nephrology and Urology

The renal system is the primary regulator of body fluid volume, osmolarity, composition, and pH. The kidneys collect and excrete many waste products of metabolism, such as urea and creatinine, and preserve the ionic equilibrium by conserving or excreting specific electrolytes as needed. Infants, in particular, are susceptible to renal challenges. Their kidneys are less effective in filtering plasma, regulating electrolytes, and concentrating urine.

Although the kidneys and urinary tract are separate systems, they are interrelated; irregularities in one system may affect the other. Abnormalities may be anatomic, infectious, cellular, inflammatory, functional, hormonal, or maturational.

RENAL DYSPLASIA

In **renal agenesis**, the kidney does not form. Bilateral renal agenesis results in Potter's syndrome. Infants with Potter's syndrome are stillborn or die shortly after birth because of pulmonary hypoplasia. Unilateral agenesis is usually an isolated defect but may be associated with other abnormalities.

A **multicystic kidney**, the most common renal dysplasia, consists of numerous noncommunicating, fluid-filled cysts. Affected kidneys are nonfunctional, but the condition is virtually always unilateral. Multicystic kidney is one of the two most common causes of renal masses in the newborn. (Note: The other is hydronephrosis resulting from ureteropelvic junction [UPJ] obstruction.) The diagnosis is confirmed by US. Most cases undergo spontaneous involution. Nephrectomy is recommended for some patients because of an increased risk of Wilm tumor in the affected kidney.

Polycystic kidney disease is an inherited disorder that occurs in two forms: the autosomal recessive type and the autosomal dominant type. In the former, the kidneys appear grossly normal but the renal collecting tubules are dilated, producing small cysts. Unaffected segments are interspersed, but in general the kidneys function poorly. The condition is usually discovered during evaluation of a palpable renal mass in an infant. Similar dilation is found in the hepatic bile ducts, with varying degrees of periportal fibrosis. Life expectancy is appreciably shortened; severely affected infants may die within weeks. The autosomal dominant form of polycystic kidney disease usually is detected in adulthood but may be diagnosed earlier on prenatal US or through workup for a positive family history. The cysts can be quite large. Hypertension and renal insufficiency develop over time. Transplant is a viable option.

URETEROPELVIC JUNCTION OBSTRUCTION

UPJ is the most common cause of hydronephrosis in childhood. Possible causes include intrinsic fibrosis at the junction of the renal pelvis and ureter, kinking of the ureter, or a crossing renal vessel. The obstruction leads to elevated intrapelvic pressure, dilation of the renal pelvis and calyces, urinary stasis, and gradual destruction of the renal parenchyma. Twenty percent of cases are bilateral.

CLINICAL MANIFESTATIONS

A palpable abdominal mass is the most common presentation in the newborn. Older infants may experience abdominal or flank pain and hematuria in addition to a mass. Urinary tract infection is not uncommon. The condition is detectable on prenatal US. In the infant, both renal US and diuretic nuclear renogram are sensitive diagnostic tests for UPJ obstruction.

TREATMENT

Surgical correction by pyeloplasty reestablishes transport of urine from the pelvis to the ureter.

VESICOURETERAL REFLUX

Vesicoureteral reflux (VUR) results from incompetence of a functional valve that normally only allows one-way (anterograde) urine flow from the ureters to the bladder. In children, the condition is usually bilateral and occurs as a consequence of insufficient tunneling of the ureters through the submucosal bladder tissue.

CLINICAL MANIFESTATIONS

The most frequent presentation is recurrent urinary tract infections (UTIs). Retrograde flow of infected urine results in pyelonephritis. Prenatal hydronephrosis may also be caused by VUR.

DIAGNOSTIC EVALUATION

A voiding cystourethrogram (VCUG) detects abnormalities at ureteral insertion sites and allows classification of the grade of reflux based on the extent of retrograde flow and associated dilatation of the ureter and pelvis (Fig. 14-1). (Note: Radionuclide cystography is an alternative in some patients.) Low grades of reflux often resolve spontaneously. High grades are associated with large, tortuous ureters and marked distortion of the renal pelvis and calyces. The associated recurrent UTIs produce progressive renal injury and scarring.

TREATMENT

First-line therapy involves antibiotic prophylaxis with amoxicillin (in the infant) or trimethoprim-sulfamethoxazole or nitrofurantoin (in the older child). Prophylaxis is recommended for all children younger than 5 years with VUR, any child with grade IV or V VUR, and patients with recurrent episodes of febrile UTIs. Most cases of low- to midgrade reflux resolve over time. Ureteral reimplantation surgery is indicated for grade V reflux or lower grades that do not resolve; the ureters are surgically tunneled through larger segments of the bladder submucosa at a more advantageous angle.

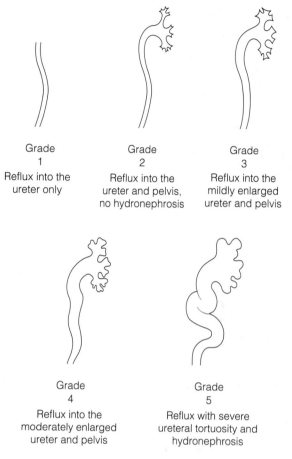

Grade 1
Reflux into the ureter only

Grade 2
Reflux into the ureter and pelvis, no hydronephrosis

Grade 3
Reflux into the mildly enlarged ureter and pelvis

Grade 4
Reflux into the moderately enlarged ureter and pelvis

Grade 5
Reflux with severe ureteral tortuosity and hydronephrosis

Figure 14-1 • Classification of vesicoureteral reflux. Severity based on level of reflux and degree of collecting system dilatation.

POSTERIOR URETHRAL VALVES

Occurring only in males, **posterior urethral valves** consist of posteriorly situated leaflets within the prostatic urethra, which result in partial bladder outlet obstruction. The increased pressure upstream causes urethral dilation, bladder neck hypertrophy, mucosal trabeculation, and, not infrequently, vesicoureteral reflux and renal dysgenesis. Posterior urethral valves are the most common cause of end-stage renal disease in childhood.

CLINICAL MANIFESTATIONS

The disorder may be suspected by detecting hydronephrosis on prenatal US or by palpating a distended bladder or renal mass during the newborn examination. In older infants, parents may note a weak or dribbling urinary stream or unexplained daytime wetting. Occasionally, the condition is diagnosed in boys during radiologic evaluation following a UTI. Posterior urethral valves are clearly visualized on VCUG.

TREATMENT

Transurethral ablation of the obstructing tissue via cystoscopy is the treatment of choice. In neonates who are too small for the procedure, temporary supravesical diversion (vesicostomy) is appropriate until ablation can be performed. Prognosis depends on the degree of renal and bladder impairment at the time of repair.

HYPOSPADIAS

Hypospadias, the most common congenital anomaly of the penis, occurs in 1 per 500 newborns. Incomplete development of the distal urethra leads to malposition of the urethral meatus along the ventral shaft of the penis, scrotum, or perineum. Proximal hypospadias may cause curving of the penis (chordee). Associated anomalies include hernias and undescended testes. Circumcision is contraindicated because surgical repair may require preputial tissue. The aims of therapy are to extend the urethral meatus to the tip of the glans penis and produce the appearance of a normal circumcised phallus. Prognosis is excellent for distal lesions; proximal lesions may require multiple revisions before an acceptable result is achieved.

CRYPTORCHIDISM

Cryptorchidism is defined as testes that have not fully descended into the scrotum and, unlike *retracted* testes, cannot be manipulated into the scrotum with gentle pressure. Testes that remain outside the scrotum develop ultrastructural changes, impaired sperm production, and an increased risk of malignancy. (Note: The contralateral descended testis also has an increased risk of malignancy.) Bilateral cryptorchidism results in oligospermia and infertility. Term infants have a 3% to 4% incidence at birth; the rate is much higher (30%) in premature infants. Cryptorchidism may occur as part of a genetic syndrome or be a spontaneous defect.

CLINICAL MANIFESTATIONS

One or both testes may be positioned in the abdomen or anywhere along the inguinal canal. Most are palpable on examination. Ninety percent of patients also have inguinal hernias.

TREATMENT

By 12 months of age, all but 0.08% of males have bilateral descended testicles. Spontaneous descent after 6 to 12 months is unlikely. Surgical repair (orchiopexy) takes place at 12 to 18 months of age and has a high success rate (99%). Orchiopexy does not appear to alter the incidence of malignant degeneration (2% to 3%), but it does render the testis accessible for regular self-examination.

TESTICULAR TORSION

Torsion is a surgical emergency, requiring prompt recognition and correction to prevent loss of the testicle. Most patients with testicular torsion lack the posterior attachment to the tunica vaginalis that keeps the testis from rotating around the spermatic cord.

CLINICAL MANIFESTATIONS

Clinical manifestations include the acute onset of unilateral scrotal pain; nausea; vomiting; a swollen, erythematous, exquisitely tender testis; scrotal edema; and absent cremasteric reflex. Epididymitis, which is more common during puberty and adolescence, presents with a similar clinical picture. Doppler US is helpful in differentiating between the two conditions but may delay appropriate treatment. Occasionally, the torsion is limited to the testicular or epididymal appendix; localized tenderness, the "blue dot" sign (on the upper aspect of the scrotum), and a normal cremasteric reflex suggest limited involvement.

TREATMENT

Early surgical intervention is critical; 90% of gonads survive when detorsion and fixation take place within 6 hours of onset. Necrotic testes must be removed. The contralateral testis is fixed to the posterior scrotal envelope during surgery to avoid subsequent torsion. Torsion of the testicular or epididymal appendix resolves spontaneously.

HYDROCELES AND VARICOCELES

Hydroceles are fluid-filled sacs in the scrotal cavity consisting of remnants of the processus vaginalis. They are often diagnosed in the newborn period or early childhood. Hydroceles that communicate with the peritoneal cavity may develop into hernias when the bowel descends along the path into the scrotum. Communicating hydroceles and scrotal hernias should be repaired as soon as possible to prevent the development of an incarcerated hernia. Most noncommunicating hydroceles involute by 12 months of age.

A **varicocele** is defined as a dilated testicular vein and enlarged pampiniform plexus resulting from the absence of the venous valves responsible for advancing the blood toward the heart. They become detectable in boys during adolescence, occur more commonly on the left, and they are usually nontender. Varicoceles are generally not visible when the patient is supine but become evident upon standing when the veins distend and produce the characteristic "bag of worms" within the scrotum. Indications for surgical repair include pain, interference with testicular hormone function, and ipsilateral testicular atrophy. Unrepaired varicoceles may place the patient at an increased risk of infertility.

URINARY TRACT INFECTIONS

PATHOGENESIS

Bacterial UTIs are a frequent cause of pediatric morbidity. Infection may be limited to the bladder **(cystitis)** or may also involve the kidney **(pyelonephritis)**. Children with pyelonephritis usually sustain damage to the infected area of the renal parenchyma, resulting in localized scarring and decreased function.

In febrile infants, the urinary tract is the most common site of bacterial infection. The source is almost always hematogenous seeding of the kidneys, which results in the high rate of renal scarring seen in this group of patients. In older children, UTIs more often result from ascent of exterior fecal flora into the urinary tract. Common pathogens include *Escherichia coli* (80%) and *Proteus* and *Klebsiella* species.

EPIDEMIOLOGY

After the first year of life (equal incidence), girls have almost a 10-fold risk over boys. Although uncircumcised male neonates are more prone to UTIs, this susceptibility alone is not a sufficient indication for universal routine circumcision.

RISK FACTORS

The most significant risk factor is the presence of a urinary tract abnormality that causes urinary stasis, obstruction, reflux, or dysfunctional voiding.

DIFFERENTIAL DIAGNOSIS

The differential diagnosis includes external genital irritation, vaginitis, vaginal foreign body, sexual abuse, and pinworm infestation. Adenovirus can cause a self-limited hemorrhagic cystitis that does not respond to antibiotics but may be mistaken for a UTI. Lower lobe pneumonia often presents with fever, chills, and flank pain.

CLINICAL MANIFESTATIONS

History and Physical Examination

In older children, the signs and symptoms of cystitis are similar to those in adults and include low-grade fever, frequency, urgency, dysuria, incontinence, abdominal pain, and hematuria. In contrast, pyelonephritis presents with high fever, chills, nausea, vomiting, and flank pain.

Infants warrant special attention because fever may be the only manifestation of a UTI in this age group, and a UTI can be the first clinical suggestion of an obstructive anomaly or vesicoureteral reflux. Ideally, the urine should be examined in all febrile patients younger than 1 to 2 years.

DIAGNOSTIC EVALUATION

Although pyuria, hematuria, and bacteriuria on urinalysis suggest a UTI, a positive **urine culture** is the gold standard for diagnosis. (Note: The absence of WBCs or RBCs in the urine does not rule out a UTI. Pyuria is often absent in febrile infants with pyelonephritis.) Urine may be obtained by suprapubic tap (in neonates), sterile catheterization of the bladder, or "clean catch" (listed in order of increasing likelihood of contamination). Bagged specimens are adequate for evaluation of cellular material but are not appropriate for culture. All febrile infants (and older patients with suspected UTIs) should receive a urine culture (results in 24 to 48 hours) and dipstick urinalysis. Patients with positive dipstick results for leukocyte esterase (with or without positive nitrites) should be treated for a presumed UTI until culture results are available. Susceptibility testing is performed on any singular bacteria isolated to ensure appropriate antibiotic treatment.

Older children are more likely to have an isolated bladder infection without kidney involvement; however, elevation of the peripheral WBC, ESR, and C-reactive protein are suggestive of upper tract involvement.

The workup of initial UTIs in children is controversial and depends on the patient's age, severity of infection, and response to treatment. Figure 14-2 provides a diagnostic algorithm for children with UTIs. Current American Academy of Pediatrics guidelines recommend that all children younger than 24 months undergo **renal US** to rule out hydronephrosis or structural lesions that predispose to infection. Those who do not respond to appropriate antibiotic therapy within 48 hours should also receive a VCUG. In prompt responders, the VCUG is optional. Other experts

argue that all children younger than a certain age (6 to 12 months) should receive a VCUG regardless of response to treatment. It is likely that further studies will result in more evidence-based recommendations.

TREATMENT

Children with suspected cystitis may be treated with an appropriate oral antibiotic such as amoxicillin, ampicillin, nitrofurantoin, or trimethoprim-sulfamethoxazole. If the culture is negative, antibiotics may be discontinued. A positive urine culture should prompt a 5- to 7-day course with an appropriate oral antibiotic (based on sensitivity results).

Non-toxic-appearing children with suspected pyelonephritis should be treated with cefixime (orally) or intravenous ampicillin plus gentamicin or cefotaxime until culture results are available. Patients who are toxic appearing, unable to tolerate oral medications, or younger than 6 months must be admitted to the hospital for 10 to 14 days of intravenous antibiotics and observation. With improvement,

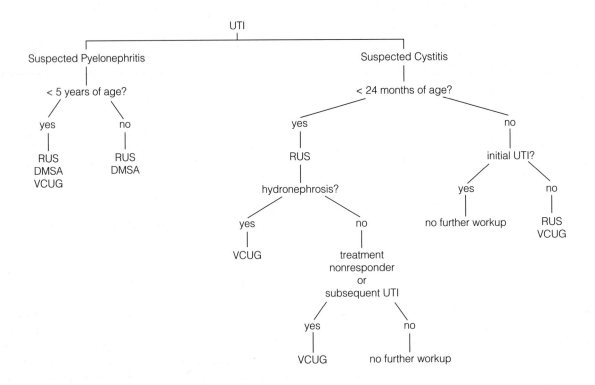

RUS, renal ultrasound; DMSA, technetium-99 dimercaptosuccinic acid renal scan; VCUG, voiding cystourethrogram.

Figure 14-2 • Diagnostic algorithm for pediatric urinary tract infection.

patients older than 6 months may be discharged on an appropriate oral antibiotic to finish the course.

The prognosis for patients with isolated cases of cystitis is excellent; morbidity increases with recurrent infection. Most UTI-related complications are caused by pyelonephritis, including perinephric abscesses, renal scarring, and renal failure.

⚷ 14-1 KEY POINTS

1. In older children, urinary tract infections (UTIs) result from contamination of the urinary tract with exterior fecal flora. Hematogenous seeding is more probable infants, particularly those younger than 2 months.
2. *Escherichia coli* is the most common pathogen in UTIs.
3. The most significant risk factor for recurrent UTIs is the presence of a urinary tract abnormality that causes urinary stasis, obstruction, reflux, or dysfunctional voiding.
4. The patient with a suspected UTI should receive a urine culture and dipstick urinalysis. If the dipstick is positive for leukocyte esterase (with or without nitrites), the patient should be presumptively treated for a UTI until culture results are available.
5. Pyelonephritis causes renal scarring and, with repeated infections, hypertension or end-stage renal disease.

NEPHROTIC SYNDROME

PATHOGENESIS

Nephrotic syndrome is a glomerular disorder characterized by proteinuria, hypoalbuminemia, hyperlipidemia, and edema.

EPIDEMIOLOGY

In children, nephrotic syndrome may be idiopathic (90%) or secondary (Table 14-1). **Minimal change disease (MCD)** is by far the most common cause of primary nephrotic syndrome in the pediatric population. Most patients present between 2 and 6 years of age, and boys outnumber girls. **Focal segmental glomerulosclerosis (FSGS)** and **membranoproliferative glomerulonephropathy** account for most of the remainder of idiopathic cases of nephrotic syndrome in children.

■ **TABLE 14-1** Agents and Conditions Associated with Pediatric Nephrotic Syndrome

Medications (ampicillin, nonsteroidal anti-inflammatory drugs)

Allergies (pollen, milk, bee stings)

Tumors (Hodgkin's disease, non-Hodgkin lymphoma, embryonal cell tumors, bronchogenic carcinoma)

Infections (viruses)

Skin disorders (contact dermatitis, dermatitis herpetiformis)

Other (Guillain-Barré's syndrome, myasthenia gravis, systemic lupus erythematosus)

Adapted from Meyers KE, Kaplan BS. Minimal change nephrotic syndrome. In Kaplan BS, Meyers KE, eds. Pediatric nephrology and urology: the requisites in pediatrics. Philadelphia: Elsevier Mosby; 2004:164.

CLINICAL MANIFESTATIONS

History and Physical Examination

Patients with early nephrotic syndrome appear quite well. Periorbital edema is commonly the first abnormality noted. This is followed by lower extremity and then generalized edema and ascites. Anorexia and diarrhea are variably present.

DIFFERENTIAL DIAGNOSIS

Edema may be renal, hepatic, nutritional, or cardiac in origin. Other conditions associated with proteinuria include exercise, trauma, UTI, dehydration, and acute tubular necrosis; however, none of these causes the degree of protein loss seen in nephrotic syndrome. Of note, glomerular filtration rate (GFR) and blood pressure are less likely to be affected in nephrotic syndrome than in the nephritic syndromes (Table 14-2).

DIAGNOSTIC EVALUATION

The hallmark of nephrotic syndrome is marked **proteinuria**. Affected children lose more than 40 mg protein/m^2/hour in their urine when averaged over a 24-hour period, a large proportion of which is albumin. Because the liver rapidly manufactures replacement proteins, large amounts of lipids are created as well.

Renal biopsy is indicated for patients outside the typical age range for MCD and those who do not

TABLE 14-2 Diseases That Present with Glomerulonephritic and Nephrotic Syndromes	
Nephritic Syndromes	**Nephrotic Syndromes**
IgA nephropathy	Minimal change disease
Acute poststreptococcal glomerulonephritis	Focal segmental glomerulosclerosis
Henoch-Schönlein purpura	Membranoproliferative glomerulonephropathy
Hemolytic-uremic's syndrome	Membranous glomerulonephritis
Systemic lupus erythematosus (SLE)	SLE
Alport's syndrome	
Bacterial endocarditis	
Membranoproliferative glomerulonephropathy	

immunosuppressant therapy. The prognosis of MCD is excellent; although up to 80% of patients relapse at least once, very few develop any long-standing renal insufficiency. Unfortunately, patients with focal segmental glomerulosclerosis and diffuse membranoproliferative glomerulonephritis do not respond well to steroid therapy, and end-stage renal disease is common. Both diseases may recur following renal transplantation.

14-2 KEY POINTS

1. Nephrotic syndrome is characterized by proteinuria, hypoalbuminemia, hyperlipidemia, and edema.
2. Minimal change disease is the most common type of pediatric idiopathic nephrotic syndrome.
3. Most cases respond to oral steroid therapy; renal biopsy is recommended for those that do not.
4. Spontaneous bacterial peritonitis is a complication of nephrotic syndrome.

respond to steroids. True to the disease's name, gross sections in MCD show few if any abnormalities; the only consistent finding is effacement of epithelial cell foot processes demonstrated by electron microscopy. Focal segmental glomerulosclerosis is characterized by focal sections of distorted glomeruli, with mesangial hypertrophy and segmental capillary loop fibrosis. Increased mesangial cellularity and glomerular basement membrane thickening are found in diffuse membranoproliferative glomerulonephritis.

TREATMENT

If the clinical presentation is consistent with uncomplicated primary nephrotic syndrome, strict dietary salt restriction and oral steroid therapy are appropriate. If symptoms do not resolve within 8 to 12 weeks or if the patient experiences frequent or severe relapses, renal biopsy is indicated to confirm the diagnosis.

Steroids result in prompt remission in most cases of MCD. Nephrotic syndrome that does not respond to oral steroids may require treatment with immune suppressants such as cyclophosphamide. Intravenous albumin (followed by a diuretic) can be used as a temporary measure to induce diuresis in the presence of incapacitating anasarca or edema-related respiratory compromise.

Bacterial infections, particularly **spontaneous peritonitis**, are the most frequent complications of nephrotic syndrome and usually occur while the patient is on

GLOMERULONEPHRITIS

The term **glomerulonephritis** implies inflammation within the glomerulus. Antigen-antibody complexes are formed or deposited in the subepithelial or subendothelial areas; immune mediators follow, resulting in inflammatory injury. **Hematuria** (overt or microscopic) with red cell casts is the hallmark of the disease. Distinguishing characteristics of the major glomerulonephritic syndromes of childhood are discussed next.

ACUTE GLOMERULONEPHRITIDES

Acute poststreptococcal glomerulonephritis (APGN), the most common glomerulonephritis in childhood, occurs sporadically in older children and is twice as common in males. Streptococcal infections involving either the throat or the skin (impetigo) precede the clinical syndrome by 1 to 3 weeks. Treating the streptococcal infection does not prevent APGN. Elevated antistreptolysin-O or anti-DNAse B titers suggest recent streptococcal infection. The C3 component of the complement pathway is low. Renal histology reveals mesangial and capillary cell proliferation, inflammatory cell infiltration, and granular "humps" of IgG and C3 below the glomerular basement membrane.

Henoch-Schönlein purpura (HSP), a systemic vasculitis characterized by purpura, crampy abdominal pain, and arthritis, may progress to a glomerulonephritis-type syndrome that is indistinguishable from IgA nephropathy. Two percent of children with HSP develop long-term renal impairment.

Rapidly progressive glomerulonephritis is the description given to a number of glomerulopathies that, for unknown reasons, deteriorate over a few weeks or months to renal failure, uremia, encephalopathy, and even death. All forms demonstrate generalized crescent formation in the glomeruli, thought to represent cellular destruction by macrophages with subsequent necrosis and fibrin deposition. Fortunately, rapidly progressive glomerulonephritis is rare in children.

CHRONIC GLOMERULONEPHRITIDES

IgA nephropathy, once thought to be a benign condition, is now known to slowly progress to renal failure in 25% of cases. C3 levels are normal. Renal biopsy alone makes the diagnosis, demonstrating mesangial deposits of IgA in the glomeruli. Glomerulonephritis associated with systemic lupus erythematosus is discussed in Chapter 11.

INHERITED GLOMERULONEPHRITIDES

Alport's syndrome, or hereditary nephritis, is caused by mutations in the gene encoding type IV collagen that result in an abnormal glomerular basement membrane. Inheritance is X-linked, although defective genes encoding other glomerular basement membrane components can cause similar disease. Because type IV collagen is important in the cochlea, Alport's syndrome is associated with sensorineural hearing loss.

Benign familial hematuria is a common cause of asymptomatic microscopic and occasionally gross hematuria. Renal function is normal, and biopsy, although unnecessary, reveals thinning of the glomerular basement membrane. Because transmission is autosomal dominant, asymptomatic microscopic hematuria is usually found in other family members.

DIFFERENTIAL DIAGNOSIS

The differential diagnosis of hematuria, the most prominent manifestation of glomerulonephritis, includes other renal conditions (infection, trauma, malignancy, stones, cystic disease) and hematologic disorders. Vaginal bleeding produces false-positive results if the specimen is collected incorrectly. Both hemoglobin and myoglobin test positive for blood on urine dipstick; however, there are no RBCs on microscopic urine examination in the presence of only myoglobin.

CLINICAL MANIFESTATIONS

The initial presentation of glomerulonephritis includes hematuria, azotemia, oliguria, malaise, abdominal pain, edema, and **hypertension**. Red cell casts are invariably present; in fact, the urine is often described as "**tea colored**" by parents. Proteinuria occurs as well but is less prominent than in nephrotic syndrome. The GFR is compromised, leading to salt and water retention and circulatory overload. Azotemia is marked by increasing serum BUN and creatinine levels. Sodium and potassium regulation may be temporarily disrupted. Important laboratory studies include UA, urine culture, hemoglobin and platelet counts, coagulation studies, serum electrolytes, BUN and creatinine, streptococcal antibody titers, and complement levels.

TREATMENT

Positive streptococcal cultures are treated with appropriate antibiotic therapy. Hypertension, when present, can be severe, requiring vasodilators, diuretics, and fluid restriction. Steroids may improve the outcome of rapidly progressive glomerulonephritis.

Although the clinical manifestations of APGN may take a few months to resolve, the overall prognosis for return to normal function is excellent. Patients with other types of glomerulonephritis fare less well. Virtually all males and 20% of females with Alport's syndrome progress to end-stage renal disease by middle adulthood. The course of rapidly progressive glomerulonephritis is particularly devastating, with most patients becoming dependent on dialysis within a few years. Many chronic glomerulonephritic syndromes eventually recur in the transplanted kidney.

✎ 14-3 KEY POINTS

1. Glomerulonephritic's syndromes are inflammatory and characterized by hematuria, azotemia, oliguria, edema, and hypertension.
2. Specific syndromes include acute poststreptococcal glomerulonephritis, IgA nephropathy, hereditary nephritis, rapidly progressive glomerulonephritis, and glomerulonephritis associated with systemic lupus erythematosus.
3. Alport's syndrome is associated with painless hematuria and sensorineural hearing loss.
4. Most syndromes recur in a transplanted kidney.

RENAL TUBULAR ACIDOSIS

All forms of renal tubular acidosis (RTA) are characterized by **hyperchloremic metabolic acidosis** resulting from insufficient renal transport of bicarbonate or acids. The nephron tubules are the site of reabsorption and secretion. Most bicarbonate filtered from the plasma is reabsorbed in the proximal tubule, along with amino acids, glucose, sodium, potassium, calcium, phosphate, and water. In the distal tubule, the remainder of the bicarbonate is reabsorbed and hydrogen ions are secreted into the tubules from the peritubular capillaries. Defects in either transport site compromise the kidney's ability to maintain pH homeostasis.

DIFFERENTIAL DIAGNOSIS

In **proximal** RTA (type 2), the proximal tubule fails to reabsorb bicarbonate from the ultrafiltrate. **Distal** RTA may result from either deficient hydrogen secretion into the filtrate (type 1) or impaired ammonia production in the face of hyperkalemia from hypoaldosteronism or pseudohypoaldosteronism (type 4). Distal RTA type 4 is the most common RTA in both children and adults. Most types of RTA are hereditary or sporadic, acute or chronic, occurring alone or as part of a disease complex. For example, most patients exhibit proximal RTA type 2 in conjunction with **Fanconi's syndrome**, a generalized disorder of proximal tubule transport resulting in excessive urinary losses of bicarbonate, amino acids, small proteins, glucose, electrolytes, and water.

CLINICAL MANIFESTATIONS

History and Physical Examination

Patients who manifest proximal RTA type 2 as part of Fanconi's syndrome present with failure to thrive; associated signs and symptoms include chronic acidosis, hypokalemia, vomiting, anorexia, polydipsia and polyuria, volume contraction, and impaired vitamin D metabolism (rickets).

Distal RTA type 1 also presents with metabolic acidosis and failure to thrive. Hypokalemia, hypercalciuria, and kidney stones are common. In contrast, the acidosis in distal RTA type 4 occurs in the presence of hyperkalemia in conjunction with primary or secondary hypoaldosteronism or end-organ resistance.

DIAGNOSTIC EVALUATION

Any patient with **hyperchloremic metabolic acidosis** of unclear etiology warrants further workup to rule out RTA (Fig. 14-3).

TREATMENT

Treatment consists of providing children with sufficient amounts of an **alkalinizing agent** (either bicarbonate or citrate) to correct the acidosis completely and restore normal growth. Thiazide diuretics are administered in proximal RTA to increase proximal tubular reabsorption of bicarbonate. Hypokalemia is treated concurrently when the alkali is coupled with potassium as a salt. Hyperkalemia is usually more difficult to correct; furosemide is prescribed unless the defect results in salt wasting. If RTA is associated with an underlying condition, the primary disorder must be treated.

🔑 14-4 KEY POINTS

1. All classifications of renal tubular acidosis (RTA) are characterized by hyperchloremic metabolic acidosis.
2. The most common type in children is distal RTA type 4, resulting from hyperkalemia (from hypoaldosteronism or pseudohypoaldosteronism) that interferes with ammonia production.
3. Fanconi's syndrome is a generalized disorder of proximal tubule transport with excessive urinary losses of bicarbonate, proteins, glucose, electrolytes, and water.
4. Alkalizing agents correct the acidosis.

NEPHROGENIC DIABETES INSIPIDUS

PATHOGENESIS

Diabetes insipidus (DI) involves a disorder in renal concentrating ability. Patients produce up to 400 mL/kg/day of very dilute urine regardless of hydration status. DI may be central or nephrogenic in origin. In **central DI**, the production or release of antidiuretic hormone is insufficient (see Chapter 6). **Nephrogenic DI** arises from end-organ resistance to arginine vasopressin (antidiuretic hormone), either from a receptor defect or from medications or other processes that interfere with aquaporin-2 protein transport of water at the renal cortical tubules.

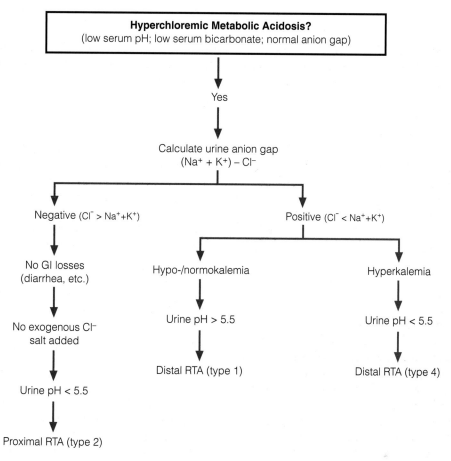

Figure 14-3 • Diagnostic workup of hyperchloremic metabolic acidosis of unknown etiology.

EPIDEMIOLOGY

Nephrogenic DI may be hereditary or acquired and usually presents within the first several years of life. Acquired nephrogenic DI has been associated with polycystic kidney disease, pyelonephritis, lithium toxicity, and sickle cell disease.

CLINICAL MANIFESTATIONS

History and Physical Examination

All patients present with polyuria and compensatory polydipsia. Other features may include intermittent fever, irritability, vomiting, and growth retardation. Most affected children also have a history of recurrent hypernatremic dehydration. Developmental delay occurs as a result of frequent hypernatremic seizures. Some patients manifest no symptoms until they are stressed with illness. Others remain completely unable to keep themselves in fluid balance without continual therapy.

DIFFERENTIAL DIAGNOSIS

Differentiating central DI from nephrogenic DI is not possible based on symptomatology alone, although the former more commonly follows head trauma or meningitis. Other conditions that may present in a similar manner include diabetes mellitus, RTA, and compulsive water drinking, which is seen in 10% to 40% of patients with schizophrenia.

DIAGNOSTIC EVALUATION

Patients with nephrogenic DI are unable to concentrate their urine. Despite significant dehydration, their urine specific gravity and osmolarity measurements remain inappropriately low. Figure 14-4 outlines the evaluation of a patient with suspected nephrogenic DI. Perinatal testing to detect arginine vasopressin receptor gene (AVPR2) mutations is now available.

TREATMENT

Acute treatment consists of rehydrating the child, replacing ongoing urinary losses, and correcting electrolyte abnormalities. A low-sodium diet (<0.7 mEq/kg/day) should be coupled with thiazide diuretics to decrease urinary sodium reabsorption. The addition of indomethacin may have an additive effect on thiazide diuretics in reducing water excretion.

Children with nephrogenic DI are at risk for poor growth. The disease is lifelong but carries a good prognosis, provided that episodes of hypernatremic dehydration are avoided.

🔑 14-5 KEY POINTS

1. Diabetes insipidus (DI) is a disorder of urine concentration and can be central or nephrogenic.
2. Clinical manifestations include polyuria, polydipsia, and growth retardation.
3. Therapy for nephrogenic DI includes a low-sodium diet, thiazide diuretics, and indomethacin.

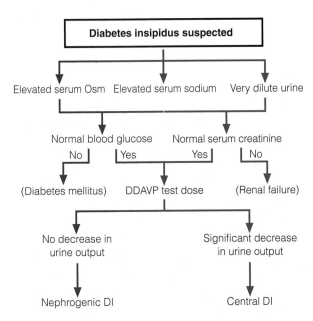

Figure 14-4 • Diagnosing nephrogenic diabetes insipidus.

HYPERTENSION

Blood pressure rises as a child grows, reaching adult values during adolescence. Hypertension in the pediatric population is defined as blood pressure **greater than 95th percentile for age, gender, and height on three separate occasions**.

DIFFERENTIAL DIAGNOSIS

Essential (primary) hypertension is the most common form in adults. Children are more likely to manifest **secondary hypertension**, usually related to renal disease. (However, because of the increase in childhood obesity and poor diet, the rate of essential hypertension in children is increasing.) Endocrine, vascular, and neurologic conditions may also be associated with increased blood pressure (Table 14-3).

CLINICAL MANIFESTATIONS

History

Stable or slowly progressive hypertension is unlikely to cause symptoms. Family history is often positive for hypertension, stroke, or premature heart attack. Patients with secondary hypertension often come to medical attention for complaints related to their underlying disease (e.g., growth failure, edema). Past medical history, state of health, recent medications, and review of systems for urinary tract symptoms provide pertinent information.

Severe hypertension or hypertension that has developed over a short period of time can cause headache, dizziness, and vision changes. **Hypertensive encephalopathy** is characterized by vomiting, ataxia, mental status changes, and seizures.

Physical Examination

The most important part of the examination is obtaining an accurate blood pressure reading. The air bladder portion of the cuff should encircle the patient's arm and be wide enough to cover 75% of the upper limb. A cuff that is too small will give a falsely elevated reading. At least once, the blood pressure should be taken in all four extremities to exclude aortic coarctation. Particular attention should be given to the heart sounds and peripheral pulses. Poor growth, flank pain, a retroperitoneal mass, large bladder, or abdominal bruit suggests a renal or renal vascular etiology. Obesity contributes to hypertension in a genetically predisposed patient.

TABLE 14-3 Differential Diagnosis of Hypertension

Factitious
  Anxiety
  Inappropriate cuff size

Primary (essential) hypertension Renal
  Glomerulonephritis
  Pyelonephritis
  Parenchymal (cystic) disease
  Obstructive uropathy
  Renal tumor
  Renal trauma
  Renal failure

Neurologic
  Pain
  Increased intracranial pressure
  Hemorrhage
  Brain injury
  Familial dysautonomia

Drugs and Toxins
  Oral contraceptives
  Corticosteroids
  Cyclosporin
  Cocaine

Endocrine
  Congenital adrenal hyperplasia
  Cushing syndrome
  Hyper- or hypothyroidism
  Pheochromocytoma
  Hyperparathyroidism
  Hyperaldosteronism
  Hypercalcemia

Vascular
  Coarctation of the aorta
  Renal vein thrombosis
  Renal artery thrombosis
  Large arteriovenous fistula
  Vasculitis

Other
  Chronic upper airway obstruction
  Malignant hyperthermia
  Acute intermittent porphyria

DIAGNOSTIC EVALUATION

The initial laboratory evaluation should include a CBC, serum electrolytes, BUN, creatinine, renin level, and UA. Doppler US of the kidneys allows assessment of anatomy as well as renal vasculature. Chest radiograph, electrocardiogram, and echocardiogram evaluate heart size and function, whether cardiac deficits are the cause or the effect of the hypertension.

TREATMENT

The best treatment for essential hypertension is **preventive health care**. High-salt diet, sedentary lifestyle, cigarette use, alcohol abuse, high serum cholesterol levels, and obesity compound the disorder and increase the morbidity and mortality. Secondary hypertension responds to treatment of the underlying disorder when possible.

Pharmacologic therapy is indicated in patients with persistent or refractory hypertension. Diuretics, β-blockers, and occasionally calcium channel blockers are used in younger children; angiotensin receptor blockers are second-line treatment in this age group but are effective first-line agents in adolescents and adults because of fewer side effects.

In patients with severe hypertension, rapid decreases in blood pressure compromise organ perfusion. Hypertensive crisis is treated with oral or sublingual nifedipine, intravenous nitroprusside, or labetalol. Hydralazine is also effective.

Stroke, heart attack, and renal disease are the most devastating complications of hypertension. Prognosis depends on the underlying disorder and degree of control.

🔑 14-6 KEY POINTS

1. Blood pressure norms are related to age, gender, and height.
2. Three blood pressure readings on separate occasions that are greater than the 95th percentile for age, height, and gender constitute hypertension.
3. Symptoms of hypertension range in severity depending on absolute value and rapidity of onset.
4. Children with hypertension should have screening tests to evaluate renal and cardiac function.
5. The first line of therapy in children with idiopathic hypertension is diet control, weight loss, and exercise.
6. Rapid drops in blood pressure, even if maintained in the normal range, may compromise cerebral perfusion in a patient with a history of sustained high blood pressure.

ACUTE RENAL FAILURE

Renal failure is an uncommon but potentially life-threatening condition in children. **Acute renal failure** (ARF) consists of an abrupt reduction in renal function, occurring over several hours to days, with retention of nitrogenous waste products (azotemia) and fluid and electrolyte imbalances.

DIFFERENTIAL DIAGNOSIS

The mechanism of ARF may be prerenal, intrarenal/intrinsic, or postrenal (Table 14-4). **Prerenal** failure results when a normal kidney experiences significant hypoperfusion through the reduction of plasma volume, hypotension, or hypoxia. The decreasing GFR produces oliguria (urine output <400 mL/m²/day) or anuria. Most patients completely recover from prerenal failure unless it is unrecognized or inappropriately treated.

By contrast, **intrinsic** renal failure results from an abnormality of the kidney itself, such as glomerulonephritis, interstitial nephritis, renal vasculitis, or acute tubular necrosis, a poorly understood condition in which damaged tubules become obstructed with cellular debris. Intrarenal conditions usually present with oliguria or anuria, although the urine output may be normal (nonoliguric renal failure). In **postrenal failure**, obstructive lesions at or below the collecting ducts produce increased intrarenal pressure and result in a rapidly declining GFR and hydronephrosis. The lesions may be congenital or acquired, structural or functional. Patients with complete obstruction are anuric. Partial obstructions may present with normal or increased urine output.

CLINICAL MANIFESTATIONS

History and Physical Examination

A history of recent dehydration, shock, cardiac surgery, treatment with nephrotoxic medications, streptococcal infection, or posterior urethral valves may help clarify the etiology. Growth failure, bony abnormalities, anemia, deafness, and previous renal conditions suggest acute deterioration superimposed on chronic renal failure. Depending on the etiology, the physical exam may reveal dehydration, cardiovascular stability, abdominal tenderness, and abdominal or suprapubic masses. Edema, oliguria, and hypertension are usually evident. Findings of congestive heart failure (hepatomegaly, diffuse crackles on lung examination) require immediate intervention.

DIAGNOSTIC EVALUATION

ARF is characterized by hyperkalemia, azotemia, and metabolic acidosis. Increased BUN and creatinine levels signal diminished renal function. Anemia is variably present. UA for hematuria, proteinuria, leukocytes, and casts also provides useful information. Urine and plasma urea nitrogen, creatinine, osmolarity, and sodium can be used to differentiate between prerenal and intrinsic failure (Table 14-5).

Renal US is the single best noninvasive radiographic test for determining the site of obstruction in postrenal failure, as well as kidney size and shape and renal blood flow. **Renal nuclear scans** delineate renal perfusion and functional differences. A voiding cystourethrogram and CT may also be helpful. **Renal biopsy** is indicated when the diagnosis remains unclear or the extent of involvement is unknown.

TREATMENT

Treatment consists of appropriate fluid management, correction of electrolyte abnormalities and pH, protein restriction, and, occasionally, short-term hemodialysis. The underlying abnormality must be corrected to achieve total resolution and prevent recurrence.

TABLE 14-4 Conditions Associated with Acute Renal Failure		
Prerenal	**Renal**	**Postrenal**
Hypovolemia syndrome[a]	Hemolytic-uremic	Obstructive uropathy
Hypotension	Glomerulonephritis	Vesicoureteral reflux
Hypoxia	Henoch-Schönlein purpura	Nephrolithiasis
	Renal vein thrombosis	
	Pyelonephritis	
	Acute tubular necrosis	
	Acute interstitial nephritis	

[a]The most common cause of acute renal failure in children.

■ **TABLE 14-5** Typical Findings in Prerenal versus Intrinsic Acute Renal Failure in Children

Diagnostic Index	Prerenal	Intrinsic
Fractional excretion of sodium (%) = $[(U_{Na} \times P_{Cr})/(P_{Na} \times U_{Cr})] \times 100$	<1	>1
Urine creatinine to plasma creatinine ratio	>40	<20
Urine urea nitrogen to plasma urea nitrogen ratio	>8	<3
Urine osmolality (mOsmol/kg H_2O)	>500	<350
Urine osmolality/Plasma osmolality	>1.5	<1.5
Urine specific gravity	>1.020	<1.020
Plasma urea nitrogen/Plasma creatinine	>20	<15

P_{Cr}, plasma creatinine concentration; PNa, plasma sodium concentration; U_{Cr}, urine creatinine concentration; U_{Na}, urine sodium concentration.

The prognosis of ARF depends on the underlying etiology, length of impairment, and severity of functional disturbance.

Medications that undergo renal clearance may require dosing adjustments in acute or chronic renal failure to avoid toxicity.

🔑 14-7 KEY POINTS

1. The cause of acute renal failure (ARF) in children may be prerenal, intrarenal, or postrenal. Hemolytic uremic syndrome (HUS) is the most common cause of acute renal failure in childhood.
2. Laboratory findings include azotemia, hyperkalemia, and metabolic acidosis.
3. In addition to managing the inciting condition, treatment consists of appropriate fluid management, correction of electrolyte abnormalities and pH, protein restriction, and, occasionally, short-term hemodialysis.

CHRONIC RENAL FAILURE

Chronic renal failure (CRF) implies that renal function has dropped below 30% of normal; function at 10% or less defines end-stage renal disease. The most common cause of CRF in the pediatric population is **obstructive uropathy**, followed by renal dysplasia, glomerulonephropathies (particularly focal segmental glomerulosclerosis), and hereditary renal conditions.

CLINICAL MANIFESTATIONS

History and Physical Examination

Growth failure frequently prompts evaluation for renal disease in the outpatient setting. Subjective complaints range from none to polyuria, episodic unexplained dehydration, salt craving, anorexia, nausea, malaise, lethargy, and decreased exercise tolerance. Hypertension and pallor are noted on examination. Long-standing CRF produces rickets.

DIAGNOSTIC EVALUATION

Patients with CRF demonstrate many of the same laboratory abnormalities seen in ARF, including azotemia, acidosis, sodium imbalance, and hyperkalemia. Anemia is usually more pronounced in CRF than ARF.

TREATMENT

Treatment for CRF includes nutritional, pharmacologic, and dialysis therapy. Close monitoring of clinical and laboratory status is required. Protein restriction prevents worsening azotemia. Sodium intake should be restricted to control hypertension. Calcium carbonate and activated vitamin D treat renal osteodystrophy. Iron and recombinant erythropoietin improve the anemia. Catch-up growth is unlikely even when optimal caloric intake and normalization of metabolic parameters occurs.

Children with less than 10% of normal renal function (a creatinine greater than 10 mg per dL) require either dialysis or renal transplant. **Peritoneal dialysis**, which can be performed at home, is the standard for children requiring long-term dialysis. Peritonitis, the most frequent complication of peritoneal dialysis, is usually caused by gram-positive organisms. Hemodialysis provides close to 10% of normal renal function but is time consuming. Hemodialysis-associated mortality is low at specialized pediatric centers, but complications of hemodialysis include **disequilibrium syndrome**, which occurs when the serum urea nitrogen level drops too rapidly, resulting in cerebral edema. Signs and symptoms of disequilibrium syndrome include headache, nausea, vomiting, abdominal pain, muscle cramps, seizures, and coma. Complications related to vascular hemodialysis include bleeding, thrombosis, and infection.

Renal transplantation is the ultimate therapy for all children with end-stage renal disease, and there are few absolute contraindications. The donated organ may come from a living related or deceased donor; living related donor transplants have better host and graft survival rates.

Children with CRF require complex and time-consuming treatment and, as a consequence, they often experience a decrease in their quality of life and are predisposed to developmental and social delays.

🔑 14-8 KEY POINTS

1. Children with growth failure should be screened for renal disease.
2. Treatment for chronic renal failure (CRF) includes peritoneal dialysis, hemodialysis, and renal transplantation.

ENURESIS

Successful bladder control is usually achieved between 24 and 36 months of age, although many developmentally normal children take significantly longer. Enuresis is the involuntary loss of urine in a child older than 5 years. It may be nocturnal or daytime, primary or secondary. **Primary** enuretics are patients who have never successfully maintained a dry period, whereas **secondary** enuretics are usually dry for several months before regular wetting recurs.

CLINICAL MANIFESTATIONS

A careful history and physical examination may suggest secondary causes for enuresis such as a UTI, developmental delay, obstruction, emotional strain, or inappropriate parental toilet training expectations. Primary nocturnal enuresis, which is far more common, is thought to be caused by delayed maturational control or inadequate levels of antidiuretic hormone secretion during sleep.

TREATMENT

Behavior modification programs are moderately effective. The most popular method of treatment is a nighttime audio alarm that sounds as soon as the child starts to urinate, eventually conditioning controlled bladder emptying before enuresis. Intranasal **desmopressin acetate** (generic name for DDAVP; analogous to endogenous vasopressin) acts to concentrate the urine. If given in the evening, less urine is produced overnight, decreasing the likelihood of wetting. With all therapies, the cure rate is 15% per year after 5 years of age; children who remain enuretic past 8 years of age have a 10% risk of never resolving their symptoms.

Additional Suggested Reading

Chan JC, Scheinman JI, Roth KS. Renal tubular acidosis. *Pediatr Rev.* 2001;22:277–287.

Chan JC, Williams DM, Roth KS. Kidney failure in infants and children. *Pediatr Rev.* 2002;23:47–60.

Christensen AM, Shaw K. Urinary tract infection in childhood. In Kaplan BS, Meyers KE, eds. *Pediatric nephrology and urology: the requisites for pediatrics.* Philadelphia: Elsevier Mosby; 2004:317–325.

Decter RM. Vesicoureteral reflux. *Pediatr Rev.* 2001; 22:205–210.

Norwood VF. Hypertension. *Pediatr Rev.* 2002;23: 197–209.

Roberts KB. A synopsis of the American Academy of Pediatrics' practice parameter on the diagnosis, treatment, and evaluation of the initial urinary tract infection in febrile infants and young children. *Pediatr Rev.*1999;20:344–347.

Roth KS, Amaker BH, Chan JC. Nephrotic syndrome: Pathogenesis and management. *Pediatr Rev.* 2002;23:237–247.

Snodgrass WT. Hypospadias. *Pediatr Rev.* 2004;25: 62–66.

Chapter

15 Neurology

NEURAL TUBE DEFECTS

Failure of neural tube closure during the third and fourth weeks of gestation results in a group of related disorders called **neural tube defects**. Maternal malnutrition, drug exposure (particularly the antiepileptics valproic acid and carbamazepine), congenital infections, radiation, and genetic factors are all associated with an increased risk of neural tube defects. (Note: There is a 3% to 4% risk of a second affected child being born to parents who already have one child with a neural tube defect.) Because failure of closure results in persistent leakage of α-fetoprotein into the amniotic fluid, the maternal serum α-fetoprotein level at 16 to 18 weeks is an excellent screening tool for identifying high-risk pregnancies. The incidence of neural tube defects is decreased in infants whose mothers receive **folic acid** supplementation prior to conception and during the early weeks of pregnancy. The overall incidence of neural tube defects is declining worldwide because of improved prenatal diagnosis and subsequent elective termination of the pregnancy; improved maternal nutrition; and other, unknown factors.

CLINICAL MANIFESTATIONS

Abnormalities may occur anywhere along the CNS; the higher the lesion, the more devastating the sequelae. Neonates with **anencephaly** are born with large skull defects and virtually no cortex. Brainstem function is marginally intact. Many are stillborn; others die within days of birth. **Encephaloceles** are projections of cranial contents through a bony skull defect, usually in the occipital region. Such patients manifest severe mental retardation, seizures, and movement disorders. Hydrocephalus is a frequent complication.

Spina bifida includes a variety of conditions (myelomeningocele, meningocele, spina bifida occulta) characterized by neural tube defects in the spinal region associated with incomplete fusion of the vertebral arches. **Myelomeningoceles** are protruding sacs of neural and meningeal tissue, whereas **meningoceles** contain meninges only. Both are most common in the lumbosacral region. Bowel and bladder sphincter dysfunction is the rule, and sensorimotor loss occurs below the lesion. In **spina bifida occulta**, the bony vertebral lesion occurs without herniation of any spinal contents. Birthmarks, dimples, or hairy tufts at the base of the back suggest an underlying defect. Although the infant may initially appear neurologically intact, the caudal end of the cord is affixed or "tethered" to the distal spine. As the vertebral column grows throughout childhood, the spinal cord is unable to ascend into the adult position, resulting in scoliosis, sphincter dysfunction, lower extremity deformities, and increasing motor deficits. Spina bifida defects have a high incidence of infectious complications and **Chiari Type II malformation** (an anatomic abnormality of the hindbrain that poses significant risk for hydrocephalus).

Children with repairable defects should have them closed as soon after birth as possible. These patients may also need subsequent CSF shunt placement, spinal cord untethering, and decompression of the Chiari Type II malformation. Fetal surgery is under investigation as a means of repairing some defects in an attempt to preserve motor and sensory function.

HYDROCEPHALUS

PATHOGENESIS

Hydrocephalus is the pathologic enlargement of the ventricles that occurs when CSF production outpaces absorption, usually secondary to outflow obstruction. In **noncommunicating** hydrocephalus, the block exists somewhere within the ventricular system, and the ventricles above the obstruction are selectively enlarged. Noncommunicating hydrocephalus is most commonly caused by narrowing at the fourth ventricle/aqueduct or malformations/enlargements of the posterior fossa. Causes include birth defects (spina bifida occulta, Chiari Type II malformation), congenital infections, and some tumors.

In contrast, all ventricles are proportionately enlarged in **communicating** hydrocephalus, which occurs when the subarachnoid villi are dysfunctional or obliterated. Subarachnoid hemorrhage and meningitis (particularly with tuberculosis, fungi, and parasites) can all cause meningeal inflammation and scarring, which result in communicating hydrocephalus.

CLINICAL MANIFESTATIONS

History and Physical Examination

The clinical manifestations of hydrocephalus depend on the rate of onset and the patency of the fontanelles. An inappropriate increase in head circumference or bulging anterior fontanelle may be the only indication in infants; poor feeding, irritability, lethargy, apnea, and bradycardia often provide additional clues. In older patients with acute courses, the signs are relatively clear and include headaches, nausea, vomiting, irritability, lethargy, papilledema, upward gaze paralysis (the "setting sun sign"), and diplopia (third or sixth cranial nerve palsies, or both). Clonus, a positive Babinski test, and excessively brisk deep tendon reflexes are additional neurologic signs. The **Cushing triad**, consisting of bradycardia, hypertension, and Cheyne-Stokes respirations, is a late and ominous development.

DIFFERENTIAL DIAGNOSIS

Conditions that lead to increased intracranial pressure without hydrocephalus include acute intraventricular bleed, diffuse brain edema (secondary to traumatic brain injury, hypoxic-ischemic encephalopathy, or encephalitis), cerebral venous sinus thrombosis, abscesses, and many tumors, all of which are easily differentiated by CT or MRI.

DIAGNOSTIC EVALUATION

The CT scan is an important adjunct in the evaluation of hydrocephalus. Anatomic malformations, ventricular size, and source of obstruction are clearly delineated. A head US may be sufficient in the young infant. If a LP is indicated, it **should not** be attempted if there is any danger of herniation. (Note: LP should not be performed in the presence of markedly increased intracranial pressure because of the risk of herniation of the brainstem contents through the foreman magnum.)

TREATMENT

Patients with hydrocephalus are at risk for developmental delay, visual impairment, and motor disturbances. If the underlying etiology cannot be corrected, surgical diversion with a ventriculoperitoneal shunt decreases intracranial pressure and relieves the symptoms. Acetazolamide decreases CSF production and may be effective in the short term if the hydrocephalus is not severe.

Indwelling shunts are fraught with complications, most commonly obstruction and infection. *Staphylococcus epidermidis* is the most frequently isolated pathogen. The management of shunt infections is currently a matter of debate. Systemic and intraventricular antibiotics are always given. Some centers remove the shunt and replace it when the infection is resolved; others replace the shunt immediately, and still others treat the shunt in place.

CEREBRAL PALSY

Cerebral palsy (CP) is a nonprogressive disorder of movement and posture that results from a fixed lesion of the immature brain. It is the most common movement disorder in children. Most cases occur in the absence of identifiable risk factors (i.e., prematurity, birth asphyxia, intrauterine growth retardation, intrauterine or maternal infection, cerebral hemorrhage with periventricular leukomalacia).

CLINICAL MANIFESTATIONS

The most common form of CP is **spastic** CP (pyramidal), which is the consequence of injury to motor tracts in the brain. It is characterized by increased muscle tone in the affected limbs. The disorder is further classified by which limbs are involved (Table 15-1). Patients with CP are generally hypotonic through the first few months of their life, only later developing the characteristic spasticity. It is usually very difficult to make the diagnosis until a patient is failing to meet motor developmental milestones or the spasticity becomes apparent on exam. As a patient's body grows and new developmental tasks are encountered, the condition may *appear* to be progressive (but is not).

Extrapyramidal CP is a rare but important disorder that results from damage to the basal ganglia, which is involved in the regulation of muscle tone and coordination. Affected patients exhibit involuntary choreoathetoid movements and postural ataxia, in addition to some spasticity. **Kernicterus** used to be a major cause; the incidence of extrapyramidal CP has decreased substantially because of advances in the management of neonatal **hyperbilirubinemia**. Unlike spastic CP, most patients with extrapyramidal CP have an identifiable brain insult (e.g., perinatal asphyxia, placental infarction, maternal toxemia).

TREATMENT

A multidisciplinary team approach, including a general pediatrician, physical and occupational therapists, nutritionist, speech-language therapist, and social support services, results in optimal therapy with the goal of maximizing function. Many medicines have been tried to reduce spasticity (including benzodiazepines, dantrolene, and baclofen) with variable success. However, significant improvements in motor function have been achieved with **botulinum toxin** motor point blocks. Many children ultimately require orthopedic surgery to correct deformities and release contractures.

Some children with CP are otherwise cognitively normal. This is generally the exception. More than half have cognitive deficits ranging from learning disabilities to mental retardation. A third develop seizure disorders. Many have hearing and vision impairments. Other frequently encountered conditions include oral-motor dysfunction, gastroesophageal reflux, and behavior problems.

SEIZURE DISORDERS

PATHOGENESIS

A **seizure** is a temporary disruption of brain function resulting from abnormal, excessive, synchronous

■ TABLE 15-1 Topographic Classification of Spastic (Pyramidal) Cerebral Palsy
Diplegia—bilateral lower extremity spasticity
Quadriplegia—all limbs severely involved
Hemiplegia—one side involved, upper extremity more than lower

cerebral neuron discharge. A patient is diagnosed with **epilepsy** when unprovoked seizures become recurrent (two or more). Many diseases, derangements, and disorders cause seizures. In approximately 50% of patients, the etiology remains undetermined.

EPIDEMIOLOGY

Approximately 5% of children have a seizure sometime during childhood. In neonates, trauma, hypoxia, and infection are the primary causes of seizures. Infections and **febrile seizures** rank high in infancy and young childhood. Systemic disease, hypoglycemia, electrolyte and metabolic abnormalities, ingestions, and congenital defects can also result in seizure activity. **Idiopathic epilepsy** is the most common form diagnosed in older children and adolescents. An estimated 1% to 2% of the general population suffers from epilepsy.

RISK FACTORS

Traumatic brain injury and meningoencephalitis are both associated with an increased risk of epilepsy. Children with a history of febrile seizures are at a minimally increased risk of epilepsy later in life, particularly those with complex or multiple febrile seizures, a family history of epilepsy, and/or a recognized neurodevelopmental abnormality.

CLINICAL MANIFESTATIONS

History, Physical Examination, and Diagnostic Evaluation

The diagnosis of a seizure disorder is primarily based on the historical account of the episode and the physical examination. The history should include questions about what the patient was doing when the seizure started, how the seizure manifestations evolved over time, how long the seizure lasted, and how the child acted following the episode. EEG studies are complementary and particularly useful in confirming the diagnosis, documenting baseline activity, and selecting effective treatment. Table 15-2 delineates the current international classification of epileptic seizures.

In **partial** seizures, only a small focus in one hemisphere is involved. The child remains conscious, and there is no postictal phase. Partial seizures may involve very specific movements or sensations that

■ TABLE 15-2 International Classification of Epileptic Seizures

Partial Seizures
Simple partial (intact consciousness)
Motor
Sensory
Autonomic
Psychic
Complex partial (impaired consciousness)
Partial seizures with secondary generalization
Generalized Seizures
Absence (typical, atypical)
Tonic
Clonic
Tonic-clonic
Myoclonic
Atonic
Infantile spasms

remain stable with recurrent episodes. The symptoms are specific to the area of the brain involved and may be motor, cognitive, affective, or somatosensory. **Jacksonian** seizures are partial motor seizures in which a rhythmic twitching begins in one extremity and "marches" proximally until the entire limb is involved. Other partial seizures, termed **complex partial seizures**, result in alteration or impairment of consciousness. Semipurposeful movement continues without direction, or the child may begin lip pursing or picking at his or her clothes. Occasionally, partial seizures progress to generalized convulsions.

Generalized seizure disorders produce a clinical syndrome indicative of bilateral hemispheric involvement, such as impaired consciousness, symmetric bilateral activity, and a postictal phase of confusion and lethargy. **Tonic-clonic** seizures are what most people think of as typical seizures. The tonic phase is characterized by sustained flexor or extensor contraction; these episodes are interspersed with clonic activity, consisting of rhythmic, symmetric, generalized contractions of the trunk and extremity muscle groups. Breathing may be irregular, although most episodes do not progress to cyanosis. Bowel or bladder incompetence is not uncommon. Seizures may also be solely tonic or solely clonic.

Absence, or **petit mal**, seizures almost always begin in children younger than 10 years. They are brief staring episodes associated with alterations in consciousness. The child is unaware and immediately returns to the task at hand with no postictal phase. Although very brief, petit mal seizures can occur hundreds of times a day and may interfere with learning and socialization. An EEG demonstrates the characteristic generalized, symmetric three-per-second spike and wave pattern.

Atonic seizures consist of abrupt, total loss of postural tone lasting several minutes. **Myoclonic** seizures are simple short jerks similar to those occasionally experienced by normal subjects while in light sleep. Consciousness is minimally impaired, and there is no postictal phase. Myoclonic seizures are common in patients with degenerative disorders.

Two particularly devastating generalized seizure syndromes are **infantile spasms** and **Lennox-Gastaut's syndrome**. Infantile spasms, which usually present between 2 and 7 months of age, are recurrent mixed flexor-extensor spasms that last only a few seconds but may repeat more than 100 times in a row. This seizure disorder may be associated with many different neurodevelopmental diseases (e.g., mental retardation, hydrocephalus, congenital malformations, tuberous sclerosis). The diagnosis is confirmed by a typical EEG pattern known as **hypsarrhythmia**. ACTH controls the seizures in many patients but does not seem to prevent developmental delay. The value of corticosteroid administration is currently unclear. Infantile spasms may evolve into Lennox-Gastaut's syndrome, characterized by the frequent occurrence of mixed, generalized seizures that are notoriously refractory to pharmacologic treatment.

DIFFERENTIAL DIAGNOSIS

Febrile seizures do not represent true epilepsy. They typically occur in children 6 months to 5 years of age with fevers greater than 39°C (102°F). The rapid rise in temperature, rather than the height of the fever, is the important determinant. A **simple** febrile seizure lasts less than 5 to 10 minutes, is generalized, and does not recur during the precipitating illness episode. **Complex** febrile seizures last longer than 10 to 15 minutes, recur within 24 hours, or have focal features. Such children should receive additional studies and close follow-up or hospitalization for observation.

Simple febrile seizures do not require evaluation beyond determining the source of the fever. Children who are toxic appearing or have meningeal signs, an abnormal neurologic examination, or an underlying brain abnormality should not be presumed to have had a febrile seizure without ruling out more serious etiologies. Significant neurologic deficits resulting from febrile seizures are exceedingly rare. In most cases, the seizures do not recur with subsequent febrile episodes. Caretakers should be counseled concerning fever avoidance and seizure precautions.

Essential tremor, spasmus nutans, tics, myoclonus, and Tourette's syndrome are various movement disorders that originate in the basal ganglia and may mimic seizures. Essential tremor begins in infancy or childhood and may involve the chin, head, neck, and hands; it usually does not interfere with normal functions. Spasmus nutans presents in infancy and includes head nodding and tilting and rapid, small-amplitude nystagmus. Myoclonic movements are sudden, involuntary jerklike motions similar to startle responses.

Tourette's syndrome consists of motor *and* vocal **tics** (sudden, involuntary behaviors that are repetitive) that persist almost daily for more than a year. Common co-morbid conditions include obsessive-compulsive tendencies and attention deficit hyperactivity disorder. Children can also have less frequent tics of one type or the other. If tics become disruptive and interfere with functioning, they can be treated with behavioral therapy or medications (including botulinum toxin) with variable success.

Other conditions that may be confused with seizures include breath-holding spells, syncope, benign paroxysmal vertigo, and temper tantrums. Pseudoseizures should be suspected in the patient with implausible findings (e.g., alert and responsive during generalized tonic-clonic movements).

TREATMENT

Effective treatment combines education and medication. Both the child and the parents should become knowledgeable about acute care and local emergency medical services.

With **medication**, approximately 50% of patients are seizure free. Another 30% have significant reductions in seizure frequency or intensity or both. There has been a dramatic increase in the number of medications available for the management of seizures. The newer medications have a

Medication	Indications	Side Effects/Toxicity
TABLE 15-3 Indications and Side Effects of Anticonvulsants		
Conventional Drugs		
Carbamazepine (Tegretol)	Partial, tonic-clonic	Diplopia, nausea and vomiting, ataxia, leukopenia, thrombocytopenia
Ethosuximide (Zarontin)	Absence	Rash, anorexia, leukopenia, aplastic anemia
Phenobarbital (Luminal)	Tonic-clonic, partial	Hyperactivity, sedation, nystagmus, ataxia
Phenytoin (Dilantin)	Tonic-clonic, partial	Rash, nystagmus, ataxia, drug-induced lupus, gingival hyperplasia, anemia, leukopenia, polyneuropathy
Valproic acid (Depakote)	Tonic-clonic, absence, partial	Hepatotoxicity, nausea and vomiting, abdominal pain, weight loss, weight gain, anemia, leukopenia, thrombocytopenia
Newer Drugs		
Gabapentin (Neurontin)	Partial	Somnolence, dizziness, ataxia, fatigue
Lamotrigine (Lamictal)	Tonic-clonic, partial, absence, and Lennox-Gastaut	Dizziness, ataxia, blurred or double vision, nausea, vomiting, rash (including Stevens-Johnson's syndrome)
Oxcarbazepine (Trileptal)	Partial, tonic-clonic	Somnolence, hyponatremia, rash
Topiramate (Topamax)	Tonic-clonic, partial, Lennox-Gastaut, infantile spasms	Somnolence, fatigue, confusion, headache, ataxia, weight loss
Zonisamide (Zonegran)	Partial, generalized, infantile spasms, myoclonic seizures	Somnolence, ataxia, confusion, irritability, renal stones

better toxicity profile. Table 15-3 lists their names, indications, and side effects. Conventional anticonvulsants require careful monitoring of serum levels; the newer drugs do not.

For patients with poor seizure control on medication (approximately 20%), additional interventions are available. By monitoring a patient's seizures with continuous EEG leads, a focus may be discovered that can be removed **surgically**. The risks and benefits of such a procedure need to be explored carefully with the patient and family. Another option is the **ketogenic diet**. Inducing ketosis through a high-fat diet may control symptoms in some children. The **vagal nerve stimulator**, approved by the Food and Drug Administration in 1997, has proven quite beneficial in some patients.

Most children with seizure disorder undergo remission, after which the medication can be tapered. Unfortunately, this is not true for children who have seizure disorders as a result of congenital or acquired brain damage.

EMERGENCY MANAGEMENT OF STATUS EPILEPTICUS

Status epilepticus is defined as a prolonged episode of seizure activity (>10 to 30 minutes) or an extended period of recurrent seizures between which the patient does not return to consciousness. Status epilepticus is dangerous, leading to hypoxia, brain damage, and death. Airway, breathing, and circulation should be evaluated and addressed as necessary. Intravenous or rectal short-acting benzodiazepines (lorazepam, diazepam) often break the seizure. Usually, fosphenytoin, midazolam, or phenobarbital loading doses are administered as well to prevent recurrence. Patients in refractory status may require induction of induction of anesthesia with thiopental.

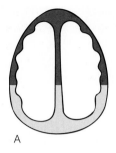 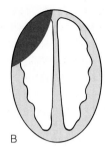

Figure 15-1 • **A:** Subdural hemorrhage. **B:** Epidural hematoma.

HEAD TRAUMA

Acute head trauma is the most common cause of pediatric death and disability in the developed world. Head injuries in children most often result from motor vehicle accidents, bicycle mishaps, falls, or child abuse. Males are twice as likely as females to sustain significant head trauma. Recovery from a head injury depends on the severity of the initial injury and factors contributing to secondary neuron injury such as hypotension and hypoxia. Severe injury is often associated with behavioral changes, motor impairment, and memory problems. Approximately 10% of children hospitalized for a traumatic brain injury have a seizure, and 35% of these go on to have a seizure disorder.

A **concussion** is defined as a brief alteration or loss of consciousness following mild head injury. Brain injury is undetectable, and the neurologic examination returns to normal within hours. In contrast, cerebral **contusions** represent a direct injury to the brain itself. **Diffuse axonal injury** results from shearing forces on the white matter of the brain that occur with rapid deceleration of the head. It frequently results in brain edema, further disruption of blood flow, inflammation, and ischemia.

Brain hemorrhages that occur because of trauma may be **epidural** or **subdural** (Table 15-4; Fig. 15-1). Some severe brain injuries may also result in subarachnoid injury and bleeding into the CSF.

CLINICAL MANIFESTATIONS

History

The source of injury should be described by the child and caretaker separately whenever possible. A history that is not consistent with a given injury is suggestive

TABLE 15-4 Differentiating Acute Subdural and Epidural Bleeds

	Subdural	Epidural
Location	Between the dura and arachnoid layers	Between the skull and the dura
Symmetry	Usually bilateral	Usually unilateral
Etiology	Rupture of bridging cortical veins or dura	Rupture of middle meningeal artery or vein or dural veins
Typical injury	Direct trauma or shaking	Direct trauma in the temporal area
Consciousness	Intact but altered	Impaired-lucid-impaired
Common associated findings	Seizures, retinal hemorrhages	Ipsilateral pupillary dilatation, papilledema, contralateral hemiparesis
Appearance on CT with contrast	Crescentic	Biconcave
Prognosis	High morbidity; low mortality	High mortality; low morbidity
Complications	Herniation	Skull fracture; uncal herniation

of child abuse. Reports of vomiting, severe headache, and mental status changes strongly suggest increased intracranial pressure. Confusion, loss of consciousness, amnesia, seizures, and visual impairment may also be present after significant injury.

Physical Examination

Patients with head injuries should receive a primary survey as soon as possible (Chapter 1). Moderate to severe injury may result in altered breathing and the need for respiratory support. The **Glasgow Coma Score** (GCS; Table 15-5) provides a rapid, widely used, easily reproducible method of quantifying neurologic function and helps guide initial therapy. Head trauma is divided into mild (GCS ≥ 13), moderate (GCS between 9 and 12), and severe (GCS ≤ 8) categories.

Bradycardia, hypertension, and irregular (Cheyne-Stokes) respirations form the **Cushing triad**, the hallmark of increased intracranial pressure. Palpation of the head may reveal step-off (depressed) skull fractures or a bulging fontanelle. Basilar skull fractures are characterized by periorbital (**"raccoon eyes"**) or postauricular (**"Battle sign"**) bruising, hemotympanum, or CSF rhinorrhea or otorrhea. Cranial nerve function, especially pupil size and reactivity, may help localize the injury. Papilledema may be evident on funduscopic exam. Sensory and motor function is difficult to assess in the patient with impaired mental status, who may respond minimally even to noxious stimuli. Deep tendon and pathologic reflexes should be assessed in all patients. Serial neurologic examinations track evolving lesions and response to interventions.

DIAGNOSTIC EVALUATION

Cervical spine films should be performed in all children with significant head trauma to rule out cervical injury. All patients with moderate or severe head trauma (as defined by GCS) should receive a head CT. Patients with mild head injury will also need imaging if they present with persistent altered mental status, focal signs on neurologic examination, signs and symptoms of increased intracranial pressure, or a history of significant injury. In patients who have sustained mild trauma, have a normal exam, and have a history of a brief alteration or loss of consciousness, the decision regarding imaging is left up to the examining physician. A CT is of little or no benefit in children with mild injury and no loss of consciousness.

TREATMENT

Treatment depends on the severity of the injury. Patients with suspected head or neck injury should be placed onto a back board with appropriate cervical spine immobilization in the field. Those with severe injury (GCS ≤ 8) generally require intubation. Hypotension is uncommon in isolated head trauma, but associated injuries may lead to shock (hypovolemic shock from hemorrhage, neurogenic shock from spinal cord injury, and cardiogenic shock from myocardial contusion). The goal of supportive therapy is to optimize the **cerebral perfusion pressure**, which is the difference between the mean arterial pressure and the intracranial pressure. Cerebral edema is the most important complication in the acute period. Normoxia, normothermia, normoglycemia, hyperosmolality, and elevation of the head of the bed are recommended to minimize intracranial hypertension and secondary brain injury. Mild hyperventilation, which

■ TABLE 15-5 Glasgow Coma Scale		
Activity	**Score**	**Activity**[a]
Eye opening		
Spontaneous	4	Spontaneous
To speech	3	To speech
To pain	2	To pain
None	1	None
Verbal		
Oriented	5	Coos, babbles
Confused	4	Irritable
Inappropriate words	3	Cries to pain
Nonspecific sounds	2	Moans to pain
None	1	None
Motor		
Follows commands	6	Normal, spontaneous movements
Localizes pain	5	Withdraws to touch
Withdraws to pain	4	Withdraws to pain
Abnormal flexion	3	Abnormal flexion
Abnormal extension	2	Abnormal extension
None	1	None

[a]Modified for infants.

reduces cerebral blood flow, is used to decrease intracranial pressure during the initial phase of therapy. Patients with evidence of impending herniation should be vigorously hyperventilated and given an osmotic agent such as mannitol to decrease intracranial pressure acutely. Patients with evidence of significant cerebral edema require intracranial pressure monitoring with a subdural bolt or intraventricular catheter.

Patients with moderate injury (GCS between 9 and 12) or a declining GCS should be admitted to an intensive care unit (ICU) for further observation, serial neurologic exams, and intervention as needed. Children with mild trauma should be observed in the hospital or at home with a reliable, competent caregiver for at least 24 hours. Any evidence of persistent headache, confusion, irritability, behavior changes, or visual disturbances should prompt further medical attention and workup.

Specific parameters exist for "return to play" for head injury that results from sports participation.

🔑 15-5 KEY POINTS

1. Subdural and epidural hemorrhages are more common than intraparenchymal bleeding when the injury is related to trauma.
2. Head trauma is divided into mild, medium, and severe categories depending on the patient's Glasgow Coma Score.
3. Basilar skull fractures are characterized by "raccoon eyes," Battle sign, hemotympanum, or CSF rhinorrhea or otorrhea.
4. Optimizing cerebral perfusion pressure is the goal of supportive care in severe brain injury.

ISCHEMIC/HEMORRHAGIC STROKES

Ischemic strokes are relatively rare in children but may be caused by sickle cell hemoglobinopathy, vasculitis, hemorrhages, emboli, trauma, hypercoagulable states, and abnormalities of lipid metabolism. Congenital vascular abnormalities, including arteriovenous malformations (AVMs), are the most common cause of intracranial hemorrhage in the pediatric population. An AVM is an abnormal collection of arteries and veins. It may present with physical findings consistent with seizures, acute hemorrhage, or a focal mass.

Occasionally, a cranial bruit is present on physical examination. Arteriography allows determination of the site of the abnormality and feeding vessels. Surgery is appropriate in some cases; however, extensive lesions are usually treated by selective embolization.

Thrombosis can occur at both arterial and venous sites. Conditions that predispose to thrombosis include sickle cell hemoglobinopathy, coagulation disorders, congenital heart disease, cardiac procedures, arrhythmias, endocarditis, trauma to the area of the internal carotid artery, bacterial meningitis, and infections leading to cavernous sinus thrombosis. Magnetic resonance angiography (MRA) can evaluate the vessels and reveal areas of ischemia. Additional laboratory tests that may prove helpful include coagulation studies, CBC and cultures, connective tissue/vasculitis profiles (ESR, C3, C4, ANA), and workups to rule out lipid and metabolic abnormalities. Low-molecular-weight heparin is useful in some conditions to dissolve thromboses and prevent recurrences. Large clots may require surgical evacuation.

HEADACHES

Headaches are a common complaint in the pediatric population. It is important to rule out dangerous conditions (e.g., tumors, intracranial bleeds, acute hydrocephalus, meningitis) before declaring the patient has more benign **tension-type** headaches.

PATHOGENESIS

Headaches may be vascular (migraines, AVMs), tension type, or result from increased intracranial pressure (classification according to the Headache Classification Committee of the International Headache Society). Other causes include some systemic illnesses (viral infections), sinusitis, dental abscess, poor vision, and temporomandibular joint disease. **Migraine headaches** are thought to be caused by vasodilation of intracranial vessels in response to a vascular or neuronal stimulus. Tension-type headaches may result from prolonged low-grade muscle contraction.

CLINICAL MANIFESTATIONS

History

Patients should be asked about the history (acute vs. chronic), onset, progression, severity, location, duration, and timing of the headaches. Response to medication and alleviating/exacerbating factors are important factors. Any weakness, visual disturbances, or abnormal sensations should be reported. Questions about stress levels, recent life changes, and precipitating factors (foods, menstruation, exercise) may assist in the diagnosis.

Headaches that wake the patient from sleep are suspicious for **increased intracranial pressure**. These headaches are usually made worse by lying flat or increasing venous pressure by bending, sneezing, or straining. Nausea and vomiting are not uncommon. The headaches usually increase in both severity and frequency over time. There may be associated personality changes, gait disturbances, and vision abnormalities.

Physical Examination

The physical exam should include examination of growth parameters, vital signs (include blood pressure), and structures of the head (sinuses, teeth). A fundu-scopic exam will allow detection of papilledema (swelling of the optic disc) in cases of increased intracranial pressure; sixth nerve palsy may also be present. Note: Poorly defined disc margins and the absence of retinal venous pulsations are consistent with papilledema. Vision acuity should be documented. Carotid bruits, which may be found in patients with AVMs, should be ruled out. A full neurologic exam including cranial nerve function, strength, sensation, deep tendon reflexes, gait, and mental status is of paramount importance.

DIAGNOSTIC EVALUATION

In most cases (migraines, tension-type headaches), no workup is needed beyond a careful history and examination. A head CT is recommended if increased intracranial pressure is suspected, the headaches are becoming progressively more frequent and severe, the patient experiences focal neurologic deficits, the headaches are persistently unilateral, or seizures develop. MRI or MRA may be necessary in suspected cases of AVMs. If a LP is indicated (in possible cases of meningitis or pseudotumor cerebri), neuroimaging should be completed before the procedure.

DIFFERENTIAL DIAGNOSIS

Migraines remain an underdiagnosed condition in the pediatric population. These severe, recurrent, pounding, often focal headaches may be precipitated by stress or specific food ingestions (e.g., chocolate). Approximately 20% of cases are preceded by an aura, usually visual. Migraines are often accompanied by other symptoms such as photophobia, nausea, vomiting, abdominal pain, and fatigue. Most patients have a family history of migraines. Sleep almost always relieves the headache. Migraines are classified as **complicated** when they are accompanied and/or followed by transient neurologic deficits such as weakness/paralysis, sensory loss, difficulty speaking, or alterations in vision or mental status.

Tension-type headaches are usually described as diffuse, constant, symmetric, and "bandlike." They occur more frequently when the patient is under stress or fatigued. There are usually no associated general (nausea) or neurologic manifestations. Tension headaches should not generally interfere with the child's normal daily activities (e.g., school attendance).

Pseudotumor cerebri, also known as idiopathic intracranial hypertension, is an uncommon but important cause of headaches that typically occurs in overweight adolescent females or in association with tetracycline or corticosteroid use. It is thought to be caused by impaired CSF resorption. The exam is positive for papilledema; however, this increased intracranial pressure is accompanied by a normal CT. Repeated LPs, which demonstrate increased opening pressure, may alleviate the headaches. Acetazolamide may also be helpful. More severe cases may require surgical intervention (optic nerve sheath fenestration).

TREATMENT

Analgesics such as acetaminophen and ibuprofen work better for children with migraines than adults. Metoclopramide is useful for some patients. Either **sumatriptan** or **ergotamine**, both vasoconstrictors, may relieve or obviate the migraine headache if administered early in its course. Patients should avoid known precipitants. Recurrent complicated migraines and migraines that substantially interfere with activities of daily living require prophylaxis therapy.

Tension headaches respond to nonprescription analgesics and rest. Stress management techniques and biofeedback training may also be beneficial.

15-6 KEY POINTS

1. In patients who present with a new, acute-onset headache, it is important to rule out tumors, intracranial bleeds, acute hydrocephalus, and meningitis. The vast majority of these patients have a more benign etiology for their headache.
2. Symptoms of increased intracranial pressure include headaches that wake the patient from sleep, are accompanied by nausea and vomiting, are made worse by maneuvers that increase venous pressure, and progress in frequency and severity over time.
3. Signs of increased intracranial pressure include sixth nerve palsy and papilledema.
4. Migraines are severe, recurrent, pounding, often focal headaches that may be preceded by an aura and may have known precipitating factors.
5. Tension-type headaches are constant, diffuse, and bandlike.
6. Pseudotumor cerebri is a syndrome of recurrent headaches caused by increased intracranial pressure in the face of normal neuroimaging.

TABLE 15-6 Causes of Encephalopathy in Children

Burns	Infection
Electrolyte disorders	AIDS encephalopathy
Hyponatremia	Encephalitis
Hypernatremia	Varicella
Hypocalcemia	Mumps
Hypercalcemia	Measles
Hypomagnesemia	Enterovirus
Hypermagnesemia	Cytomegalovirus
Hypertension	Herpes simplex encephalitis
Hypoxia/ischemia	Lyme's disease
Toxins	Tuberculosis
Lead	Reye's syndrome
Illicit drugs	Metabolic disorders
Carbon monoxide	Uremia
Sedatives	Hypoglycemia
Anticholinergics	Ketoacidosis
Salicylates	Environmental toxins
	Parainfectious syndromes

ENCEPHALOPATHY

To function normally, the brain needs adequate blood flow, oxygen, energy substrates, removal of metabolic waste, and appropriate electrolyte balance. Disruption of any of these will lead to generalized cerebral dysfunction, termed **encephalopathy**.

DIFFERENTIAL DIAGNOSIS

Table 15-6 lists the conditions that may lead to encephalopathy. Recent or concurrent febrile illness is consistent with **infectious** encephalitis. Focal findings (hemiparesis, ataxia, cranial nerve defects) on examination and seizures are more common with **herpes simplex (HSV) encephalitis** than other viral etiologies. **Reye's syndrome**, a rare mitochondrial disorder characterized by acute-onset encephalopathy and degenerative liver disease, may follow a viral illness, especially when aspirin has been administered. Signs and symptoms include severe vomiting, delirium, stupor, hypoglycemia, and elevated transaminase and ammonia levels. **Metabolic's disorders** typically present with recurrent episodes of mental status changes that clear when the acute process is corrected. A careful history may suggest environmental exposures or drug use.

CLINICAL MANIFESTATIONS

History and Physical Examination

Encephalopathy is characterized by mental status changes, odd or inappropriate behavior, disorientation, a shortened attention span, cognitive deficits, lethargy, stupor, and/or coma. The onset may be rapid or insidious. Particular areas of interest on exam include vital signs, liver size, pupil and funduscopic exams, and neurologic findings (cranial nerves, reflexes, strength, sensation, and cerebellar function).

DIAGNOSTIC EVALUATION

Electrolyte abnormalities, uremia, hypoglycemia, acidemia, and hyperammonemia can be ruled out with simple blood tests. The WBC count is elevated in the presence of infection. Urine and blood should be sent for toxicologic screening. An emergency head CT scan is indicated in patients with evidence of increased intracranial pressure or focal neurologic signs. A LP is appropriate when meningitis or encephalitis is suspected and increased intracranial pressure has been ruled out. HSV encephalitis is characterized by focal mediotemporal spikes superimposed on a diffuse slow wave pattern on EEG and temporal lobe abnormalities on CT and MRI.

TREATMENT

Treatment depends on the cause and whether or not increased intracranial pressure is present. Patients with severe disease require intubation and close intracranial pressure monitoring in an ICU. Antibiotics are added in cases of bacterial infection; acyclovir or foscarnet is recommended for patients with HSV. Metabolic's disorders are discussed in Chapter 9. Ingestions are discussed in Chapter 2.

🔧 15-7 KEY POINTS

1. Reye's syndrome is a mitochondrial disorder characterized by acute-onset encephalopathy and degenerative liver disease. It has occasionally been observed in children with viral illnesses who receive aspirin.
2. Encephalitis caused by herpes simplex virus may present with focal neurologic findings and seizures. The characteristic EEG shows focal spiking in the mediotemporal area, and temporal inflammatory lesions are demonstrated on MRI.

WEAKNESS

Abnormalities leading to weakness or paralysis, or both, may occur at any level of the neuromotor axis, from the motor cortex and pyramidal tracts to the anterior horn cell, peripheral nerve, neuromuscular junction, and muscle.

DIFFERENTIAL DIAGNOSIS

Guillain-Barré's syndrome (GBS) is an acute-onset, progressive, ascending weakness caused by autoimmune-mediated demyelination of the peripheral nerves. More than half of cases develop 7 to 21 days after an acute viral illness (usually respiratory). Sensory and autonomic impairments are often present but not prominent. Initial symptoms include numbness of the distal extremities followed by progressive (usually) ascending weakness. Deep tendon reflexes wane and disappear. Severity varies from mild weakness to progressive involvement of the trunk and cranial nerves. Respiratory muscle involvement may necessitate mechanical ventilation. A significantly increased CSF protein level is consistent with GBS. Motor nerve conduction studies may be helpful, particularly early in disease. Symptoms may progress for up to 4 weeks, and resolution typically begins approximately 4 weeks thereafter. Recovery is usually complete in children, although the rare patient experiences permanent lingering disability. Plasmapheresis or intravenous immune globulin may hasten resolution.

Tick paralysis resembles GBS, although ocular palsies and pupillary abnormalities are more commonly seen. Certain ticks in the Appalachian and Rocky Mountains are capable of producing a neurotoxin that blocks acetylcholine release. The patient recovers completely when the tick is removed from the skin.

Myasthenia gravis (MG) is an autoimmune disorder of the neuromuscular junction. Auto-antibodies bind to the postsynaptic acetylcholine receptor and block its activity. The rate of receptor breakdown also increases, so fewer receptors are present. The principal symptoms are easy fatigability and weakness that is exacerbated by sustained activity and improves with rest. Juvenile MG typically presents in late childhood or adolescence; the onset may be rapid or insidious, and symptoms wax and wane over time. Almost half of patients experience ocular muscle involvement, resulting in ptosis or diplopia or both. Bulbar weakness leads to dysarthria and difficulty swallowing. Administration of an intravenous anticholinesterase (edrophonium chloride) results in a transient increase in muscle strength by blocking the breakdown of acetylcholine in the synaptic cleft. Repetitive electrical nerve stimulation studies demonstrate a significant fall in response strength over several rapid-fire trials. Acetylcholine receptor antibodies are measurable in the serum. MG may go into complete or partial remission after several years; however, most patients continue to experience periodic exacerbations throughout adulthood. Anticholinesterase therapy (pyridostigmine bromide) may relieve all or most of the symptoms in patients with mild involvement. Corticosteroids and other immune suppressants help curb the autoimmune response. Finally, thymectomy is recognized as a potential method of treatment, presumably because the thymus is thought to sensitize the lymphocytes producing the offending antibodies.

Duchenne-type muscular dystrophy (DMD), an X-linked recessive disease of muscle tissue, is the classic myopathy. The disease presents in early childhood with motor delay. Weakness is greatest in the proximal muscle groups, so the patient must rise from sitting on the floor in two steps: first leaning on the hypertrophied calves, and then pushing the trunk up with the arms (**Gower sign**). Eventually, ambulation is lost, the muscles atrophy, and contractures develop. Cardiac and cognitive abnormalities are often present as well. Treatment is supportive. Most children become wheelchair bound early in the second decade, with death in adolescence or early adulthood from respiratory failure or cardiomyopathy.

Spinal muscle atrophy (SMA) is an inherited disorder involving degeneration of the anterior horn cells and cranial nerve motor nuclei. The most severe form, SMA type I (Werdnig-Hoffmann's disease), becomes evident in early infancy with generalized hypotonia and weakness. SMA type 2 presents between 6 and 12 months of age and is usually less severe. Cognitive abilities remain unaffected in both forms of the illness. No specific therapy is available; death occurs from repeated aspiration or lung infections. Both SMA and DMD are suggested by characteristic changes on EMG and muscle biopsy and confirmed by specific gene tests.

Poliomyelitis is a viral illness affecting primarily the anterior horn cells of the spine. There have only been a few cases of polio in the last several years, and they seem to have been related to reversion of the live oral polio vaccine to wild type. As a result, killed virus in the form of an injected vaccine is now recommended. The oral vaccine still has an important role in world health efforts because it contributes to herd immunity by being passively spread.

Tumors that compress the spinal cord result in weakness and paralysis below the lesion and constitute a surgical emergency. **Cervical spinal cord injuries** produce sudden-onset paresthesias and paralysis. **Environmental toxin exposure** may induce acquired neuropathies or myopathies. For example, infants in certain endemic areas (or those fed honey) may be exposed to spores of *Clostridium botulinum* and develop progressive paralysis from the elaborated toxin, which irreversibly blocks release of acetylcholine at the motor endplate.

CLINICAL MANIFESTATIONS

Diagnostic workup is tailored by findings on history and physical examination. Patients with asymmetric weakness or signs of increased intracranial pressure should receive neuroimaging to rule out mass or hemorrhage. Findings localized to a particular level of the spinal cord require evaluation for cord compression or injury. An LP is helpful when infection is suspected. Supportive treatment may be required at some point; more definitive treatment, if available, is disease specific.

🔑 15-8 KEY POINTS

1. Guillain-Barré's syndrome is an acute-onset, ascending, progressive weakness caused by peripheral nerve demyelination.
2. Myasthenia gravis is an autoimmune disorder of the neuromuscular junction characterized by easy fatigability and weakness.
3. The Gower sign is classically observed with DMD.

NEURODEGENERATIVE DISORDERS

Neural tissue degeneration can occur at any level of the nervous system, from the brain cell bodies to the peripheral nerves. Many of the diseases are inherited; most are progressive and debilitating.

CLINICAL MANIFESTATIONS AND TREATMENT

Neurodegenerative disorders may be divided into *gray matter* disorders, *white matter* disorders, and *system* disorders. Gray matter disorders, which include Tay-Sachs, Gaucher, and Niemann-Pick's diseases, result from lipid buildup in neuronal cell bodies. Hypotonia, mental retardation, seizures, retinal degeneration, and ataxia are common.

White matter disorders (**leukodystrophies**) are inherited progressive degenerative diseases resulting from abnormally formed myelin, impaired conduction, and rapid myelin breakdown. They present in younger patients with spasticity and developmental milestone loss; older children and adolescents experience visual disturbances (optic atrophy), changes in personality, and dropping school grades. **Adrenoleukodystrophy**, so named because of its frequent association with adrenal insufficiency, is characterized by areas of demyelination coupled with an intense perivascular inflammatory reaction. Psychomotor retardation progresses to spasticity, extensor posturing, and death by early adulthood.

Dietary therapy is controversial; no curative treatment is available.

System diseases are categorized according to the particular neural pathway affected. **Rett's syndrome** is an *X-linked* but usually sporadic disorder of cerebral atrophy, which appears to occur primarily in *girls*. These patients initially show normal development; however, after 1 year of age, microcephaly and developmental milestone regression occur. Persistent hand wringing, seizures, ataxia, mental retardation, and autistic behavior are the rule. Life expectancy is appreciably shortened.

🔑 15-9 KEY POINT

1. Adrenoleukodystrophy is the classic white matter degenerative disease.

ATAXIA

Ataxia is the inability to coordinate purposeful movement and control balance. Conditions that affect the cerebellum, connected sensory/motor pathways, or the inner ear are likely to cause ataxia in children. The two most common causes in children are drug ingestion (e.g., phenytoin, carbamazepine, sedatives, hypnotics, phencyclidine) and acute postinfectious cerebellar ataxia.

DIFFERENTIAL DIAGNOSIS

Viral infections have been known to cause ataxia during attacks of acute labyrinthitis. **Acute cerebellar ataxia** may follow some viral infections (particularly varicella) by 2 to 3 weeks and is thought to be autoimmune in origin. These children present with horizontal nystagmus, postural ataxia, vomiting, and occasionally dysarthria. Headache and nuchal rigidity are absent, and the CSF is sterile.

Ataxia that is slowly progressive is more likely to be caused by a brain tumor or a degenerative spinocerebellar disease such as ataxia-telangiectasia or Friedreich ataxia. **Ataxia-telangiectasia** is an autosomal recessive neurodegenerative disorder that presents in toddlers and progresses to wheelchair dependence. The ataxia is associated with extensive telangiectasias and immunodeficiency (see Chapter 11). The genetic defect is located on chromosome 11.

Friedreich ataxia presents later in childhood with progressive ataxia, weakness, and muscle wasting. Skeletal deformities invariably follow. Most patients die of cardiomyopathy-related heart disease before 30 years of age. Inheritance is autosomal recessive, linked to a defect on chromosome 9.

Intoxications and ingestions, metabolic derangements, hydrocephalus, head trauma, and cerebellar hemorrhages may also cause ataxia.

CLINICAL MANIFESTATIONS

History and Physical Examination

The history should include questions concerning disease onset (acute vs. chronic) and progression (slow vs. rapid). Associated symptoms may include fever, headache, vomiting, vertigo, photophobia, and altered mental status. Recent precipitating events (seizures, infections, head trauma) and exposures (medications, heavy metals, solvents, gases) should be documented. Some ataxias have a genetic basis, so the family history may be positive for neurologic illnesses.

The examination includes evaluation of truncal balance, mental status, gait, deep tendon reflexes, and muscle tone and strength. An abnormal gait may be caused by weakness (reduced reflexes and muscle strength) rather than imbalance. The examiner should note the presence of any nystagmus and/or signs of increased intracranial pressure (bradycardia, hypertension, papilledema, meningismus). If the child is old enough and cooperative, tests such as heel-to-knee, finger-to-nose, and rapid alternating movement, along with the Romberg test, help evaluate cerebellar function. (Note: The Romberg test is performed with the patient's feet together and eyes closed. The examiner briefly pushes the patient in various directions to see whether he or she can compensate and maintain an upright posture. Excessive swaying [or falling] is considered the Romberg sign.)

DIAGNOSTIC EVALUATION

Neuroimaging can rule out hydrocephalus, mass lesions, and cerebellar hemorrhages. A brain MRI is preferable to head CT, given its superior detail of posterior fossa structures. Patients with a fever should receive a LP to evaluate for infection; the procedure may be delayed until after neuroimaging in most cases. Toxicologic screens of blood and urine should be obtained in all cases of acute ataxia. Chronic or recurrent ataxia warrants metabolic and genetic workup.

🔑 15-10 KEY POINT

1. The differential diagnosis for ataxia (incoordination) includes labyrinthitis, acute ingestion, acute postinfectious cerebellar ataxia, ataxia-telangiectasia, and Friedreich ataxia.

PHAKOMATOSES

Phakomatoses are neurocutaneous diseases characterized by lesions in the nervous system, skin, and eyes. Three autosomal dominant conditions are described: neurofibromatosis, tuberous sclerosis, and von Hippel-Lindau disease. Sturge-Weber's disease, a purely sporadic disorder, is traditionally included as well.

CLINICAL MANIFESTATIONS AND TREATMENT

Neurofibromatosis

Of the several variants of neurofibromatosis, types 1 (**von Recklinghausen's disease**; Table 15-7) and 2 (bilateral acoustic neurofibromatosis) are the most common in children. Neurofibromatosis type 1 is a clinical diagnosis based in part of the presence of six or more café-au-lait spots of a certain size. The genetic defect is mapped to chromosome 17. Patients with von Recklinghausen's disease should receive treatment for the associated seizures, learning disorders, renovascular hypertension, and scoliosis. Neurofibromas that cause impairment may be surgically removed; however, most will recur.

Bilateral acoustic neuromas are the hallmark of type 2 neurofibromatosis. Complications include hearing loss and vestibular disorientation. Brain MRI demonstrates bilateral eighth cranial nerve masses. Neurofibromas, meningiomas, schwannomas, and astrocytomas are also associated with type 2 neurofibromatosis. Cataracts and retinal hamartomas are not uncommon. Surgical debulking is appropriate when hearing impairment becomes pronounced. Cochlear implants have restored hearing in some patients. The genetic abnormality occurs on chromosome 22.

Tuberous Sclerosis

Tuberous sclerosis, like neurofibromatosis, is a progressive autosomal dominant neurocutaneous disorder.

■ TABLE 15-7 Diagnosis of Neurofibromatosis Type 1

Two of the following must be present:.

1. Six or more café-au-lait spots, >5 mm in size in children and >15 mm in adolescents or adults

2. Axillary or inguinal freckling

3. Two or more Lisch nodules (hamartomas) in the iris

4. Two or more neurofibromas or one plexiform neurofibroma

5. A distinctive osseous lesion, such as sphenoid dysplasia

6. Optic gliomas

7. Affected first-degree relative diagnosed based on the preceding criteria

A genetic abnormality exists at chromosome site 9q34 or 16p13. The normal genetic product is tuberin, a protein thought to suppress the development of tumors. Sporadic cases are more common than inherited ones. Disease severity varies greatly from patient to patient.

Typical skin lesions include **ash-leaf spots** (flat, hypopigmented macules), **shagreen patches** (areas of abnormal skin thickening), sebaceous adenomas, and uncal fibromas. Ash-leaf spots are the earliest manifestation and are best seen under Wood lamp examination. Neuroimaging demonstrates the distinctive periventricular knoblike areas of localized swelling, or "tubers." Subependymal nodules and giant cell astrocytomas may also be present. Mental retardation and seizures (including infantile spasms) are common. Tumors also have a predilection for the kidney, heart (particularly cardiac rhabdomyomas), and retina. Treatment consists of antiepileptic therapy and surgical removal of related tumors when indicated.

Von Hippel-Lindau's Disease

Von Hippel-Lindau's disease is characterized by retinal angiomas (abnormal masses of thin-walled capillaries), cerebellar hemangioblastomas, and associated neoplasms, including renal cell carcinoma and pheochromocytoma. Ocular lesions respond to laser therapy; no specific treatment exists for the CNS growths. The genetic abnormality occurs on chromosome 3p25 and exhibits variable penetrance. It generally does not present until adolescence or beyond.

Sturge-Weber's Disease

Sturge-Weber's disease is a disorder of neurologic deterioration associated with a port-wine stain (nevus flammeus) over the area innervated by the **first division of the trigeminal nerve**. Affected children manifest progressive mental retardation, seizures, hemiparesis, and visual impairment; approximately a third develop glaucoma. Laser therapy may "fade" the port-wine stain but does not address the underlying neurologic dysfunction. Optimal control of seizures may limit subsequent developmental delay. Hemispherectomy is controversial; if performed in the first year of life, it may prevent progression to mental retardation by controlling recalcitrant seizures.

⚕15-11 KEY POINTS

1. Neurofibromatosis type 1 is characterized by multiple café-au-lait spots on examination.
2. In contrast, the typical skin lesions of tuberous sclerosis include ash-leaf spots and shagreen patches.
3. Sturge-Weber's disease is associated with a port-wine stain over the area innervated by cranial nerve V, first division (CNV_1).

SKULL ABNORMALITIES

Microcephaly describes a head circumference that is greater than 2 standard deviations below mean head size for age. It often results from genetic abnormalities (e.g., trisomy 21, Prader-Willi's syndrome) or congenital insults (maternal drug ingestions, congenital infections, or insufficient placental blood flow). Affected children demonstrate both cognitive and motor delay; associated seizure disorders are not uncommon.

Macrocephaly, in contrast, refers to a head circumference greater than 2 standard deviations above the mean. Macrocephaly may be the result of a large brain; however, cranioskeletal dysplasias, storage diseases, and hydrocephalus should be explored as possible causes, particularly if the growth rate crosses percentile lines over time.

Craniosynostosis is the premature fusion of one or more cranial sutures. It may be idiopathic or occur as part of a syndrome. Bony growth continues along the open sutures, resulting in an abnormally shaped head. If early obliteration of the sagittal suture occurs (most common), the child has a long head and a narrow face (scaphocephaly). In contrast, premature closure of the coronal sutures results in a very wide face with a short, almost boxlike, skull. The need for and timing of surgical intervention, which consists of reopening the sutures and retarding their subsequent fusion, is controversial. Most defects are repaired before 2 years of age for cosmetic reasons. Craniosynostosis with associated hydrocephalus, subnormal brain growth, and development issues is addressed sooner.

Additional Suggested Reading

Coombs JB, David RL. A synopsis of the American Academy of Pediatrics' practice parameter on the management of minor closed head injury in children. *Pediatr Rev.* 2000;21:413–415.

Dias MS. Neurosurgical management of myelomeningocele (spina bifida). *Pediatr Rev.* 2005;26:50–59.

Dinolfo EA. In brief: evaluation of ataxia. *Pediatr Rev.* 2001;22:177–178.

Gedeit R. Head injury. *Pediatr Rev.* 2001;22:118–124.

Iqpal MM. Prevention of neural tube defects. *Pediatr Rev.* 2000;21:58–66.

Mackay MT, Weiss SK, Adams-Webber T. Practice parameter: Medical treatment of infantile spasms. *Neurology.* 2004;62:1668–1681.

Pellock JM. New pharmacotherapies for pediatric seizures. *Pediatr Ann.* 2004;33:385–391.

Rich J. In brief: degenerative central nervous system disease. *Pediatr Rev.* 2001;22:175–176.

Shinnar S, O'Dell C. Febrile seizures. *Pediatr Ann.* 2004;33:395–401.

Wheless JW. Treatment of status epilepticus in children. *Pediatr Ann.* 2004;33:377–384.

Zinner SH. Tourette's syndrome: much more than tics. *Contemp Pediatr.* 2004;21:22–49.

16 Nutrition

Good nutrition is necessary for optimal physical growth and intellectual development. A healthy diet protects against disease, provides reserve in times of stress, and contains adequate amounts of protein, carbohydrates, fats, vitamins, and minerals. Children with vegetarian diets are at risk for vitamin B_{12} and trace mineral deficiencies. Infant feeding intolerance, failure to thrive, and obesity are the most common pediatric conditions associated with malnutrition.

To assess a patient's nutritional status and growth, pediatricians rely on following a patient's **growth chart**. Growth charts represent cross-sectional data from the National Center for Health Statistics. The patient's weight and height are recorded as points on the chart at each well child visit. Separate growth charts are generated for premature infants and infants with certain genetic disorders, including Down syndrome and Turner syndrome. Increasing attention is being given to using the **body mass index (BMI**; weight in kilograms divided by height in meters squared) as a more useful assessment of growth. The major drawback (difficulty of rapid calculation) has been overcome by the availability of BMI wheels and printed charts. BMI charts that track growth over time, similar to standard growth charts, are becoming increasingly widespread.

INFANT FEEDING ISSUES

Infant feeding addresses the physical and emotional needs of both mother and child. Babies **triple in weight** and double in length during the first year. Although breast-feeding is strongly recommended, many commercially prepared iron-fortified formulas provide appropriate calories and nutrients. Premature infants (<32 weeks) need formulas specifically designed for them or breast milk with added fortifier. Newborns feed on demand, usually every 1 to 2 hours.

Neonates normally lose up to 10% of their birth weight over the first several days; formula-fed babies regain their birth weight by the second week of life, whereas breast-fed babies may take approximately a week longer. Healthy infants automatically regulate intake to meet caloric demand.

All infant formulas contain the recommended amount of vitamins and minerals. However, at 4 to 6 months of age, iron-fortified cereals should be added to the infant diet. (Note: Iron fortification is particularly important in breast-fed infants: maternal stores are depleted by 6 months of age, and the iron in human breast milk, although well absorbed, is low.) After 6 months of age, other baby foods may be started, including fruits and vegetables. When introducing new foods, only one new product should be introduced at a time to evaluate for potential adverse reactions. Infants 6 months of age and older (possibly sooner in breast-fed infants) may require fluoride supplementation, depending on the concentration of fluoride in their tap water. Whole cow milk may be introduced at 12 months and should continue until 24 months when skim milk should be substituted. Infants and children sent to bed with a bottle containing anything but water are at risk for **milk-bottle teeth caries**.

BREAST-FEEDING

The American Academy of Pediatrics recommends **exclusive breast-feeding** during the first 6 months of life and continuation of breast-feeding during the second 6 months for optimal infant nutrition. Studies have shown that breast-fed infants have a lower incidence of infections, including otitis media, pneumonia, sepsis, and meningitis. Human milk contains bacterial and viral antibodies (secretory IgA) and macrophages.

■ **TABLE 16-1** Clinical and Laboratory Manifestations of Rickets
Craniotabes (thinning of the outer skull layer)
Rachitic rosary (enlargement of the costochondral junctions)
Epiphyseal enlargement at the wrists and ankles
Delayed closing of abnormally large fontanelle
Bowlegs
Delayed walking
Normal-to-low serum calcium
Low serum phosphorus
Elevated serum alkaline phosphatase
Low serum 25-hydroxycholecalciferol

Lactoferrin is a protein found in breast milk that increases the availability of iron and has an inhibitory effect on the growth of *Escherichia coli*. Breast-fed infants are less likely to experience feeding difficulties associated with allergy (eczema) or intolerance (colic).

Breast-fed infants with dark skin and/or rare sunlight exposure should receive **vitamin D supplementation** beginning in the weeks after birth to prevent **rickets**, a condition in which developing bone fails to mineralize because of inadequate 1,25-dihydroxycholecalciferol. Rickets in breast-fed infants becomes clinically and chemically evident in late infancy (Table 16-1). Rickets attributable solely to vitamin D deficiency begins to respond to supplementation within weeks.

In developed countries, mothers with HIV infection, untreated active tuberculosis, or those who are using illegal drugs should not breast-feed. Other contraindications include infants with galactosemia and some maternal medications, including antithyroid medications, lithium, chemotherapy agents, and isoniazid.

INFANT FEEDING INTOLERANCE

Feeding intolerance may lead to food aversion and failure to thrive; the most significant cause is cow milk protein intolerance or allergy.

Clinical Manifestations

History and Physical Examination

Feeding intolerance may present with any number of clinical manifestations. **Malabsorption** is characterized by poor growth and chronic diarrhea. **Colitis**, indicated by anemia or obvious blood in the stools, can occur. **Allergy** may be accompanied by eczema or wheezing. Other possible symptoms include vomiting, irritability, and abdominal distention.

Differential Diagnosis

Infectious gastroenteritis, necrotizing enterocolitis, intussusception, intermittent volvulus, celiac disease, cystic fibrosis, chronic protein malnutrition, aspiration, and eosinophilic enteritis should be considered. The most common condition mistaken for milk protein intolerance is **colic**, which is generally limited to infants younger than 3 months. Colic is a syndrome of recurrent irritability that persists for several hours, usually in the late afternoon or evening. During the attacks, the child draws the knees to the abdomen and cries inconsolably. The crying resolves as suddenly and spontaneously as it begins.

Treatment

Exclusive breast-feeding during the first year of life eliminates the problem posed by milk protein intolerance, except in severely allergic infants. If there is no evidence of any underlying disease, many pediatricians recommend a trial of casein hydrolysate formulas because as many as 25% of children with milk protein allergy are also intolerant of soy protein.

🔑 **16-1 KEY POINTS**
1. Newborns initially lose weight but should regain to birth weight by the third week of life.
2. Cow's milk protein intolerance can lead to feeding intolerance and aversion.
3. The sporadic nature and sudden onset of colic usually distinguish this condition from feeding intolerance.
4. The American Academy of Pediatrics recommends exclusive breast-feeding during the first 6 months of life, with continued breast-feeding through 12 months of age.

FAILURE TO THRIVE

Failure to thrive (FTT) is defined here as persistent weight below the third percentile or falling off the patient's previously established growth curve. (Note: Many children cross percentiles between 9 and 18 months of age as growth begins to be based more on genetic potential than on maternal nutrition prior to birth.) Risk factors include low birth weight, lower socioeconomic status, physical or mental disability, and caretaker neglect. FTT is often associated with developmental delay, particularly if it occurs during the first year of life when brain growth is maximal.

DIFFERENTIAL DIAGNOSIS

FTT may be caused by inadequate caloric intake, excessive caloric losses, or increased caloric requirements. **Most cases of FTT in developed countries are nonorganic or psychosocial in origin**; that is, there is no coexistent medical disorder. The list of organic diagnoses predisposing to FTT is extensive, and virtually all organ systems are represented (Table 16-2). **Organic** FTT virtually never presents with isolated growth failure; other signs and symptoms are generally evident with a detailed history and physical exam.

CLINICAL MANIFESTATIONS

History

The caretaker must be questioned in detail about the child's diet, including how often the child eats, how much at each feeding, what the child is fed, how the formula is prepared, and who feeds the child. Information regarding diarrhea, fatty stools, irritability, vomiting, food refusal, and polyuria should be documented. Recurrent infections suggest congenital or acquired immunodeficiency. Constitutional growth delay can usually be diagnosed by family history alone. Foreign and domestic travel, source of water, and developmental delay are occasionally overlooked topics. The psychosocial history includes questions concerning the caretaker's expectations of the child, parental and sibling health, financial security, recent major life events, and chronic stressors.

Physical Examination

Weight, height, and head circumference should be plotted out on an appropriate **growth chart**. Relatively recent growth failure is usually limited to weight alone, whereas height and (late) head circumference are also affected in chronic deficiency. Severely deprived children may present with lethargy, edema,

■ TABLE 16-2 Differential Diagnosis of Failure to Thrive

Nonorganic
- Neglect
- Psychosocial
- Abuse
- Inadequate amount fed
- Incorrect preparation of formula

Cardiac
- Congenital heart malformations

Gastrointestinal
- Malabsorption
- Milk protein intolerance/allergy
- Gastroesophageal reflux
- Pyloric stenosis
- Inflammatory bowel disease
- Celiac disease
- Hirschsprung disease

Pulmonary
- Cystic fibrosis
- Bronchopulmonary dysplasia
- Chronic aspiration
- Respiratory insufficiency

Infectious
- HIV
- Tuberculosis
- Chronic gastroenteritis
- Intestinal parasites
- UTI

Neonatal
- Prematurity
- Low birth weight
- Congenital or perinatal infection
- Congenital syndromes

Endocrine
- Diabetes mellitus
- Hypothyroidism
- Adrenal insufficiency or excess
- Growth hormone deficiency

(Continued)

■ TABLE 16-2 Differential Diagnosis of Failure to Thrive (*continued*)

Neurologic

   Cerebral palsy

   Mental retardation

   Degenerative disorders

   Oral-motor dysfunction

Renal

   Renal tubular acidosis

   Chronic renal insufficiency

Other

   Inborn errors of metabolism

   Malignancy

   Cleft palate

   Immunodeficiency syndromes

   Collagen vascular disease

scant subcutaneous fat, atrophic muscle tissue, decreased skin turgor, coarsened hair, dermatitis, and distended abdomen.

Observation of caretaker-to-child interaction and feeding behavior is critical. Children who are listless, minimally responsive to the examiner and/or caretaker, withdrawn, or excessively fearful often have contributing psychosocial issues. Findings suggestive of physical abuse or neglect (see Chapter 2) should be sought and documented.

A complete physical examination, with careful attention to dysmorphism, pallor, bruising, cleft palate, rales or crackles, heart murmurs, and muscle tone, may suggest the etiology.

DIAGNOSTIC EVALUATION

Information obtained from the history and physical determine the direction of further diagnostic workup. Any child with FTT should receive a CBC, serum electrolytes, BUN and creatinine, protein and albumin measurements, UA, and urine culture. Bone age films may also be helpful in children beyond infancy. Severely malnourished children and patients with suspected nonorganic FTT should be admitted to the hospital. Adequate catch-up growth during hospitalization on a regular diet is virtually diagnostic of psychosocial FTT.

⚒ 16-2 KEY POINTS

1. Consistent weight below the third percentile and falling off a previously established growth curve are both evidence of failure to thrive (FTT).
2. Most cases of FTT in developed countries are nonorganic.
3. Any organ system may be implicated in organic FTT; the history, physical exam, and screening tests should help focus the search.

OBESITY

Pediatric **obesity**, defined as BMI greater than the 95th percentile for age, is at epidemic proportions in many developed countries today. A child whose BMI falls between the 85th and 95th percentiles is considered at risk for the development of obesity. It is currently estimated that 10% of children 2 to 5 years of age and 15% of older children are overweight. A period of adipose cell proliferation occurs from 2 to 4 years of age and again during puberty, placing pediatricians in the position to affect their patients' health well into adulthood.

Although the root cause is simply caloric intake in excess of expenditure, the presence of certain gene markers results in increased risk. Factors associated with an increased risk of obesity in children include genetic, parental, family, and lifestyle issues (Table 16-3). The social and psychological consequences of being a "fat" child may be particularly damaging to self-esteem at a critical age. The workup of an obese child should include consideration of endocrine disorders (hypothyroidism, Cushing syndrome), genetic syndromes, and hypothalamic tumors.

■ TABLE 16-3 Risk Factors for Obesity in Children

Overweight parent(s)

Large birth weight

Diabetic mother

Low parental education level

Poverty

Overweight child at 3 years of age

Increased length of TV viewing

Poor dietary choices

Lower activity levels

A condition termed "**metabolic syndrome X**" has been described that consists of **obesity, insulin resistance, hypertension, and dyslipidemia**. (Note: Examples of dyslipidemia include elevated serum cholesterol, elevated low-density lipoprotein [LDL] cholesterol, elevated triglycerides, and decreased high-density lipoprotein [HDL] cholesterol levels.) The incidences of both type 2 diabetes and cardiovascular disease are increased in patients with this syndrome. Other potential complications of obesity include depression, sleep apnea, gallbladder disease, slipped capital femoral epiphysis, and early-onset puberty in females.

Obesity is treated by altering dietary habits (limiting intake of high-calorie, high-fat foods), developing a regular exercise program, and behavioral modification (setting goals and monitoring self-control). Careful attention must be paid to maintaining the patient's growth and development while at the same time decreasing BMI over time. Surgical options currently are limited to the adult population.

🔑 16-3 KEY POINTS

1. Children with body mass indexes (BMIs) greater than the 95th percentile for age are considered obese.
2. Metabolic syndrome X (obesity, insulin resistance, dyslipidemia, and hypertension) increases the risk for development of type 2 diabetes and cardiovascular disease.

Additional Suggested Reading

Binns HJ, Ariza AJ. Guidelines help clinicians identify risk factors for overweight children. *Pediatr Ann.* 2004;33:18–24.

Hall RT, Carroll RE. Infant feeding. *Pediatr Rev.* 2000;21:191–200.

Schneider MB, Brill SR. Obesity in children and adolescents. *Pediatr Rev.* 2005;26:155–162.

Schwartz ID. Failure to thrive: an old nemesis in the new millennium. *Pediatr Rev.* 2000;21:257–264.

Oncology

LEUKEMIA

The leukemias account for the greatest percentage of cases of childhood malignancies. There are more than 3,000 new cases of leukemia each year in the United States, and approximately 35 to 40 children per million are affected. Table 17-1 lists types of childhood cancer (0 to 14 years of age) and the fraction of the total childhood malignancies that each accounts for annually.

PATHOGENESIS

Leukemia results from malignant transformation and clonal expansion of hematopoietic cells at an early stage of differentiation that are unable to undergo further maturation. Leukemias are classified on the basis of leukemic cell morphology into **lymphoblastic leukemias** (lymphoid lineage cell proliferation) and **nonlymphoblastic leukemias** (granulocyte, monocyte, erythrocyte, or platelet lineage cell proliferation). **Acute leukemias** constitute 97% of all childhood leukemias and are subdivided into acute lymphoblastic leukemia (ALL) and acute nonlymphocytic leukemia, also known as acute myelogenous leukemia (AML). If untreated, they are rapidly fatal within weeks to a few months of diagnosis, but with treatment they are curable. **Chronic leukemias** make up only 3% of childhood leukemias, the majority of which are chronic myelogenous leukemia (CML) seen in adolescents. Unlike patients with acute leukemias, CML is indolent and patients may survive without treatment for months to years. If left untreated, the chronic leukemias undergo an acute transformation that requires immediate therapy to survive. Because CML is so rare in children, a discussion of the chronic leukemias goes beyond the scope of this review text. The following discussion focuses on ALL and AML of childhood and adolescence.

CLASSIFICATION

ALL is classified by both morphologic and immunologic methods. **Morphologic classification** is based on the appearance of the lymphoblasts. The L1 type lymphoblast is the most common (85%), followed by the L2 morphology (14%), with L3 lymphoblasts the rarest form. Therapy and outcome is not different for L1 versus L2 lymphoblasts. L3 blasts, or Burkitt or mature B leukemia is treated more like Burkitt lymphoma with spread to the bone marrow. **Immunologic classification** is based on immunophenotype, which is described by CD surface antigens and flow cytology. The most frequent childhood ALL immunophenotype, precursor B cell, accounts for 80% of cases and is associated with a good prognosis. T-cell ALL, which is responsible for 19% of childhood ALL, has a worse prognosis, but outcome is improving with more intensive therapy. Mature B-cell ALL or Burkitt leukemia, which accounts for 1% of cases, is treated like Burkitt lymphoma with a good outcome.

AML is classified into eight subtypes by morphologic and histochemical information using the French-American-British (FAB) classification system: M0 is undifferentiated stem cell leukemia, M1 is myeloblastic leukemia without differentiation, M2 is myeloblastic leukemia with differentiation, M3 is promyelocytic leukemia, M4 is myelomonocytic leukemia, M5 is monoblastic leukemia, M6 is erythroleukemia, and M7 is megakaryoblastic leukemia.

■ TABLE 17-1 Distribution of Childhood Cancer by Diagnosis, Age 0 to 14 Years

Cancer	Percentage of Total Pediatric Malignancies Annually
ALL	23.3
CNS	23.2
Wilms tumor	6.6
Neuroblastoma	6.0
Non-Hodgkin lymphoma	5.9
Hodgkin lymphoma	4.7
Rhabdomyosarcoma	4.6
AML	4.2
Osteosarcoma	2.5
Ewing sarcoma	2.3
Retinoblastoma	1.8
Other	14.9

ALL, acute lymphocytic leukemia; AML, acute myelogenous leukemia.
Adapted from Gurney JG, Severson RK, Davis S, et al. Incidence of cancer in children in the United States. Sex-, race-, and 1-year age-specific rates by histologic subtype. Cancer. 2000;80:2321–2332.

EPIDEMIOLOGY AND RISK FACTORS

Table 17-2 compares the epidemiology of ALL and AML. ALL, the most common pediatric neoplasm, accounts for 75% of all cases of childhood acute leukemia. ALL is 1.3 times more common in boys than in girls and more common in white children than in African American children. The incidence of ALL peaks between 2 and 5 years of age. AML accounts for 20% of all cases of childhood acute leukemia. There is no race or gender predilection in patients with AML. The incidence of AML, in contrast to ALL, is increased in adolescence.

Syndromes with an increased risk for leukemia include trisomy 21, Fanconi anemia, Bloom syndrome (a chromosomal breakage disorder), ataxia-telangiectasia, X-linked agammaglobulinemia, and severe combined immunodeficiency. Twins have an increased risk of leukemia if one twin develops ALL or AML during the first 5 years of life. Children who have undergone chemotherapy or radiation therapy for a first malignancy have an increased risk of developing a secondary leukemia 1 to 7 years after treatment. Children with congenital bone marrow failure states, such as

■ TABLE 17-2 Epidemiology of Acute Lymphocytic Leukemia and Acute Myelogenous Leukemia

Characteristic	ALL	AML
Incidence	2,500–3,000 cases/yr (75%)	350–500 cases/yr (15%–20%)
Peak age	4 yr	Increased in adolescence
Race	White > African American	Equal (APML more common in Hispanic population)
Gender	Male > female	Equal
Genetics	Trisomy 21, Bloom syndrome, Fanconi anemia, ataxia telangiectasia, Shwachman's syndrome, neurofibromatosis, twins, siblings at increased risk	Trisomy 21 (AML much more likely <3 yr), Bloom syndrome, Fanconi anemia, ataxia telangiectasia, Kostmann's syndrome, NF-1, Diamond-Blackfan's syndrome, Li-Fraumeni's syndrome
Noninherited		Aplastic anemia, Myelodysplastic's syndromes (MDS), PNH
Pathogenesis		
• Environment	Ionizing radiation	Ionizing radiation, benzene, epipodophyllotoxins, alkylating agents (nitrogen mustard, melphalan, cyclophosphamide)
• Viral	Epstein-Barr virus and L3 ALL	None
• Immunodeficiency	Wiskott-Aldrich, congenital hypogammaglobulinemia, ataxia telangiectasia	

APML, acute promyelocytic leukemia; MDS, myelodysplastic syndrome ; PNH, paroxysmal nocturnal hemoglobinuria.
Frank G, Shah SS, Catallozzi M, et al., eds. The Philadelphia guide: inpatient pediatrics. Malden, Mass Blackwell; 2005:303.

Shwachman-Diamond's syndrome (exocrine pancreatic insufficiency and neutropenia) and Diamond-Blackfan's syndrome (congenital red cell aplasia), have an increased risk of developing AML.

CLINICAL MANIFESTATIONS

History and Physical Examination

Symptoms usually develop days to weeks before diagnosis. Nonspecific constitutional symptoms include lethargy, malaise, and anorexia. Children may complain about bone pain or arthralgias caused by leukemic expansion of the marrow cavity. Progressive bone marrow failure may lead to pallor from anemia and ecchymoses or petechiae from thrombocytopenia. The anemia is normochromic and normocytic. Decreased marrow production of RBCs leads to a low reticulocyte count. The WBC count is low (<5,000 per mm^3) in a third of patients, normal (5,000 to 20,000 per mm^3) in a third of patients, and high (>20,000 per mm^3) in a third of patients. Many children have hepatosplenomegaly and cervical lymphadenopathy at diagnosis. Extramedullary involvement is also seen in the CNS, skin, and testicles. CNS infiltration causes neurologic signs and symptoms, such as headache, emesis, papilledema, and sixth cranial nerve palsy. Patients with AML may develop a soft-tissue tumor called a **chloroma** in the spinal cord or on the skin. Table 17-3 shows compares the presentation of ALL and AML.

▦ **TABLE 17-3** Comparison of the Clinical Presentation of Acute Lymphocytic Leukemia and Acute Myelogenous Leukemia		
Characteristic	**ALL**	**AML**
Marrow failure:		
• Anemia (g/dL)	Hb < 7 (43%)	Hb < 9 (50%)
• Thrombocytopenia (per mm^3)	Hb 7–11 (45%)	Plt < 100,000 (75%)
	Hb > 11 (12%)	WBC > 100,000 (20%)
• Neutropenia (per mm^3)	Plt < 20,000 (20%)	
	Plt 21,000–99,000 (47%)	
	Plt > 100,000 (25%)	
	WBC < 10,000 (53%)	
	WBC 10,000–49,000 (30%)	
	WBC > 50,000 (17%)	
Fever	60%	30%–40%
Mediastinal mass	10% (mostly in T cell)	
CNS involvement	5%	2%
Chloromas		Common in M4, M5 subtype
		Common in periorbital area
Testicular involvement	2%–5%	Rare
Disseminated intravascular coagulation		Common (esp. in APML)
Bone pain	20%	20%
Hepatosplenomegaly	60%–65%	50%
Other		Leukemia cutis (10%)
		• Neonates
		• Blueberry muffin spots
		Gingival hypertrophy (15%)

APML, acute promyelocytic leukemia.
Frank G, Shah SS, Catallozzi M, et al., eds. The Philadelphia guide: inpatient pediatrics. *Malden, Mass: Blackwell; 2005:304.*

DIFFERENTIAL DIAGNOSIS

The differential diagnosis includes aplastic anemia, idiopathic thrombocytopenic purpura, Epstein-Barr virus infection, other malignancies, rheumatologic diseases such as lupus or juvenile rheumatoid arthritis, and viral-induced or familial hemophagocytic syndrome.

DIAGNOSTIC EVALUATION

A CBC with manual differential and review of the blood smear to look for blast cells should be obtained on any child with suspected leukemia. Bone marrow biopsy is critical, even if there are blasts in the peripheral blood, because the morphology of the peripheral blasts may not reflect the true bone marrow morphology. Biopsy material is sent for morphology, immunophenotype, and cytogenetics. A comprehensive metabolic panel, LDH, uric acid, calcium, magnesium, and phosphorus are obtained to define baseline values prior to chemotherapy and possible tumor lysis syndrome. Coagulation studies are sent to exclude DIC. Blood, urine, and viral cultures are obtained if infection is suspected. A chest radiograph is sent to evaluate for mediastinal mass. If mediastinal mass is suspected, an echocardiogram is needed. No sedation should be used in the patient with mediastinal mass until an echocardiogram is performed and an anesthesia consultation is acquired. A LP is performed to evaluate for CNS disease. If the patient has thrombocytopenia or coagulation abnormalities, the LP may not be advisable.

TREATMENT

The treatment strategy for both ALL and AML is to stabilize the patient at diagnosis, put the leukemia in remission, and manage the complications of therapy. Managing leukemic complications at presentation involves blood product transfusions, empirical treatment of potential infection, prevention of the sequelae of hyperviscosity, and metabolic abnormalities and renal insufficiency from tumor lysis syndrome. Neutropenia, defined as an absolute neutrophil count less than 500 per mm^3, predisposes children to serious bacterial and fungal infection. The development of fever in a child with neutropenia warrants careful evaluation for bacteremia or sepsis.

Acute Lymphocytic Leukemia Therapy

Patients with ALL have a high risk of **tumor lysis syndrome**, a triad of metabolic abnormalities (hyperuricemia, hyperphosphatemia, and hyperkalemia) resulting from spontaneous or treatment-induced tumor cell death, with rapid release of intracellular contents into the circulation that exceeds the excretory capacity of the kidneys. Tumor lysis' syndrome is generally seen in tumors with high growth rates such as T-cell ALL or Burkitt lymphoma, and patients with mediastinal mass or high WBC count. Tumor lysis syndrome is rarely seen in solid tumors. Rapid release of intracellular contents leads hyperphosphatemia, hyperkalemia, and hyperuricemia. Hyperkalemia can cause cardiac arrhythmias. Phosphate, especially at high serum levels, binds to calcium, resulting in precipitation of calcium phosphate in renal tubules, hypocalcemia, and tetany. Purines are processed to uric acid. Hyperuricemia can result in precipitation of uric acid in renal tubules and renal failure. Prevention and management of tumor lysis syndrome includes vigorous hydration, urine alkalinization, uric acid reduction with allopurinol, and potassium and phosphate reduction. The risk for tumor lysis is greatest during the first 3 days of chemotherapy.

Hyperleukocytosis (WBC count >200,000 per mm^3) occurs in 9% to 13% of patients with ALL. Hyperleukocytosis can cause significant vascular stasis. This is often seen in patients with ALL whose WBC count is greater than 300,000 per mm^3. Symptoms include mental status changes, headache, blurry vision, dizziness, seizure, and dyspnea. Without therapy, hyperleukocytosis may cause hypoxemia and secondary acidosis or stroke from sludging in the lungs and CNS, respectively. The WBC count may be lowered using hyperhydration or leukophoresis. It is recommended to keep the hemoglobin concentration at approximately 10 g per dL to minimize viscosity and to maintain a platelet count more than 20,000 to minimize the risk of hemorrhage.

Large collections of malignant cells in the mediastinum, common in T-cell leukemia, compress vital structures, causing tracheal compression or superior vena cava syndrome. Superior vena cava syndrome is characterized by distended neck veins; swelling of the face, neck, and upper limbs; cyanosis; and conjunctival injection. The mass and the compressive symptoms it creates usually resolve with chemotherapy and radiation.

The ALL treatment regimen includes induction, consolidation, interim maintenance, and maintenance therapies. At diagnosis children with ALL undergo **induction therapy**, during which maximum log kill is achieved. If remission is achieved, all blasts disappear from the bone marrow, and the CBC values return to normal. Induction therapy occurs over 28 days with vincristine, steroids, intrathecal methotrexate, and asparaginase. For high-risk patients, daunomycin is added. The disease response is generally re-evaluated every 7 to 14 days. Failure to achieve adequate response requires intensification of therapy. More than 95% of patients with ALL achieve remission after induction therapy. The goals of **consolidation** are to kill additional leukemic cells with further systemic therapy and to prevent leukemic relapse within the CNS by giving intrathecal methotrexate. The objectives of maintenance therapies are to continue the remission achieved in the previous phases and to provide additional cytoreduction to cure the leukemia. **Interim maintenance**, which follows induction and consolidation, is less intense and includes vincristine, 6-mercaptopurine, and methotrexate. **Maintenance** therapy completes the therapeutic course and includes intrathecal methotrexate every 3 months, monthly vincristine and steroid therapy, weekly oral methotrexate, and daily oral 6-mercaptopurine. Leukemia can recur while the child is on therapy, or after the completion of maintenance therapy. The earlier the relapse the worse the prognosis, although isolated extramedullary (CNS, testes) relapses have better outcomes than bone marrow relapses. Radiation is utilized for CNS and testicular disease. Discontinuation of chemotherapy occurs when the patient has remained in remission throughout the prescribed course of maintenance therapy. The total length of therapy is approximately 2 years for females and 3 years for males.

Factors associated with poor prognosis in patients with ALL include age greater than 10 years or less than 1 year at diagnosis, WBC count greater than 50,000 per mm^3 at diagnosis, and failure to respond to induction therapy. In addition, hypodiploidy and certain translocations noted in the leukemic cells put patients at higher risk.

Acute Myelogenous Leukemia Therapy

Hyperleukocytosis occurs in 5% to 22% of patients with AML. The most common symptoms for patients with AML-induced hyperleukocytosis include dyspnea and hypoxemia, from pulmonary leukostasis, and mental status change or seizure, from stroke. Patients may require hyperhydration or leukophoresis similar to ALL. In contrast to ALL, patients with AML and hyperleukocytosis are treated at a lower WBC count (200,000 per mm^3) because AML cells are larger and stickier than the lymphocytes found in ALL. Similar to ALL treatment, a hemoglobin concentration of 10 g per dL is recommended to reduce

viscosity and a platelet count of more than 20,000 is advisable to minimize the risk of CNS hemorrhage.

AML chemotherapy is more intensive than that used for ALL. Induction therapy includes an anthracycline with Ara-C. Although 70% to 85% of patients with AML achieve remission with induction therapy, many patients relapse within a year. Myelosuppression is severe, and good supportive care is essential. If remission can be achieved for at least 3 months, matched sibling bone marrow transplant is recommended, although only 40% have a matched related donor. If no donor is available, patients continue on a standard chemotherapeutic regimen.

Acute promyelocytic leukemia (APML), M3 subtype, has a higher overall survival rate (80%) than the other AML subtypes. Similarly, patients with AML and trisomy 21 also have an excellent overall survival. Factors associated with a poor prognosis in AML include a WBC count greater than 100,000 at diagnosis, secondary AML/myelodysplastic syndrome, M4 and M5 subtype, and monosomy 7.

🔨 17-1 KEY POINTS

1. The leukemias account for the greatest percentage of cases of childhood malignancies.
2. Leukemias are classified on the basis of leukemic cell morphology into lymphoblastic leukemias, which are proliferations of cells of lymphoid lineage, and nonlymphocytic or myelogenous leukemias, which are proliferations of cells of granulocyte, monocyte, erythrocyte, or platelet lineage.
3. Acute leukemias constitute 97% of all childhood leukemias and are subdivided into acute lymphoblastic leukemia (ALL) and acute myelogenous leukemia (AML).
4. ALL is the most common pediatric neoplasm and accounts for 85% of all cases of childhood acute leukemia.

NON-HODGKIN LYMPHOMA

PATHOGENESIS

Non-Hodgkin lymphomas (NHLs) are a heterogeneous group of diseases characterized by neoplastic proliferation of immature lymphoid cells, which, unlike the malignant lymphoid cells of ALL, accumulate outside the bone marrow. NHLs can be divided into T- and B-cell categories. Histopathologic subtypes in childhood NHL include lymphoblastic (pre-T or pre-B cell), Burkitt lymphoma or large B cell lymphoma (B cell), and anaplastic large cell lymphoma (T or null cell). Other peripheral T-cell lymphomas are under the category of NHL but very uncommon in children. Burkitt lymphoma is interesting in that the presentation and pathogenesis in equatorial Africa is different than in developed countries because it almost uniformly presents as a rapidly expanding jaw lesion and 95% of these tumors carry EBV genomes in their cells, whereas 15% to 20% of North American tumors are associated with EBV.

EPIDEMIOLOGY

Lymphomas are the third most common malignancy in childhood and account for 10% of childhood cancer. There is a distinct geographic frequency of NHL, and in equatorial Africa, NHL accounts for 50% of childhood cancer. Approximately 60% of pediatric lymphomas are non-Hodgkin lymphomas; the remainder is Hodgkin lymphoma. Lymphoblastic lymphoma accounts for 50% of cases, and Burkitt and anaplastic large cell lymphomas account for approximately 35% and 15%, respectively. NHL occurs at least three times more frequently in boys than in girls and has a peak incidence between 7 and 11 years of age.

RISK FACTORS

Children with congenital immunodeficiency (e.g., Wiskott-Aldrich's syndrome, X-linked lymphoproliferative disease, severe combined immunodeficiency) and acquired immunodeficiency (e.g., AIDS, iatrogenic immunosuppression in organ and bone marrow transplant recipients) have an increased incidence of NHL. Patients with Bloom syndrome and ataxia-telangiectasia also have a higher incidence of NHL than the general pediatric population.

CLINICAL MANIFESTATIONS

T-cell lymphoblastic lymphoma is most often associated with a mediastinal mass (50% to 70%), whereas B-cell lymphoblastic lymphoma often involves bone, isolated lymph nodes, and skin. Superior vena cava syndrome may be associated with the T-cell type secondary to mediastinal mass. Burkitt lymphoma often exhibits rapid growth and can be associated with tumor lysis syndrome after chemotherapy is started. The sporadic form of Burkitt lymphoma can present as an abdominal tumor associated with nausea, emesis, or intussusception. Other Burkitt locations may include tonsils, bone marrow (20%), and the CNS. The endemic form of Burkitt lymphoma involves the jaw, orbit, and/or maxilla. Anaplastic large cell lymphoma is a slowly progressive disease with fever, and weight loss involvement is rare.

DIAGNOSTIC EVALUATION

The evaluation before therapy should include a CBC to look for leukocytosis, thrombocytopenia, and anemia. A comprehensive metabolic panel includes calcium, phosphorus uric acid, and LDH to evaluate for tumor lysis syndrome. Chest radiograph should be performed to assess for mediastinal mass prior to sedation and biopsy of accessible affected nodes. An echocardiogram and anesthesia consultation is required prior to sedation in the patient with a mediastinal mass. A bone marrow aspiration and biopsy with flow cytometry, cell markers/immunophenotyping, and cytogenetics should be performed to isolate the type of lymphoma. An LP with cytology is performed to evaluate for CNS involvement. CT scan of neck, chest, abdomen, and pelvis help assess the extent of disease, and gallium or PET scan is useful for diagnostic purposes and follow-up for residual disease or recurrence.

TREATMENT

Similar to ALL therapy, lymphoblastic non-Hodgkin lymphoma is generally treated with combination chemotherapy. ALL and lymphoblastic non-Hodgkin lymphoma therapy are immuno-phenotypically similar but with a different distribution of disease (nodal vs. marrow).

Chemotherapy is the mainstay of treatment for Burkitt lymphoma unless the tumor is localized and complete surgical resection is possible. Therapy is quite intense and given over a short period of time (4 to 6 months) using drugs including cyclophosphamide, prednisone, vincristine, methotrexate, cytarabine, doxorubicin, and etoposide. Patients with CNS involvement are known to have a poorer prognosis. Patients with tumor lysis syndrome require extremely careful management with increased fluid intake, alkalinization of the urine, frequent electrolyte observation, and allopurinol.

Anaplastic large cell lymphoma is treated with combination chemotherapy. Children are most commonly treated on B-cell lymphoma protocols.

HODGKIN LYMPHOMA

PATHOGENESIS

The cause of **Hodgkin's disease (HD)** is unknown, and a number of studies investigating potential etiologies have shown that age, ethnicity, socioeconomic status, and geographic distribution of HD suggest both environmental and genetic components and a multifactorial etiology. There is increased risk in siblings, twins, and an association with EBV, although the EBV genome is not universally found in tumor tissue. Additionally, there is an increased risk of HD in patients with ataxia-telangiectasia, Wiskott-Aldrich, and Bloom syndromes. Histopathologic subtypes in childhood Hodgkin's disease include nodular sclerosing (40% to 55%), lymphocyte predominant (10% to 15%), mixed cellularity (30%), and lymphocyte depleted (5%).

EPIDEMIOLOGY

Hodgkin's disease accounts for 5% of all cases of childhood cancer prior to 15 years of age and 9% prior to 20 years of age. Epidemiologic studies have identified three distinct forms of Hodgkin's disease: a childhood form (younger than 14 years); a young adult form (15 to 34 years of age); and an older adult form (55 to 74 years of age). Its incidence has a bimodal distribution with peaks occurring at 15 to 30 years of age and after the age of 50. It rarely occurs in children younger than 10 years. There is a 3:1 male predominance in the childhood form of Hodgkin's disease.

CLINICAL MANIFESTATIONS

History and Physical Examination

The most common presentation is painless, rubbery, cervical lymphadenopathy in 80% of patients. Two thirds of patients also have mediastinal lymphadenopathy, and this presentation is more common in adolescent patients. Systemic symptoms ("B" symptoms) are present in 20% to 30% of patients and include unexplained fever, drenching night sweats, and unintentional weight loss of more than 10% over the preceding 6 months. Other common presenting symptoms include anorexia, fatigue, and extreme pruritus.

DIFFERENTIAL DIAGNOSIS

The differential diagnosis for HD includes other diseases that can result in lymphadenopathy with or without systemic symptoms. Reactive or inflammatory nodes as a result of bacterial lymphadenitis, infectious mononucleosis, tuberculosis, atypical mycobacterial infection, cat-scratch disease, HIV, histoplasmosis, and toxoplasmosis should be considered. Other primary or metastatic malignant processes resulting in cervical adenopathy or a mediastinal mass include leukemia, non-Hodgkin lymphoma, head/neck rhabdomyosarcoma, and germ cell tumors.

DIAGNOSTIC EVALUATION

Evaluation for HD should include a detailed history and physical exam with attention to the signs and symptoms that require a more urgent evaluation including cough, dyspnea, orthopnea, chest pain, bleeding, bruising, jaundice, or pallor. The physical examination should include a careful evaluation of all lymph node groups including the tonsils. Lymphadenopathy in the upper anterior and posterior cervical chains tends to be more commonly associated with childhood infections, whereas nodes in the supraclavicular area are consistent with malignancy. Enlargement of the liver or spleen is consistent with more advanced disease.

Evaluating a child for HD necessitates imaging and should begin with chest radiograph prior to any biopsy or procedure to determine whether or not there is clinically significant mediastinal involvement. The presence and size of a mediastinal mass and whether there is airway compromise or cardiac compression influences the way in which the biopsy is performed and the type of anesthesia required. Patients with a mediastinal mass should have pulmonary function testing and an echocardiogram before undergoing general anesthesia. Node biopsy is required to make the diagnosis, preferably excisional lymph node biopsy. The hallmark of diagnosis is the identification of Reed-Sternberg cells in tumor tissue.

Recommended basic tests include a CBC, ESR, chemistry panel including LFTs, direct antibody testing (DAT) if there is evidence of jaundice or anemia and ferritin. Eosinophilia is seen in 15% to 30% of patients, and anemia is seen either secondary to advanced disease or hemolysis. Global immune defects are common at diagnosis of HD, and anergy is seen in 25% of patients. This immune dysregulation seen at diagnosis predispose patients to opportunistic infections during their treatment. Imaging studies include a CT scan of the neck, chest, abdomen, and pelvis. The gallium scan is quite useful and has a role in diagnosis and in following for residual or recurrent disease. Positron emission tomography (PET) is becoming standard for adult patients and may soon be incorporated into pediatric care. Although uncommon, evidence of cytopenias should prompt bone marrow aspirate and biopsy, which is routinely performed in patients with extensive disease and "B" symptoms. Bone scan is only recommended for patients with bone pain.

■ TABLE 17-4 Staging for Hodgkin lymphoma	
Stage	**Definition**
I	Involvement of single lymph node region or single extralymphatic site
II	Involvement of two or more lymph node regions on the same side of diaphragm or localized involvement of an extralymphatic site and one or more lymph node regions on the same side of the diaphragm
III	Involvement of lymph node regions on both sides of the diaphragm with involvement of the spleen or localized involvement of an extralymphatic site
IV	Disseminated involvement of one or more extralymphatic organs with or without lymph node involvement
"B" symptoms:	Fever higher than 38 degrees for 3 consecutive days
	Drenching night sweats
	Unexplained weight loss >10% during the prior 6 mo
	Those without "B" symptoms have stage [number] A disease.

TREATMENT

Treatment depends on the histologic subtype of disease, staging, and response to therapy (Table 17-4).

Most pediatric protocols involve multiagent chemotherapy given in a risk-adapted and response-based manner. Involved field radiation therapy is used for patients with bulky mediastinal disease with residual tumor after initial chemotherapy. Vincristine, prednisone, cyclophosphamide, and procarbazine were used commonly in the past, although newer chemotherapy combinations are being used in patients with low- or intermediate-risk disease, given the certain infertility for males with the use of cyclophosphamide and procarbazine together. Prognosis varies from 70% to 90% depending on the extent of disease and response to therapy. As in adults, lymphocyte predominance has the most favorable prognosis. There are many late effects secondary to therapy including second malignant neoplasms (breast, thyroid, sarcomas); cardiac toxicity (anthracyclines and XRT); pulmonary (bleomycin); hypothyroidism (XRT); infertility (alkylating agents as above, pelvic radiation); and musculoskeletal/growth (XRT).

🔑 17-3 KEY POINTS

1. The incidence of Hodgkin's disease has a bimodal distribution with peaks occurring at 15 to 30 years of age and after 50 years of age.
2. Hodgkin lymphoma must be considered in an otherwise healthy adolescent with persistent cervical lymphadenopathy.
3. A diminished cellular immunity seen in patients at diagnosis can result in opportunistic infections in these patients.
4. The overall prognosis for HD is 70% to 90%, and this is one of the few diseases where treatment is being tailored to decrease the risk of late effects of therapy, given the large number of survivors.

CENTRAL NERVOUS SYSTEM TUMORS

CNS tumors are the most common solid tumors in children and are second to leukemia in overall incidence of malignant diseases. In contrast to adults, in whom supratentorial brain tumors are more common, brain tumors in children are predominantly infratentorial, involving the cerebellum and brainstem. Table 17-5 denotes the location, clinical manifestations, and prognosis of CNS tumors in children. Childhood brain tumors are differentiated further from those in adults in that they are usually low-grade astrocytomas or malignant neoplasms such as medulloblastomas,

■ **TABLE 17-5** Location and Manifestations of Primary CNS Tumors

Tumor	Age at Onset (yr)	Manifestations[a]	5-Year Survival (%)	Comments
Infratentorial				
Cerebellar astrocytoma	5–8	Ataxia; nystagmus; head tilt; intention tremor	90	20% of all primary CNS tumors
Medulloblastoma	3–5	Obstructive hydrocephalus; ataxia, CSF metastasis	50	Acute onset of symptoms; 20% of all primary CNS tumors
Ependymoma	2–6	Obstructive hydrocephalus; rarely seeds spinal fluid	50	25%–40% supratentorial
Brainstem glioma (intrinsic pontine glioma)	5–8	Progressive cranial nerve dysfunction; gait disturbance; pyramidal tract and cerebellar signs	<10	Worst prognosis of all childhood CNS tumors
Supratentorial				
Cerebral astrocytoma	5–10	Seizures; headache; motor weakness; personality changes	10–50	Survival for high-grade glioma is poor
Craniopharyngioma	7–12	Bitemporal hemianopsia; endocrine abnormalities postoperative diabetes insipidus common	70–90	Calcification above sella turcica; postoperative diabetes insipidus common
Optic glioma	<2	Poor visual acuity; exophthalmos; nystagmus; optic atrophy; strabismus	50–90	Neurofibromatosis in NF-1 in 70% of patients
Germ cell tumor (pineal or pituitary)	—	Paralysis of upward gaze (Parinaud's syndrome); lid retraction (Collier sign); precocious puberty; may seed spinal fluid	75	Germ cell line: may secrete BhCG or α-fetoprotein

[a]All CNS tumors may cause increased intracranial pressure.
hCG, human chorionic gonadotropin.

whereas most CNS tumors in adults are malignant astrocytomas or metastases from non-CNS cancers.

CLINICAL MANIFESTATIONS

The presenting signs and symptoms of CNS tumors depend on the age of the child and location of the tumor (Table 17-5). Any CNS tumor may cause increased intracranial pressure (ICP) by obstructing CSF flow. Symptoms of increased ICP include early morning headaches, vomiting, and lethargy. The headache is usually present upon awakening, improves with standing, and worsens with coughing or straining. It is intermittent but recurs with increasing frequency and intensity. Obstructive hydrocephalus may produce macrocephaly if it occurs before the sutures have fused. Strabismus with diplopia can result from a sixth nerve palsy induced by ICP. Papilledema may be detected on funduscopic examination. The Cushing triad (hypertension, bradycardia, and irregular respirations) is a late finding.

Children with **infratentorial tumors** often present with deficits of balance or brainstem function (truncal ataxia, problems with coordination and gait, cranial nerve dysfunction). Because it can result from increased ICP, a sixth nerve palsy is not considered a localizing focal neurologic deficit, whereas other cranial nerve deficits, by definition, localize the lesion to the brainstem. Head tilt, as a compensation for loss of binocular vision, is noted with focal deficits of cranial nerve III, IV, or VI, which cause extraocular muscle weakness. Nystagmus is usually caused by cerebellovestibular pathway lesions, but it may also be seen with a marked visual deficit (peripheral or cortical blindness).

Children with **supratentorial tumors** commonly present either with signs of increased ICP (discussed earlier) or seizures. Although most seizures are generalized, less dramatic episodes with incomplete loss of consciousness (complex partial seizures) and transient focal events without loss of consciousness (partial seizures) are also seen. Personality changes, poor school performance, and change in hand preference suggest a cortical lesion. Endocrine abnormalities are noted with pituitary and hypothalamic tumors. Babinski reflex, hyperreflexia, spasticity, and loss of dexterity occur with either brainstem or cortical tumors.

DIFFERENTIAL DIAGNOSIS

The differential diagnosis includes arteriovenous malformation, aneurysm, brain abscess, parasitic infestation, herpes simplex encephalitis, granulomatous disease (tuberculosis, cryptococcal, sarcoid), intracranial hemorrhage, pseudotumor cerebri, primary cerebral lymphoma, vasculitis, and, rarely, metastatic tumors.

DIAGNOSTIC EVALUATION

CT and MRI are the procedures of choice for diagnosing and localizing tumors and other intracranial masses. A head CT can be performed much faster than a head MRI, and in the case of the unstable patient is safer. CT is useful as an initial screen, and to assess for hydrocephalus, hemorrhage, or calcification. MRI is the gold standard for localization of brain tumors to assist with surgical planning. Brain MRI is especially helpful in diagnosing tumors of the posterior fossa and spinal cord. Examination of CSF cytology is essential to determine the presence of metastasis in medulloblastoma and germ cell tumors.

TREATMENT

Table 17-6 outlines the general principles of treatment of primary CNS tumors.

🔑 17-4 KEY POINTS

1. CNS tumors are the most common solid tumors in children and second to leukemia in overall incidence of malignant diseases.
2. In contrast to brain tumors in adults, in whom supratentorial tumors are more common, brain tumors in children are predominantly infratentorial (posterior fossa), involving the cerebellum, midbrain, and brainstem.

NEUROBLASTOMA

PATHOGENESIS

Neuroblastoma is a childhood embryonal malignancy of the postganglionic sympathetic nervous system. Neuroblastoma can be located in the abdomen, thoracic cavity, or head and neck. Abdominal tumors account for 70% of tumors, a third of which arise from the retroperitoneal sympathetic ganglia and two thirds from the adrenal medulla itself. Thoracic masses, accounting for 20% of the tumors, tend to arise from paraspinal ganglia in the posterior mediastinum. Neuroblastoma of the neck occurs in 5% of cases and often involves the cervical sympathetic ganglion.

■ TABLE 17-6 Approach to Treatment of Childhood CNS Tumors

Treatment	Goals
Surgery	Establish diagnosis
	Debulk and/or resect tumor
	Treat increased ICP (ventricular shunt, if required)
Radiation	Control residual disease
	Control tumor dissemination
	Cure
Chemotherapy	Adjuvant therapy for malignant tumors
	Minimize radiation exposure
	Delay and/or obviate need for radiation
New approaches	Immunotherapy to scavenge for minimal residual disease
	Antiangiogenic therapy to suppress abnormal tumor blood vessel development
	Molecularly targeted therapy to suppress abnormal growth factor pathways

ICP, intracranial pressure.

EPIDEMIOLOGY

Neuroblastoma accounts for 6% of all childhood cancers, and, in children, it is the most common solid tumor outside the CNS and the most common malignancy of infancy. The median age at diagnosis is 19 months; more than 50% of children are diagnosed before 2 years of age, 90% are diagnosed before 5 years of age, and 97% are diagnosed by 10 years of age. There is a slight male predominance. Neuroblastoma accounts for 15% of the pediatric cancer-related deaths each year.

RISK FACTORS

The prevalence is approximately 1 case per 7,000 live births, and there are approximately 600 new cases of neuroblastoma per year. The etiology is unknown in most cases, and no causal environmental factor has been isolated. No prenatal or postnatal exposure to drugs, chemicals, viruses, electromagnetic fields, or radiation has been associated strongly or consistently with an increased incidence of neuroblastoma. A family history of the disease can be found in 1% to 2% of cases. Neuroblastoma has been reported in patients with Hirschsprung disease, congenital central hypoventilation syndrome (Ondine curse), pheochromocytoma, and/or neurofibromatosis type 1, suggesting the existence of a global disorder of neural-crest derived cells.

CLINICAL MANIFESTATIONS

The clinical manifestations are extremely variable because of the widespread distribution of neural crest tissue and the length of the sympathetic chain.

History and Physical Examination

Abdominal tumors are hard, smooth, nontender abdominal masses that are most often palpated in the flank and displace the kidney anterolaterally and inferiorly. Abdominal pain and systemic hypertension occur if the mass compresses the renal vasculature. Respiratory distress is the primary symptom seen in thoracic neuroblastoma tumors. Sometimes the thoracic variant is asymptomatic, and the tumor is discovered as an incidental finding on chest radiograph obtained for an unrelated reason. Neuroblastoma of the neck presents as a palpable tumor causing Horner syndrome (ipsilateral ptosis, miosis, and anhidrosis) and heterochromia of the iris on the affected side. Sometimes thoracic or abdominal tumors invade the epidural space posteriorly in a dumbbell fashion, compromising the spinal cord and resulting in back pain and symptoms of cord compression.

The signs and symptoms vary according to location of primary disease and degree of dissemination. Metastatic extension occurs in lymphatic and hematogenous patterns. Nonspecific symptoms of metastatic disease include weight loss and fever. Specific metastatic sequelae include bone marrow failure, resulting in pancytopenia; cortical bone pain, causing a limp (Hutchinson's syndrome); liver infiltration, resulting in hepatomegaly (Pepper syndrome); periorbital infiltration, resulting in proptosis and periorbital ecchymoses ("raccoon eyes"); distant lymph node enlargement; and skin infiltration, causing palpable nontender subcutaneous bluish nodules in infants with International Neuroblastoma Staging System (INSS) stage IVS tumors. Paraneoplastic effects, such as watery diarrhea in patients with differentiated tumors that secrete vasoactive intestinal peptide and opsoclonus-myoclonus (chaotic eye movements, myoclonic jerking, and truncal ataxia), have been noted.

DIFFERENTIAL DIAGNOSIS

The differential diagnosis of abdominal neuroblastoma includes benign lesions such as hydronephrosis, polycystic kidney disease, and splenomegaly and malignant tumors such as renal cell carcinoma, Ewing sarcoma, Wilms tumor, hepatoblastoma, lymphoma, retroperitoneal rhabdomyosarcoma, and ovarian tumors.

DIAGNOSTIC EVALUATION

The presence of a mass can be confirmed by CT of chest, abdomen, and pelvis. Diagnosis of neuroblastoma can be made by pathologic identification of tumor tissue or by the unequivocal presence of tumor cells on bone marrow aspirate combined with elevated urinary catecholamines (VMA and homovanillic acid). Tissue biopsy for histology, DNA ploidy, and MYCN analysis is helpful with prognosis. Measurement of urinary catecholamines, which are breakdown products of epinephrine and norepinephrine, is also useful for following response to therapy and for detecting recurrence. For tumors arising from the adrenal medulla, intravenous pyelogram shows displacement of the kidney with minimal distortion of the calyceal system. Conversely, Wilms tumor generally results in distortion of the calyceal system. Enhanced sensitivity and specificity for detecting bone metastases and occult soft-tissue masses can be afforded by metaiodobenzyl-guanidine (MIBG) scintigraphy.

TREATMENT

Treatment involves surgery and chemotherapy because 50% of patients have distant metastases at diagnosis. After surgical resection of the primary tumor and any lymph nodes or selected metastases, surgical and radiologic data are gathered to stage the tumor based on the **International Neuroblastoma Staging System (INSS)**. See Table 17-7.

Several biological variables have prognostic values and are used in addition to INSS staging for patients with neuroblastoma. These include age at diagnosis, stage as per INSS criteria, Shimada histopathology, DNA index of the tumor, and MYCN gene amplification.

Treatment modalities traditionally employed in the management of neuroblastoma include surgery, chemotherapy, and radiotherapy. Depending on stage

■ **TABLE 17-7 Staging for Neuroblastoma. International Neuroblatoma Staging System (INSS)**

Stage	Definition
I	Localized tumor with complete gross excision
II	Localized tumor with incomplete gross excision; ipsilateral lymph node sampling (LNS) negative for tumor (IIA), or ipsilateral nodes positive for tumor (IIB)
III	Tumor extends beyond the midline, with or without regional lymph node involvement, or localized unilateral tumor with contralateral regional lymph node involvement
IV	Dissemination of tumor to distant lymph nodes, bone, bone marrow, liver, and/or other organs (except as defined in stage IVS)
IVS	Age younger than 1 year with dissemination of tumor to liver, skin, or bone marrow without bone involvement and with a primary tumor that would otherwise be stage I or II

and biological features, treatment can range from observation or surgery alone to multimodal therapy with chemotherapy, stem cell transplantation, radiation, and biotherapy.

Postsurgical radiation is used to treat residual local disease and selected metastatic foci, whereas chemotherapy varies in duration and intensity depending on the stage and biologic features. Regimens usually include vincristine, cyclophosphamide, doxorubicin (Adriamycin), and cisplatin. Spontaneous regression is common in stage IVS tumors. In stage IVS, surgical removal of the small primary tumor is indicated to prevent late local recurrence. Bone marrow transplantation is often the best therapy for extensive stage III and IV disease.

Infants younger than 1 year have the best prognosis. Stages I, II, and IVS have a good prognosis, whereas stages III and IV have a poor prognosis. Serum markers associated with a poor prognosis include elevated neuron-specific enolase, ferritin, and lactic dehydrogenase. Certain genetic features, such as N-myc oncogene amplification within the tumor cells, are associated with a poor prognosis. Respective 5-year survival rate for low-, intermediate-, and high-risk groups are as follows: low-risk disease (stages 1 and II): 90% to 95% event-free survival; intermediate-risk disease (stage III, MYCN single-copy): 85% to 90% event-free survival; high-risk disease (stage IV): 35% event-free survival.

WILMS TUMOR

PATHOGENESIS

Wilms tumor results from neoplastic embryonal renal cells of the metanephros. The most often cited genetic anomaly in Wilms tumor is partial deletion of chromosome 11p13.

EPIDEMIOLOGY

This tumor accounts for 6.6% of all childhood cancers. It is predominantly found in the first 5 years of life (mean 3 years of age) and has equal occurrence in both boys and girls.

RISK FACTORS

Associated anomalies include sporadic aniridia, hemihypertrophy, cryptorchidism, hypospadias, and other genitourinary anomalies. Associated syndromes include Beckwith-Wiedemann (hemihypertrophy, macroglossia, omphalocele, and genitourinary abnormalities); Denys Drash; Wilms tumor, aniridia, genitourinary abnormalities, and mental retardation (WAGR) and PERLMAN (unusual facies, islet cell hypertrophy, macrosomia, hamartomas).

CLINICAL MANIFESTATIONS

History and Physical Examination

Most children (85%) are diagnosed after incidental detection of an asymptomatic abdominal mass by the child's parents while bathing or dressing the child or by the pediatrician during a routine physical examination. Abdominal pain or fever may develop after hemorrhage into the tumor. Other associated findings include microscopic or gross hematuria (33%) and hypertension (25%). Hypertension occurs as a result of either renin secretion by tumor cells or compression of the renal vasculature by the tumor. Additionally, varicocele can be present on physical examination if there is spermatic vein cord compression of the tumor. Von Willebrand disease is present in 8% of patients. It is important to evaluate the patient for the associated anomalies and syndromes associated with Wilms tumor.

DIFFERENTIAL DIAGNOSIS

The differential diagnosis of Wilms tumor includes benign lesions such as hydronephrosis, polycystic kidney disease, and splenomegaly, as well as malignant tumors such as renal cell carcinoma, neuroblastoma, lymphoma, retroperitoneal rhabdomyosarcoma, and ovarian tumors.

DIAGNOSTIC EVALUATION

Screening tests include a CBC with differential, LFTs, electrolytes, BUN, creatinine, and UA. Radiologic studies include abdominal US to establish the presence of an intrarenal mass, assess the renal vasculature, and examine the contralateral kidney. An abdominal CT scan assesses the degree of local extension and involvement of the inferior vena cava. CT scan of the abdomen is routinely performed to detect hematogenous metastases, which are present at diagnosis in 10% to 15% of patients. The most common patterns of spread include the renal capsule, extension through adjacent vessels (inferior vena cava), regional nodes, lung, and liver. The lung is the most common site of metastatic spread. Chest radiograph continues to be the radiographic standard for evaluation of pulmonary metastases, although the use of chest CT is controversial. Bone scan and MRI of the head are only indicated for clear cell sarcoma or rhabdoid tumor of the kidney. These are not Wilms tumor variants.

TREATMENT

Treatment may involve surgery, chemotherapy, or radiation. Surgical therapy involves thorough abdominal exploration including the contralateral kidney to provide accurate assessment of tumor spread for staging. Removal of the primary tumor without spill/rupture through an anterior approach may then be performed. If the whole tumor is not safely resectable (massive size or intravascular invasion), a biopsy only should be performed. Table 17-8 notes chemotherapeutic and radiation guidelines.

If tumor histology demonstrates anaplasia, clear cell sarcoma of the kidney, or rhabdoid tumor, the treatment can differ from that just described. Favorable prognostic factors include small tumor size, patient older than 2 years, favorable histology, and no lymph node metastases or capsular/vascular invasion. The 4-year overall survival of patients with stages II through IV favorable histology disease is approximately 90%.

■ TABLE 17-8 Chemotherapeutic and Radiation Guidelines

Chemotherapy for favorable histology tumors

Stage I: Tumor limited to kidney and completely excised. Dactinomycin/vincristine × 6 mo.

Stage II: Regional tumor extension, but completely resected. Dactinomycin/vincristine × 6 mo.

Stage III: Residual tumor present, but confined to the abdomen. Dactinomycin/vincristine/doxorubicin × 6 mo and XRT as below.

Stage IV: Metastatic disease. As stage III.

Stage V: Bilateral disease. Special considerations depending on extent of disease in each kidney.

Radiation

Stage III: XRT to tumor bed and extends across vertebral column to avoid scoliosis

Stage III as a result of peritoneal spill: Whole abdominal XRT

Stage IV: XRT to primary disease site (only if stage III and to lung, liver, or other metastases)

⚒ 17-6 KEY POINTS

1. Staging is done after exploratory laparotomy, and the therapy involves surgery, chemotherapy, and sometimes radiation.
2. The tumor's histology and stage are important for prognosis because the overall survival for stage IV or better with favorable histology is 90%.

BONE TUMORS

Primary malignant bone tumors account for 5% of childhood cancers. Two forms predominate: Ewing sarcoma and osteosarcoma.

EWING SARCOMA

Pathogenesis

Ewing sarcoma is an undifferentiated sarcoma that arises primarily in bone. The clonal nature of the disease is revealed by the consistent translocation from chromosome 11 to chromosome 22 in affected cells. Ewing sarcoma is thought to arise from a pluripotent neural crest cell of the parasympathetic nervous system. Other tumors with the same or similar translocations occurring outside of bone are known as peripheral primitive neuroectodermal tumors, and they are also members of the Ewing family of soft-tissue tumors.

Epidemiology

Ewing sarcoma is seen primarily in adolescents and is 1.5 times more common in males than females. It is an extremely rare occurrence in African Americans. Like osteosarcoma, it is twice as likely to occur in adolescents than in young children.

Clinical Manifestations

Pain and localized swelling at the site of the primary tumor are the most common presenting complaints. Unlike osteosarcoma, in which the long bones are predominantly involved, flat and long bones are equally represented. The most commonly involved sites are the femur (20%), pelvis (20%), fibula (12%), and humerus and tibia (10%). Other sites include ribs, clavicle, and scapulae. In the long bones, Ewing sarcoma often begins midshaft, rather than at the ends as in osteosarcoma. Systemic manifestations are more common in children with metastases and include fever, weight loss, and fatigue.

Differential Diagnosis

The differential diagnosis for Ewing sarcoma includes osteomyelitis, eosinophilic granuloma (Langerhans cell histiocytosis), and osteosarcoma. Metastasis to the bone by neuroblastoma or rhabdomyosarcoma should be considered in younger children with a solitary bone lesion.

Diagnostic Evaluation

Leukocytosis and an elevated ESR are often seen. Radiographs characteristically reveal a lytic bone lesion with calcified periosteal elevation ("onion skin") or a soft-tissue mass, or both. Biopsy confirms the diagnosis.

Treatment

Treatment involves both global (chemotherapy) and local control (radiation therapy or surgery). Chemotherapy is critical to both reduce the size of the primary tumor and treat metastases, even if overt metastases are not seen, because almost all patients with Ewing sarcoma have microscopic metastatic disease at the time of diagnosis. Specific agents used include vincristine, doxorubicin, cyclophosphamide, etoposide, and ifosfamide. If the tumor affects an expendable bone (proximal fibula, rib, or clavicle), complete surgical excision may be warranted.

The prognosis is excellent for patients with distal extremity nonmetastatic tumors; the 5-year survival rate is greater than 50% in patients without metastatic disease. Children with metastatic disease at diagnosis or tumors of the pelvic bones or proximal long bones have less favorable outcomes. Other less favorable features include soft-tissue extension, low lymphocyte count, and elevated serum LDH.

🗝 17-7 KEY POINTS

1. Ewing sarcoma is an undifferentiated sarcoma that arises primarily in bone.
2. It affects young children and adolescents but is extremely rare in African Americans.
3. Pain and localized swelling are the most common presenting complaints.
4. The most common sites for Ewing sarcoma are the femur and the bones of the pelvis, which have the least favorable prognosis.

OSTEOGENIC SARCOMA

Pathogenesis

Osteosarcoma, also called osteogenic sarcoma, is a malignant tumor of the bone-producing mesenchymal stem cells. Osteosarcoma arises in either the medullary cavity or the periosteum. The primary tumor is usually located at the metaphyseal portion of bones that are associated with maximum growth velocity, which include the distal femur, proximal tibia, and proximal humerus.

Epidemiology

Osteosarcoma is seen mainly in adolescence, with a male-to-female ratio of 2:1. Peak incidence occurs during the maximum growth velocity period.

Clinical Manifestations

Similar to Ewing sarcoma, pain and localized swelling are the most common presenting complaints, but in contrast to Ewing sarcoma, systemic manifestations are rare. Because these tumors occur most frequently in adolescents, initial complaints may be attributed to trauma. The most common tumor sites are the distal femur (40%), proximal tibia (20%), and proximal humerus (10%). Metastases are present at diagnosis in 20% of cases, the majority of which are in the lungs. Gait disturbance and pathologic fractures also may be present.

Differential Diagnosis

The differential diagnoses for osteosarcoma are similar to Ewing sarcoma, and include Ewing sarcoma, benign bone tumors, and chronic osteomyelitis.

Diagnostic Evaluation

The ESR and CBC are generally normal, and the serum alkaline phosphatase level may be elevated at diagnosis. Lytic bone lesion with periosteal reaction is characteristic on radiograph. The periosteal inflammation has the appearance of a radial "sunburst" that results as the tumor breaks through the cortex and new bone spicules are produced. A CT scan of the chest is essential to detect pulmonary metastases, which appear as calcified nodules.

Treatment

At diagnosis, 20% of patients have clinically detectable metastatic disease, and most of the remaining patients have microscopic metastatic disease. Management of the primary tumor is surgical, either with amputation or limb-sparing surgery. Unlike Ewing sarcoma, osteosarcoma is relatively resistant to radiation therapy. The addition of both neoadjuvant (before surgery) and adjuvant (after surgery) chemotherapy has raised the survival rate substantially; before chemotherapy, survival from osteosarcoma was 20%. Currently, with aggressive chemotherapy, long-term relapse-free survival is greater than 70%. Specific chemotherapeutic agents include cisplatin, doxorubicin, and methotrexate. Aggressive treatment of metastatic disease is indicated because some patients can be cured with high-dose chemotherapy and surgical resection of all pulmonary metastases. Poor prognostic findings include age younger than 10 years, metastatic disease, undifferentiated cell type, involvement of the axial skeleton, elevated serum LDH at diagnosis, and presence of symptoms for less than 2 months.

🔑 17-8 KEY POINTS

1. Osteogenic sarcoma is a malignant tumor of the bone-producing cells of the mesenchyma.
2. Osteosarcoma arises most often during maximum growth velocity in the distal femur, proximal tibia, or proximal humerus.
3. Similar to Ewing sarcoma, pain and localized swelling are the most common presenting complaints, but in contrast to Ewing sarcoma, systemic manifestations are rare.
4. Treatment consists of surgery and chemotherapy.

Additional Suggested Reading

Golden CB, Fenusner JH. Malignant abdominal masses in children: quick guide to evaluation and diagnosis. *Pediatr Clin North Am.* 2002;49: 1369–1392.

Hughes WT, Armstrong D, Bodey GP, et al. 2002 Guidelines for the use of antimicrobial agents in neutropenic patients with cancer. *Clin Infect Dis.* 2002;34:730–751.

Pearce JM, Sills RH. Consultation with the specialist: childhood leukemia. *Pediatr Rev.* 2005;26: 96–104.

Ulrich NJ, Pomeroy SL. Pediatric brain tumors. *Neurol Clin.* 2003;2:897–909.

Velez MC. Consultation with the specialist: lymphomas. *Pediatr Rev.* 2003;24:380–386.

VISION SCREENING

Vision screening in children is critical because the young eye is part of a dynamic system that may be quickly damaged by visual deprivation. The development of normal vision requires the production of *clear retinal images* and *proper eye alignment*. Table 18-1 lists the American Academy of Ophthalmology's recommendations for vision screening and referral. Children older than 8 years can be screened according to adult guidelines. Patients with a history of prematurity, intrauterine infection, CNS disease, or family history of ocular disease are at higher risk for eye pathology and require more extensive follow-up by a pediatric ophthalmologist.

STRABISMUS

Strabismus, or misalignment of the eyes, occurs in approximately 4% of children. When strabismus occurs in a child younger than 4 to 6 years, the child's brain begins to "suppress" the image from the deviating eye. Certain neurologic diseases are associated with an especially high incidence of strabismus, including cerebral palsy, Down syndrome, hydrocephalus, and brain tumors. Unilateral visual deprivation (e.g., ptosis) may also lead to strabismus.

CLINICAL MANIFESTATIONS

The deviating eye of a patient with strabismus may turn inward (esotropia), outward (exotropia), upward, or downward. Diagnosis is made using the corneal light reflex and cover tests. (Note: With one eye covered, the patient fixes vision on an object. When the obscured eye is quickly uncovered, no eye movement should be detectable. The test is repeated on the other side. If eye drift is noted when either eye is uncovered, this is considered a "positive" cover test.)

TREATMENT

The most important consequences of untreated strabismus, aside from the cosmetic deformity, are **amblyopia** (discussed later in the chapter) and reduced stereopsis (depth perception). Treatment is aimed at eliminating or preventing amblyopia, realigning the eyes, and addressing any underlying/predisposing condition (if present). Some causes of strabismus respond to corrective lenses and occlusion, but usually surgery is needed as well. **Early intervention results in an improved chance for establishing normal vision**.

🔑 18-1 KEY POINTS

1. Screening for strabismus by means of cover testing should be included in every pediatric health maintenance examination.
2. Early recognition and treatment offer the best chance for avoiding permanent visual abnormalities.

AMBLYOPIA

Amblyopia, literally meaning "dull sight," describes the development of reduced vision in an otherwise normal eye. The condition occurs in 2% to 5% of the general population. Children are most susceptible between birth and 7 years of age. The earlier amblyopia develops, the more severe the visual defect. Amblyopia resulting from strabismus (the most common cause in

■ **TABLE 18-1** Pediatric Vision Screening Recommendations of the American Academy of Ophthalmology

Age	Examination	Referral
Newborn	Corneal light reflex test	Abnormal red reflexes
	Red reflexes	Any other ocular abnormality
By age 6 mo	Fixation to light or small toys	Aversion to occlusion
	Monocular occlusion	Strabismus
	Corneal light reflex test	Nystagmus
	Cover/uncover test	Abnormal red reflexes
	Red reflexes	Any other ocular abnormality
Age 3–4 yr	Visual acuity	Visual acuity less than 20/40 in either eye and/or no more than one-line difference between the two eyes on vision testing
	Corneal light reflex test	
	Fundus examination	Strabismus
		Any other ocular abnormality
Age 5 or older	Visual acuity	Visual acuity of 20/40 or less in one or both eyes
	Corneal light reflex test	Strabismus
	Cover/uncover test	Any other ocular abnormality
	Fundus examination	

Source: Communication of the American Academy of Ophthalmology, San Francisco, 2001.

children) is caused by suppression of retinal images from a misaligned eye. Visual deprivation or image blurring because of opacities of the optical axis (corneal opacity, cataracts) or to unequal refractive errors in the two eyes (anisometropia) also results in amblyopia. Other risk factors include premature birth and a family history of amblyopia or strabismus.

CLINICAL MANIFESTATIONS

Subnormal vision is the only sign of amblyopia. Untreated amblyopia leads to permanent vision loss and diminished stereopsis.

TREATMENT

The first step in treating amblyopia involves correcting any refractive errors with glasses. Visual opacities such as cataracts, if present, should be removed. Proper alignment must be restored. Finally, **occlusion** of the better-seeing eye forces development of the affected eye and the visual centers in the brain corresponding

with that eye. Early intervention is crucial to promote normal vision; **beyond 8 years of age, treatment is unlikely to be successful.**

🔑 18-2 KEY POINTS

1. Amblyopia represents a common and potentially reversible cause of vision loss in children.
2. Strabismus is the most common cause of amblyopia in children.
3. Successful treatment depends on early recognition and referral for occlusion therapy and elimination of predisposing conditions.

LEUKOCORIA

Leukocoria (white pupil, or absence of the red reflex) in an infant or child may be caused by a number of entities, ranging from isolated ocular abnormalities to life-threatening systemic disease. All cases of leukocoria require prompt ophthalmologic referral.

DIFFERENTIAL DIAGNOSIS

Retinoblastoma, the most common intraocular malignancy of childhood, is a life-threatening cause of leukocoria. The disease occurs in approximately 1 in 20,000 live births, resulting in 300 new cases in the United States each year. The associated genetic defect is found on the q14 band of chromosome 13. Untreated retinoblastoma leads to death from brain and visceral metastasis in almost all cases.

Cataracts (opacities of the crystalline lens) occur in 1 of every 250 newborns, thus making cataracts the most common cause of leukocoria. They may be congenital or acquired and may be unilateral or bilateral. Cataracts are often genetically determined but may result from metabolic diseases or intrauterine infections.

Retinopathy of prematurity (ROP) is a retinal vascular disease of premature infants that can also lead to leukocoria. Risk factors include birth weight less than 1,250 g, gestational age less than 32 weeks, mechanical ventilation, and need for supplemental oxygen.

Other causes of leukocoria include congenital glaucoma and ocular toxocariasis (a parasitic infection most frequently acquired in infancy or young childhood).

CLINICAL MANIFESTATIONS

Leukocoria is detectable by routine screening of the **red reflex** in all neonates. Infants at high risk for the development of ROP should be examined by an ophthalmologist when discharged from the nursery and again at 3 to 6 months of age.

TREATMENT

Successful therapy combines treatment of the underlying condition with attention to associated amblyopia. Treatment for retinoblastoma includes **enucleation** (removal of the eye), radiation therapy, chemotherapy, and/or cryotherapy. Small localized tumors may not require enucleation. Prognosis is directly related to the size of the tumor at diagnosis, and cure rates approach 90%. If retinoblastoma is not bilateral at presentation, the patient should be closely followed because 20% will develop another tumor in the previously unaffected eye.

Unilateral or bilateral congenital cataracts may be surgically removed. The visual prognosis for children requiring cataract extraction is not as good as that seen in adults because amblyopia or associated ocular abnormalities may limit the ultimate level of visual acuity.

Cataracts that are not removed by 3 to 4 months of age result in significant, often irreversible, amblyopia.

Most cases of ROP regress spontaneously; however, cryotherapy performed at an intermediate stage of ROP reduces progression to the vision-threatening stages of disease. Infants with treated or regressed ROP remain at risk for the development of amblyopia, strabismus, myopia, and glaucoma.

✎ 18-3 KEY POINTS

1. The most common cause of leukocoria is a congenital cataract.
2. All cases of leukocoria require prompt ophthalmologic referral.
3. All children at high risk for retinopathy of prematurity should be seen by an ophthalmologist before discharge from the nursery.
4. Retinoblastoma should be diagnosed early and treated aggressively to secure a favorable outcome.

NASOLACRIMAL DUCT OBSTRUCTION

Congenital nasolacrimal duct obstruction (dacryostenosis), a common cause of overflow tearing, occurs in 6% of neonates. Obstruction is usually caused by failure of the distal membranous end of the nasolacrimal duct to open.

CLINICAL MANIFESTATIONS

Chronic tearing in the absence of conjunctival injection is the hallmark of nasolacrimal duct obstruction. The presence of mucopurulent discharge and tenderness over the medial aspect of the lower lid suggests superimposed infection of the nasolacrimal sac (dacryocystitis). Other causes of excess tearing include chronic irritation from allergens and congenital glaucoma.

TREATMENT

Treatment varies according to the severity of symptoms. The obstruction resolves spontaneously by 1 year of age in 96% of infants. Referral to an ophthalmologist is indicated if symptoms persist. **Probing** of the nasolacrimal duct system is performed at 12 to 15 months of age unless severe symptoms warrant earlier intervention. Superimposed dacryocystitis should be treated with warm compresses, nasolacrimal massage, and systemic antibiotics (i.e., a first-generation cephalosporin) in select cases.

🔧 18-4 KEY POINTS

1. Nasolacrimal duct obstruction is a common cause of tearing in infants and neonates and typically resolves spontaneously.
2. Referral is indicated if symptoms persist beyond 9 to 12 months of age and for infants with recurrent dacryocystitis.

OPHTHALMIA NEONATORUM

Ophthalmia neonatorum refers to conjunctivitis occurring within the first month of life. Any ocular discharge in the neonate requires evaluation because tears are usually absent in the first few weeks of life.

DIFFERENTIAL DIAGNOSIS

Common causes of ophthalmia neonatorum include chemical irritation, *Chlamydia trachomatis*, and *Neisseria gonorrhoeae*. Chemical conjunctivitis can be caused by birth trauma or by antibiotic prophylaxis given at birth to prevent gonococcal infection. Less common infectious causes, including herpes simplex virus (HSV), *Staphylococcus aureus*, *Haemophilus influenzae*, and *Pseudomonas aeruginosa*, typically manifest after the first week of life. Nasolacrimal duct obstruction should be considered in neonates with persistent conjunctival discharge.

CLINICAL MANIFESTATIONS

Infants usually present with eyelid edema, conjunctival hyperemia, and ocular discharge. Age at onset and clinical features may suggest the diagnosis, but appropriate laboratory evaluation is required (Table 18-2).

TREATMENT AND PREVENTION

Infants with suspected gonococcal, HSV, or *P. aeruginosa* conjunctivitis should be referred to an ophthalmologist. Infants with conjunctivitis related to other causes require referral if signs worsen or symptoms persist after 3 days of treatment. Parents and their sexual partners should be treated for *Chlamydia* and gonococcal infections in the usual manner.

■ TABLE 18-2 Distinguishing Features of Ophthalmia Neonatorum			
Features	**Chemical**	**N. gonorrhoeae**	**C. trachomatis**
Age at onset	24 hours	2–4 days	4–10 days
Clinical features	Bilateral	Bilateral	Unilateral or bilateral
	Serous discharge	Purulent discharge	Mucopurulent discharge
	Conjunctival hyperemia	Marked eyelid edema	Conjunctival hyperemia
		Chemosis	
Complications	Self-limited	Sepsis	Corneal scarring
		Meningitis	Pneumonia
		Arthritis	
		Corneal ulceration	
		Blindness	
Diagnosis	Exclude serious causes	Conjunctival culture on chocolate or Thayer-Martin agar	Conjunctival *Chlamydia* culture
			Direct immunofluorescent antibody test
Treatment	None	Topical erythromycin; intravenous cefotaxime; treat parents	Oral plus topical erythromycin; treat parents

The incidence of neonatal conjunctivitis has decreased dramatically since the introduction of ocular prophylaxis with silver nitrate. **Erythromycin**, effective against both *C. trachomatis* and *N. gonorrhoeae*, currently is preferred.

🔑 18-5 KEY POINTS

1. Conjunctivitis in the neonate may represent chemical irritation or acquired infection.
2. *Chlamydia trachomatis* and *Neisseria gonorrhoeae* are the most common infectious agents.
3. Suspected gonococcal infection requires emergent treatment to prevent blindness.
4. Patients with chlamydial infections should be treated with topical and systemic antibiotics; chlamydial pneumonia may develop later in the neonatal period if the patient is not treated orally.

INFECTIOUS CONJUNCTIVITIS

Non-neonatal infectious conjunctivitis ("**pink eye**") is very common in childhood and may be bacterial or viral in origin. The infection causes inflammation in the conjunctiva, the outer covering of the eye over the sclera. Adenovirus in particular is a frequent cause of viral conjunctivitis.

DIFFERENTIAL DIAGNOSIS

Inflammation of the conjunctiva may be precipitated by exposure to allergens, toxins, chemicals, or irritants. Some systemic diseases may also have "red eyes" as part of the presentation.

Corneal abrasions may present with a red, painful, tearing eye that is sensitive to light. Examination of the eye with a blue-filtered light following instillation of **fluorescein** reveals the denuded area. Corneal abrasions are treated with eye patching (to decrease pain and promote healing) and topical antibiotics. Most heal within 24 hours.

CLINICAL MANIFESTATIONS

Table 18-3 compares and contrasts the clinical manifestations of viral, bacterial, and allergic conjunctivitis.

TREATMENT

In practice, most cases of infectious conjunctivitis are treated with a trial of antibiotic drops or ointment for 5 to 7 days. Choices include polymyxin-bacitracin, trimethoprim-polymyxin B, sodium sulfacetamide, gentamicin, or ofloxacin. Refractory cases require culture results to guide therapy. Although both viral and most bacterial conjunctivitis are usually self-limited diseases, antibiotics limit infectivity and decrease disease duration by approximately 2 days. (Notable exceptions include *Neisseria gonorrhoeae* conjunctivitis, which must be treated with parenteral ceftriaxone, and *Haemophilus influenzae* conjunctivitis that occurs in conjunction with same-sided otitis media, which must be treated with appropriate oral agents.)

Antibiotic drops that contain steroids (to decrease inflammation) must **not** be given if HSV-1 is thought to be the cause of the infection because there is an increased risk of more severe disease and visual impairment.

TABLE 18-3 Comparison of Viral, Bacterial, and Allergic Conjunctivitis			
Symptom	Viral	Bacterial	Allergic
Pain	Mild	Mild to moderate	None
Discharge	Clear	Mucopurulent	Clear
Mild to copious	Mild to copious	Mild to moderate	
Prone to crusting	Definite crusting	No crusting	
Itching	Usually absent	Absent	Present
Injection	Diffuse	Diffuse	Diffuse
Vision	Normal	Normal	Normal
Possible Etiologies	Adenovirus, ECHO virus, coxsackievirus	*Haemophilus influenzae*, *Streptococcus pneumoniae*, *Neisseria gonorrhoeae*	Seasonal pollen (or other) allergen exposure

🔑 18-6 KEY POINTS

1. Conjunctivitis can be caused by infectious agents (bacteria, viruses) as well as systemic disease, irritants, and allergen exposure.
2. Corneal abrasions may be diagnosed by examining the surface of an eye that has been exposed to fluorescein drops under a blue-filter light.
3. Some cases of bacterial conjunctivitis require systemic therapy both for resolution and to prevent other manifestations of the infectious disease.
4. Steroid drops must **not** be given if herpes simplex virus 1 is thought to be the cause of the conjunctival infection because there is an increased risk of more severe disease and visual impairment.

HORDEOLUM AND CHALAZION (STYES)

A **hordeolum** is an acute infection of the meibomian glands, small fluid-secreting structures in the tarsal plate of the lid. *Staphylococcus aureus* is the usual culprit. Localized tender swelling progresses to a point, which ruptures to the outside. Treatment involves warm compresses; the value of ophthalmic antibiotics is questionable. Occasionally, incision and drainage or systemic antibiotics may be indicated.

Chalazions are areas of sterile lipogranulomatous reaction within the meibomian glands that may progressively enlarge. The affected area is typically firm but nontender. Excision may be required for cosmetic purposes or if the area becomes irritated or obscures vision. The condition tends to be chronic and recurrent.

PERIORBITAL CELLULITIS

Periorbital cellulitis is caused by bacterial infection of the eyelids and surrounding skin anterior to the orbital septum, a fibrous band that separates the subcutaneous lid from the orbit itself.

PATHOGENESIS

Bacteria gain access to the area around the eye through breaks in the skin (*Staphylococcus aureus*, group A *streptococcus*), hematogenous dissemination (*Streptococcus pneumoniae*, *Haemophilus influenzae*), or via extension from infected sinuses or other upper respiratory structures (*S. pneumoniae*, *H. influenzae*, *Moraxella catarrhalis*). Both the Hib vaccine and the pneumococcal conjugate vaccine have contributed to a measurable decline in the incidence of periorbital infections.

DIFFERENTIAL DIAGNOSIS

Orbital cellulitis, in which the infection extends behind the orbital septum, is a true emergency. Severe pain with eye movement, proptosis, vision changes, and decreased ocular mobility accompany this disease. A CT scan should be obtained to confirm the diagnosis, identify any coinfected structures (e.g., sinuses), and delineate extension. Associated orbital abscesses require surgical drainage. Empirical parenteral antibiotic therapy should provide coverage against *S. aureus*, *S. pyogenes*, *S. pneumoniae*, *H. influenzae*, *M. catarrhalis*, and anaerobic bacteria found in the upper respiratory tract. Suggested regimens include cefuroxime (with clindamycin added if anaerobic infection is suspected) or ampicillin/sulbactam. When the patient appears recovered, he or she may be released with oral antibiotics to complete a 3-week course. Brain abscesses, meningitis, and cavernous sinus thrombosis are known complications of orbital cellulitis.

Other causes of a swollen eye include trauma, edema, allergies, and tumor.

CLINICAL MANIFESTATIONS

In periorbital cellulitis, the skin around the eye is indurated, warm, and tender, although there is no true eye pain. Fever is variably present in cases of localized skin trauma. In the young child with hematogenous seeding or extension as the source, the fever is generally quite high, with rapid progression of the swelling. The physical examination may reveal sinus tenderness, sore throat, or a point of entry on the skin. It is important to mark the area of induration to assist in documenting subsequent resolution (or lack thereof). Any child with signs or symptoms consistent with meningitis (Chapter 12) should receive an LP.

TREATMENT

Intravenous antibiotics should be begun as soon as possible and continued until resolution of induration. For periorbital cellulitis that follows a break in the skin, a penicillinase-resistant penicillin or a first-generation cephalosporin is appropriate. Vancomycin may be required depending on local resistance patterns. Cefuroxime is the antibiotic of choice in other cases; occasionally, a third-generation cephalosporin is used to prevent extension to the meninges in the young child. The patient may be released with oral antibiotics to complete a 10-day course when symptoms abate.

⚿ 18-7 KEY POINTS

1. Orbital cellulitis, characterized by (a combination of) eye pain, decreased mobility, vision changes, and proptosis, is a true emergency. Surgical drainage of associated abscesses may be required.
2. Periorbital cellulitis may originate from a break in the skin, hematogenous spread, or by extension of respiratory or sinus bacteria.

Additional Suggested Reading

Wald ER. Periorbital and orbital infections. *Pediatr Rev.* 2004;25:312–320.

Wright KW. *Pediatric ophthalmology for primary care.* 2nd ed. Elk Grove Village, Ill: American Academy of Pediatrics; 2003.

Pediatricians and family practitioners require a basic knowledge of orthopedic principles to treat injuries, facilitate rehabilitation, and recognize the musculoskeletal manifestations of many systemic illnesses. The timely diagnosis and management of genetic, congenital, developmental, and infectious bone and joint conditions in children can minimize potential deformities and loss of function.

DEVELOPMENTAL HIP DYSPLASIA

PATHOGENESIS

Developmental dysplasia of the hip (DDH) refers to an abnormal relationship between the head of the femur and the acetabulum that results in instability and/or dislocation at the hip joint. The condition is thought to develop when contact between the acetabulum and the head of the femur is lost during intrauterine development, most likely because of positioning of the fetus or restriction of fetal movement in utero.

EPIDEMIOLOGY

DDH is more common in females, first-born children, breech presentations, and patients with a positive family history of DDH. There is also an association with other anomalies, including clubfoot, congenital torticollis, metatarsus adductus, and infantile scoliosis. The severity of dysplasia ranges from **subluxtable** (partial dislocation induced on examination) to **dislocatable** (full dislocation induced on examination) to **dislocated** (abnormally positioned most of the time).

CLINICAL MANIFESTATIONS

Early diagnosis results in a better outcome; therefore, a careful newborn examination is critical. First the examiner should look for any asymmetry in the gluteal folds. Then, with the examiner's fingers on the greater and lesser trochanters, both the **Barlow test** (posterosuperior dislocation of the hip with adduction and posterior pressure) and the **Ortolani maneuver** (abduction with a resulting "clunk" as the head relocates into the joint) are essential parts of every newborn evaluation (Fig. 19-1). DHH can evolve over time, so children should be screened at regular intervals until they are ambulatory. In examining a somewhat older infant, a Galeazzi sign should be sought. By holding the ankles with the knees bent and hips flexed, the examiner looks for any foreshortening of the (affected) limb. Older infants may also present with limited hip abduction and apparent shortening of the involved extremity.

The diagnosis rests with the demonstration of a "false" acetabulum in the lateral ileum on US or hip radiographs. The true acetabulum will be distorted and shallow. Because most of the hips and pelvis are not ossified at birth, radiographs are not helpful until 4 to 6 months of age. US becomes accurate much earlier, at approximately 4 to 6 weeks of age.

TREATMENT

When an abnormal "clunk" is elicited at the newborn exam (or thereafter), the patient should receive an orthopedic consult. Most subluxtable and dislocatable hips stabilize without intervention within the first 4 weeks of life. If treatment is indicated in children younger than 6 months, a **Pavlik harness** (which keeps the hip abducted and flexed) may be prescribed. Body casting is used in older patients. Cases that do not

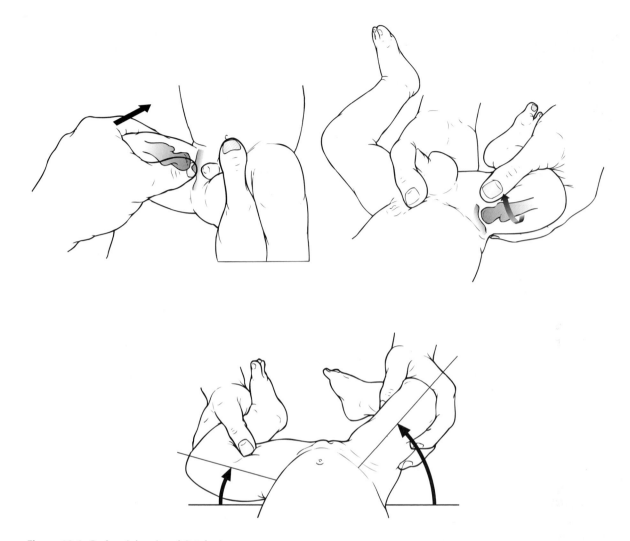

Figure 19-1 • Barlow (*above*) and Ortolani maneuvers.

respond to conservative measures require open reduction.

Avascular necrosis of the femoral head is the most serious complication and more likely to occur when the child has been left untreated for longer than 6 months. Patients with DDH are at risk for degenerative hip arthritis later in life.

🔑 19-1 KEY POINTS

1. Developmental dysplasia of the hip (DDH) may be demonstrated on physical examination by performing the Barlow test and the Ortolani maneuver as well as looking for asymmetry of the gluteal folds and the Galeazzi sign.
2. DDH must be discovered and treated early in life to obtain a favorable outcome.

FOOT DEFORMITIES

Foot deformities predispose children to difficulty walking, poor shoe fit, and pain. Some disorders correct themselves as the child begins to ambulate; others require bracing or surgical correction. In general, any congenital orthopedic condition of the foot that can be molded by the examiner's hands to its anatomically correct position requires minimal intervention.

CLINICAL MANIFESTATIONS AND TREATMENT

Metatarsus Adductus

Metatarsus adductus (in-toeing of the forefoot without hindfoot abnormalities) is a common, relatively benign condition caused by intrauterine positioning. As opposed to clubfoot, dorsiflexion and plantar flexion at the ankle joint are unrestricted. Mild metatarsus adductus occurs when the infant is able to straighten the foot actively when tickled along the lateral border. In cases of moderate deformity, the foot can be straightened with gentle pressure; these cases respond well to stretching exercises. More severe cases (those that are not correctable with manipulation by the examiner) are treated with serial bracing or casting. Surgery is rarely indicated.

Idiopathic Talipes Equinovarus (Congenital Clubfoot)

Talipes equinovarus, or clubfoot, is a more rare but more debilitating deformity that includes medial rotation of the tibia, *fixed* plantar flexion at the ankle, inversion of the foot, and forefoot adduction (metatarsus adductus). Dorsiflexion at the ankle is impossible in patients with clubfoot. Without treatment, the foot becomes progressively more deformed, and ulcerations develop when the child is old enough to limp. Early intervention is essential for subsequent normal function and development. Initial treatment consists of bracing or serial casting; patients with unsatisfactory improvement require surgical repair, preferably before the age of anticipated ambulation. One in seven children with this condition also has other congenital malformations.

19-2 KEY POINT

1. Plantar and dorsiflexion are intact in metatarsus adductus, whereas in talipes equinovarus, the hindfoot is fixed in plantar flexion.

LIMP

Limp is probably the most common musculoskeletal complaint prompting medical evaluation in children. Pain, weakness, decreased range of motion, and leg-length discrepancy all disrupt the normal gait.

DIFFERENTIAL DIAGNOSIS

The list of conditions that present with limp is extensive (Table 19-1); some are benign and self-limited, whereas others result in significant morbidity. **Trauma** is the most common cause of limp at any age.

■ TABLE 19-1 Differential Diagnosis of Limp by Disease Category

Trauma or overuse
  Fracture
  Soft-tissue injury
Infectious
  Septic arthritis
  Osteomyelitis
  Lyme arthritis
  Discitis
Inflammatory
  Transient synovitis
  Rheumatic disease
  Reactive arthritis
Developmental/Acquired
  Developmental dysplasia of the hip
  Avascular necrosis
  Slipped capital femoral epiphysis
Neurologic
  Muscular dystrophy
  Peripheral neuropathy
Neoplasia
  Bone tumors
  Leukemia
  Spinal cord tumors
Metabolic
  Rickets
Hematologic
  Sickle cell disease
  Hemophilia
Other
  Appendicitis
  Pelvic inflammatory disease
  Testicular torsion

The patient's age affects the differential diagnosis. Infection, inflammation, and paralytic syndromes are common etiologies in children from 1 to 3 years of age. From 3 to 10 years of age, **Legg-Calvé-Perthes' disease**, **toxic synovitis**, and JRA become more common. **Slipped capital femoral epiphysis** is a consideration in older patients.

Legg-Calvé-Perthes' disease is defined as avascular necrosis (ischemic compromise) of the femoral head. The etiology is unknown. Eventually (over approximately 2 years), the ischemic bone is resorbed and reossification occurs, with continued (but not necessarily normal) growth. Legg-Calvé-Perthes' disease occurs more often in males and younger children (4 to 8 years of age). A painless or mildly painful limp that develops insidiously is the most common presenting complaint. The pain is often referred to the knee or thigh, clouding the diagnostic picture. Range of motion is limited upon abduction, flexion, and internal rotation. Initial radiographic studies may appear normal; subsequent films demonstrate epiphyseal radiolucency (Fig. 19-2). A bone scan may be helpful to detect early impairment in the blood supply and fragmentation and flattening of the femoral head. Treatment involves containing the fragile femoral head within the acetabulum, preserving its spherical contour, and maintaining normal range of motion. Younger children with minimal involvement and full range of motion may be observed. Orthotic bracing or surgery is necessary in older patients with significant changes in the femoral head. The amount and area of ischemic damage affect the prognosis. Collapse of the femoral head is the most serious acute complication; long-term disability is related to abnormal or asymmetric growth.

Slipped capital femoral epiphysis (SCFE) is the gradual or acute separation of the proximal femoral growth plate, with the femur head slipping off the femoral neck and rotating into an inferior/posterior position. The cause is unknown but may be hormonal (the condition is most common during puberty) in origin or related to excessive weight bearing (SCFE is more common in overweight individuals). It occurs slightly more often in males. Antecedent trauma is **not** a contributing factor. Although usually asymmetric at presentation, 25% of cases eventually progress to bilateral involvement. The typical patient presents with a limp and pain, which may be centered in the hip or groin but often is referred to the knee. Limited internal rotation and limb shortening are present on examination. Radiographs with the child's hips in the **frog-leg lateral position** are the study of choice for noting epiphyseal displacement (Fig. 19-3). Radiographs may show physeal plate widening, decreased epiphyseal height, and a Klein line (line drawn along the femoral neck) that does not intersect the lateral epiphysis. The primary goal of treatment is prevention of further misalignment. Pin fixation is effective in the acute setting. Chronic cases generally require osteotomy. Long-term complications include avascular necrosis and late degenerative changes similar to those seen with osteoarthritis.

CLINICAL MANIFESTATIONS

History

The history should include questions about the onset, timing, and evolution of the limp. Pain may be severe (fracture, infection), constant, associated with activity (injury), acute, or chronic. The absence of pain suggests weakness or instability. Swelling and stiffness are common in rheumatologic disease. Toxic synovitis may follow a recent viral illness. Any history of bowel or bladder incontinence suggests spinal cord compression.

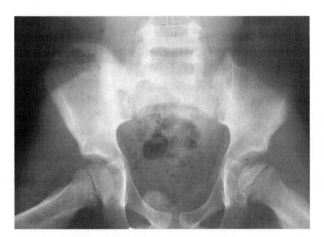

Figure 19-2 • Legg-Calve-Perthes' disease of left hip. Epiphysis is narrowed and radiodense. A subchondral fracture is also visible. From: Fleisher GR, Ludwig S, Baskin MN. *Atlas of pediatric emergency medicine.* Philadelphia: Lippincott Williams & Wilkins; 2004.

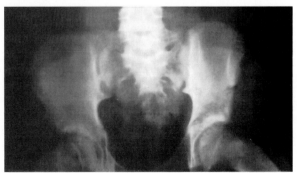

Figure 19-3 • Radiograph of a slipped capital femoral epiphysis. Frog-leg view in this 13-year-old boy demonstrates increased radiolucency of the left femoral epiphysis with medial and perhaps posterior angulation of the femoral head on the neck.

Physical Examination

Watching the child walk is particularly important because certain gaits are associated with specific disorders. Each joint should be examined for range of motion, swelling, warmth, erythema, and tenderness. Fractures produce point tenderness and occasionally angulation. Neurologic evaluation includes deep tendon reflexes, strength, and sensation. Extremities are assessed for adequate perfusion and deformities. Muscle atrophy and fasciculation may be present in neuromuscular disease.

DIAGNOSTIC EVALUATION

All patients with significant limp should have **plain films**. An elevated WBC may indicate infection; if greater than 30,000 per μL, malignant marrow invasion should be considered. The ESR is increased in both infection and rheumatologic disease. A bone scan reveals areas of increased blood flow consistent with inflammation. US is useful to evaluate for the presence of an effusion, especially when a septic joint is considered. A CT scan of the limb is rarely helpful. However, MRI is a great modality for evaluating joints, cartilage, and soft tissue. Patients with weakness should have electrolytes, calcium, serum creatinine kinase, and urine myoglobin studies done; electromyography and nerve conduction studies may also be helpful. If the weakness is progressive and limited to the lower extremities, spinal cord compression must be ruled out with imaging studies (i.e., MRI).

✎ 19-3 KEY POINTS

1. Trauma is the most common cause of limp in all age groups.
2. Plain films are helpful screening tools.
3. Any evidence of neurologic involvement (weakness, bowel, and/or bladder incontinence) necessitates aggressive workup to rule out spinal cord compression.
4. The typical patient with Legg-Calvé-Perthes' disease is a young male child who presents with a painless or moderately painful limp and knee pain.
5. Trauma is not a cause of slipped capital femoral epiphysis (SCFE).
6. The typical SCFE patient is an obese adolescent male who presents with hip or knee pain and no history of trauma.

OSGOOD-SCHLATTER DISEASE

Osgood-Schlatter's disease involves inflammation, swelling, and tenderness over the tibial tuberosity. It is caused by tendonitis of the distal insertion of the infrapatellar tendon caused by mechanical forces. Osgood-Schlatter' disease typically occurs between 10 and 17 years of age, during the adolescent growth spurt. Repetitive stress and trauma may be contributing factors. Pain is worsened with kneeling, running, jumping, or squatting but is relieved by rest. Radiographs reveal irregularities of the tubercle ossification center and possibly haziness of the adjacent tibial epiphysis. Most cases are mild and treated with activity modification and stretching exercises. Severe cases may require casting for up to 6 weeks. Long-term morbidity is quite low; the disorder disappears when skeletal maturity is reached.

IDIOPATHIC SCOLIOSIS

PATHOGENESIS

Idiopathic scoliosis is found in otherwise healthy children with normal bones, muscles, and vertebral discs. The cause is unknown, but heredity definitely plays a role. **Scoliosis**, or lateral curvature with rotation, is the most common.

EPIDEMIOLOGY

Five percent of children display some degree of spinal deformity. Routine screening is very important. Severe scoliosis requiring intervention occurs more often in **females**. Progression of the curve is most rapid during the adolescent growth spurt.

CLINICAL MANIFESTATIONS

History and Physical Examination

Idiopathic scoliosis is **not** associated with back pain or fatigue; such symptoms warrant further investigation. The physical examination consists of two parts. First, the child is examined from the rear while standing up. Shoulder girdle and iliac crest areas are noted for symmetry and height. Then, the Adam forward bending test is performed. The child bends forward from the waist with the arms hanging freely. The examiner should watch from in front and behind the patient to look for alignment of the spinous processes and asymmetry of rib height.

DIFFERENTIAL DIAGNOSIS

Occasionally, scoliosis may be caused by neuromuscular abnormalities or congenital deformities. Scoliosis should not be confused with **kyphosis**, an increase in the **posterior** convexity of the thoracic spine. Kyphosis is usually postural and responds well to specific daily exercises; inflexible kyphosis may be caused by wedge-shaped vertebral bodies (Scheuermann disease) and requires bracing.

DIAGNOSTIC EVALUATION

Patients with evidence of curvature on exam should receive standing posteroanterior (PA) and lateral spine radiographs to allow angular measurement of the deformity.

TREATMENT

Treatment depends on the degree of curvature and the skeletal maturation and gender of the child. Premenarchal females are the most likely to experience progression of their curvature and should be treated more aggressively. Curvatures less than 25 degrees need only be followed. More pronounced deformity (25 to 45 degrees) in a child who is still growing should be treated with **external bracing** until the growth spurt is completed. Bracing does not reduce the curve, but it does halt progression and is 85% effective if used correctly. Unfortunately, compliance tends to be low. Curvature greater than 40 to 50 degrees after the growth spurt will continue to progress; such patients require spinal fusion to reduce the curve and stabilize the spine. Curves of 50 degrees or greater are associated with decreased vital capacity and low functional pulmonary reserve.

⚓ 19-4 KEY POINTS

1. Scoliosis is more common in adolescent females than in males.
2. Idiopathic scoliosis does not result in back pain or fatigue.
3. Bracing is recommended for curves from 25 to 45 degrees until the growth spurt is complete.
4. Bracing halts curve progression; it does **not** correct the curvature already there.

ACHONDROPLASIA

Achondroplasia is a disorder of cartilage calcification and remodeling. Inheritance is autosomal dominant. The physical appearance is strikingly characteristic: These patients are very short with proportionally large heads. Long bones tend to be wide, short, and curved, and digits are short and stubby. Kyphoscoliosis and lumbar lordosis may be quite pronounced. Heterozygotes have fairly normal intelligence, sexual function, and life expectancy. Homozygotes fare less well, given their increased susceptibility to pulmonary complications and an abnormally small foramen magnum that predisposes to brainstem compression.

COMMON FRACTURES IN CHILDREN

Fractures in children deserve special attention because their bones are characteristically different from those of adults. For one thing, they are more porous, which limits fracture propagation. The periosteum is more substantial in children, so "buckle" and greenstick fractures are more common than displaced fractures. Ligaments and tendons are relatively stronger than bones; injuries that would cause sprains or tears in adults can fracture bones in children. Fractures through the epiphyseal growth plate require particular care because they may result in deformity or limb-length discrepancy.

DIFFERENTIAL DIAGNOSIS

Greenstick fractures occur when the force applied breaks one side of a bone and bends the other. A fracture is complete if the bone is broken through both sides. **Spiral fractures** are particularly common in toddlers because of twisting forces on the tibia during falling. (At one time spiral fractures were thought to be suggestive of injuries of abuse. It is now known that any twisting force—abusive or nonabusive—can result in a spiral fracture [see Chapter 2].)

Epiphyseal fractures disrupt the growth plate, the weakest portion of the child's skeletal system. Epiphyseal fractures are categorized according to the Salter-Harris classification (Fig. 19-4). **Torus fractures** or "buckle" fractures occur at the metaphysis because of a compressive load that causes a buckle in a small area. **Stress fractures** are hairline cracks related to repetitive activity and are usually seen in athletes. **Pathologic fractures** result when underlying

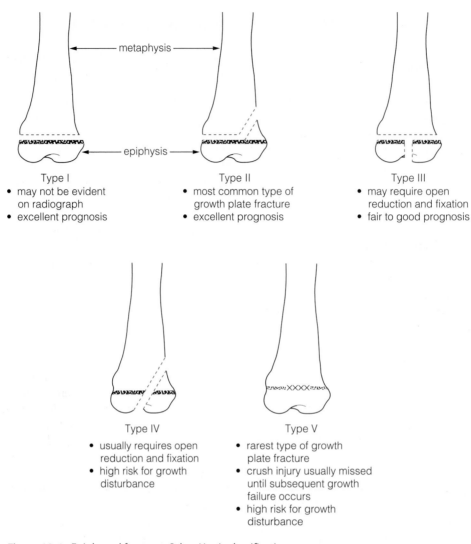

Figure 19-4 • Epiphyseal fractures: Salter-Harris classification.

disease weakens the bone, as may occur in osteogenesis imperfecta, malignancies, long-term steroid use, infection, endocrine disorders, and some inborn errors of metabolism.

CLINICAL MANIFESTATIONS

History and Physical Examination

The history is positive for trauma in virtually all cases of nonpathologic fractures; caretakers who have abused a child may not offer this information. Isolated point tenderness occurs over the site of the fracture. Angulation is variably present and may be quite subtle. Point tenderness directly over a growth plate should raise suspicion for a possible fracture.

DIAGNOSTIC EVALUATION

Radiographs should include AP and lateral view of the involved bone as well as the joints immediately adjacent to the injury. Salter-Harris types I and V may not be seen on these views; oblique views or serial radiographs may be needed to confirm the diagnosis.

TREATMENT

Most fractures can be adequately treated with external stabilization. Fractures that are unstable, misaligned, or through the growth plate often require operative reduction (and fixation). In younger children, bony overgrowth at the site of the fracture may produce limb angulation or asymmetric limb length if not correctly set.

🔑 19-5 KEY POINTS

1. Fractures through the growth plate may result in deformity or leg-length discrepancy.
2. Epiphyseal fractures categorized as Slater-Harris type IV or V have the greatest risk of disruption of growth.

OSTEOGENESIS IMPERFECTA

Osteogenesis imperfecta (OI) describes a group of closely related genetic disorders resulting in fragile, brittle bones. The common denominator in all variants is the abnormal synthesis of type I collagen, which normally constitutes approximately 90% of the bone matrix but is also dispersed in the teeth, ligaments, skin, ears, and sclerae. The most severe form is type II, or fetal OI, which results in multiple intrauterine and birth fractures and is uniformly fatal in the perinatal period.

CLINICAL MANIFESTATIONS

Clinical severity depends on the subclass of OI (Table 19-2). Some variants cause death early in life; others present with only moderately increased susceptibility to fractures. **Blue sclerae** are a characteristic feature in some forms of the disease. Short stature is not uncommon as a result of frequent recurrent fractures. Fractures associated with OI occasionally raise the suspicion of child abuse.

TREATMENT

Treatment involves standard fracture care, pneumatic bracing, and careful avoidance of even minor trauma. Patients with severe disease may benefit from pamidronate therapy, which inhibits osteoclastic resorption.

🔑 19-6 KEY POINTS

1. Type II osteogenesis imperfecta (OI) is the most severe form, resulting in intrauterine or perinatal death.
2. Patients with OI types I and II typically have blue sclerae.

SUBLUXATION OF THE RADIAL HEAD

Subluxation of the radial head, or "nursemaid's elbow," is a common injury seen in young children. The history is often remarkable for a sudden strong jerking of the child's pronated hand, resulting in rapid extension at the elbow. The patient holds the arm close to the body and slightly flexed with the hand pronated. Motion at the elbow is limited. Treatment consists of holding the patient's elbow at 90-degree flexion and firmly manipulating the forearm into supination. A successful reduction is usually accompanied by a "click" as the radial head pops back into place. Usually the child begins to move the arm normally within minutes.

■ TABLE 19-2 Classification of Osteogenesis Imperfecta

Syndrome	Mode of Inheritance	Orthopedic Manifestations	Nonorthopedic Manifestations	Life Expectancy
Type I	Autosomal dominant	Neonatal fractures; bow legs; kyphoscoliosis; joint laxity; mild short stature	Blue sclerae; conductive hearing loss	Generally shortened
Type II	Autosomal recessive	Short, deformed limbs; severe bone fragility	Intrauterine growth retardation; stillbirth; blue sclerae	Days
Type III	Autosomal recessive	Neonatal fractures; severe bone fragility; lower limb deformities; short stature	Normal or mildly blue sclerae	Infancy/ childhood
Type IV	Autosomal dominant	Increased susceptibility to fractures	Normal sclerae	Near normal

OSTEOMYELITIS

PATHOGENESIS

Bone infections require early recognition and aggressive treatment to bring about a favorable outcome. Hematogenous seeding is the usual source of origin; trauma seems to increase susceptibility. The femur and tibia account for two thirds of cases. Infection usually begins in the metaphysis, an area of relative blood stasis and few phagocytes. Fifty percent of neonates have an associated septic joint.

EPIDEMIOLOGY AND RISK FACTORS

Incidence peaks in the neonatal period and again in older children (9 to 11 years of age) when it becomes more common in males. The predominant organism in all age groups is **Staphylococcus aureus**. Osteomyelitis caused by group A streptococcus, Kingella kingae, and *Haemophilus influenzae* infection occurs in children as well. Group B streptococci and *Escherichia coli* are important pathogens in the neonate. Patients with sickle cell disease are particularly susceptible to **Salmonella** osteomyelitis. Occasionally, osteochondritis of the foot may result from puncture wounds through sneakers. In these cases, the organism involved is *Pseudomonas aeruginosa* or *S. aureus*.

CLINICAL MANIFESTATIONS

History and Physical Examination

Infants present with a history of fever and refusal to move the involved limb. Older patients also complain of localized bone pain and often are febrile. The physical examination may reveal soft-tissue swelling, limited range of motion, erythema, and point tenderness. Occasionally, sinus tracts drain purulent fluid onto the skin surface.

DIFFERENTIAL DIAGNOSIS

Traumatic injury and malignant invasion of the bone may present with similar symptoms. Range of motion generally remains intact in patients with osteomyelitis as opposed to those with septic arthritis and epiphyseal disorders.

DIAGNOSTIC EVALUATION

The WBC is often within the normal range. Only 50% to 60% of blood cultures are positive. **Aspiration** of the involved bone is imperative for recovery, identification, and sensitivity testing of the causative organism, especially if initial blood cultures are negative. Radiographs are initially normal but demonstrate periosteal elevation or radiolucent necrotic areas in 2 to 3 weeks. Bone scans are positive within 24 to 48 hours. MRI may be required in sickle cell patients or in cases of vertebral osteomyelitis. Serum markers of inflammation are usually elevated. An elevated C-reactive protein value is seen in 98% of cases and returns to normal within 7 days of effective treatment. The ESR is elevated in 90% of cases but requires longer (3 to 4 weeks) to return to normal.

TREATMENT

Treatment consists of intravenous or high-dose oral antibiotics for 4 to 6 weeks. Initially, broad-spectrum antistaphylococcal agents, such as oxacillin, are appropriate. Second- or third-generation cephalosporins may be chosen if immunization against *H. influenzae* type b is incomplete. Treatment of neonates requires coverage for group B streptococci and gram-negative bacilli. Patients with sickle cell should initially receive a third-generation cephalosporin for salmonella coverage. When the organism has been recovered and sensitivities are available, therapy may be narrowed. Most patients do not require surgery.

Abscess formation within the metaphyseal shaft is not uncommon. If the infection extends to the epiphyseal plate, growth deformities may occur. Septic arthritis is also a known complication.

🔑 19-7 KEY POINTS

1. The peak incidence of osteomyelitis is bimodal (neonatal period and 9 to 11 years of age).
2. Only approximately half of blood cultures are positive, so aspiration of the bone yields invaluable information.
3. The bone scan is more sensitive than plain films early in the disease process.
4. *S. aureus* is the most common pathogen in all age groups. It is also the most common pathogen in sickle cell patients, who are also particularly susceptible to *Salmonella*.

SEPTIC ARTHRITIS

PATHOGENESIS

Septic arthritis (purulent infection of the joint space) is more common and potentially more debilitating than osteomyelitis. Pathogens are theorized to enter the joint during episodes of bacteremia.

EPIDEMIOLOGY

The incidence is highest in infants and young children. Neonates may be infected with group B streptococcus, *E. coli*, *Streptococcus pneumoniae*, and *S. aureus*. In infants older than 6 weeks and young children, the hip is the most common site. The knee is more frequently affected in older children. *S. aureus* is the most likely pathogen outside the neonatal period. Other bacteria with a predilection for joints in younger children include *K. kingae*, *S. pneumoniae*, and *H. influenzae*, although the latter has declined precipitously in incidence because of vaccination. In older children, streptococci and gram-negative bacteria are not uncommon. *Neisseria gonorrhoeae* must be considered in the sexually active adolescent, especially if multiple joints are involved.

CLINICAL MANIFESTATIONS

History and Physical Examination

Septic arthritis presents as a painful joint, often accompanied by fever, irritability, and refusal to bear weight. On examination, range of motion is clearly limited. The joint is tender and may be visibly swollen.

DIFFERENTIAL DIAGNOSIS

Osteomyelitis and arthritis should be considered in the differential diagnosis. In addition, many causes of reactive or postinfectious arthritis may present in a similar manner. **Toxic synovitis** is a frequent cause of joint pain in children. It has not been definitively proven to be an infectious condition, although it often follows a viral illness. The hip is most commonly involved. In contrast to septic arthritis, range of motion is minimally limited, the child is generally afebrile and will usually bear weight, the ESR is less than 40 mm per hour, and the WBC count is less than 12,000 per mm^3.

DIAGNOSTIC EVALUATION

The standard of care for septic arthritis involves **aspiration of the joint**. The synovial fluid usually yields a WBC count in excess of 25,000 and a pathologic organism. The exception is *N. gonorrhoeae*, which is difficult to recover; blood, cervical, rectal, and nasopharyngeal cultures may be additionally helpful.

TREATMENT

Delay in treatment may result in permanent destructive changes and functional impairment. A septic hip is an orthopedic emergency. Intravenous antibiotic therapy remains the treatment of choice; conversion to oral therapy is appropriate when sensitivities are known and symptoms substantially improve. Ceftriaxone is an appropriate initial choice in the young child; a semisynthetic penicillin or (first- or second-generation) cephalosporin are preferred in older children because of the overwhelming presence of *S. aureus* arthritis in this age group. Cefotaxime is a better choice in the neonate. Antibiotic therapy can be specifically targeted to the pathogen when culture results become available.

⚒ 19-8 KEY POINTS

1. The most common cause of septic arthritis in infants and children is *S. aureus*.
2. *N. gonorrhoeae* must be considered in the sexually active adolescent.
3. Children with toxic synovitis have lower ESRs and WBCs and, generally, although the joint is tender, do not refuse to bear weight.

Additional Suggested Reading

Dinolfo EA. In brief: fractures. *Pediatr Rev.* 2004;25: 218–219.

Goldberg MJ. Early detection of developmental hip dysplasia: Synopsis of the AAP Clinical Practice Guideline. *Pediatr Rev.* 2001;22:131–134.

Roye BD, Hyman J, Roye DP. Congenital idiopathic talipes equinovarus. *Pediatr Rev.* 2004;25:124–129.

Sachs HC. In brief: dislocations. *Pediatr Rev.* 2000;21: 433–434.

Scherl SA. Common lower extremity problems in children. *Pediatr Rev.* 2004;25:52–61.

Sharif I. In brief: current treatment of osteomyelitis. *Pediatr Rev.* 2005;26:38–39.

Pulmonology

Respiratory diseases rank as the second leading cause of death in children younger than 4 years of age in the developed world. Optimal exchange of oxygen and carbon dioxide depends on the adequate function of the many components of pulmonary physiology. Clinically significant pulmonary disease can result from *obstruction* in the upper or lower airways, compliance changes (*restrictive* lung diseases), *ventilation-perfusion* mismatch, or abnormalities in the *control of ventilation*.

Respiratory diseases specific to the topic of the newborn (including bronchopulmonary dysplasia) are discussed in Chapter 13.

UPPER AIRWAY OBSTRUCTIVE DISEASE

The upper airway extends from the nose to the carina. Some of these structures are intrathoracic (distal trachea and below), and some are extrathoracic (nose, pharynx, larynx, proximal trachea). Obstruction or dysfunction of any of the structures in the upper airway can lead to disease.

THE NEONATE

Choanal atresia is the most proximal abnormality of the upper airway. In this disorder, a bony or membranous septum between one or both of the nasal passages and the pharynx prevents airflow through (part or all of) the nose. Trauma during vaginal delivery can lead to recurrent laryngeal nerve damage with **vocal cord paralysis** (and partial obstruction at the level of the cords). Prolonged intubation may result in significant long-term **subglottic stenosis** (narrowing of the upper airway). Immature cartilage can leave the larynx

and (less frequently) trachea floppy (and prone to closure), referred to as **laryngomalacia** or **tracheal malacia**. The upper airway may also be obstructed by congenital malformations such as hemangiomas, laryngeal webs, or vascular rings. A small hypopharynx (associated with Pierre-Robin's syndrome) or a big tongue (in Down syndrome) can also cause obstruction. **Apnea of infancy** (discussed later in the chapter) may be partially obstructive.

Clinical Presentation

Upper airway obstruction usually presents with evidence of difficulties with inspiration. Signs and symptoms include stridor, tachypnea, respiratory distress, inspiratory retractions, or occasionally apnea. It is important to remember that most young infants are obligate nose breathers. As a result, *bilateral* choanal atresia can lead to significant cyanosis in the delivery room and is life-threatening. Unilateral obstruction may only cause symptoms during feeding. A hoarse or absent cry may indicate vocal cord dysfunction.

Diagnostic Evaluation

Pulse oximetry can quickly assess the level of oxygen saturation, but an ABG measurement is necessary to evaluate the true degree of respiratory compromise in an infant in distress. Inability to pass a NG tube is suggestive of choanal atresia. Lateral neck radiographs may demonstrate subglottic stenosis, but bronchoscopy is usually needed to confirm vocal cord abnormalities or laryngotracheal malacia. A chest radiograph demonstrating a right aortic arch should prompt consideration of a vascular ring. A barium swallow may help delineate congenital abnormalities in the thoracic cavity including vascular rings, tracheoesophageal fistulas, subglottic stenosis, and other forms of central airway compression.

Treatment

Mild to moderate congenital stridor may be followed with close observation, but any degree of obstruction is exacerbated by respiratory infections. Severe respiratory distress mandates immediate endotracheal intubation. Some disorders require a surgical tracheostomy to bypass the obstruction long term. Choanal atresia and vascular rings are repaired surgically.

OLDER CHILD

Obstruction of the upper airway in the older child may result from incomplete resolution of congenital conditions, but additional processes need to be considered. A number of infectious etiologies, including epiglottitis, peritonsillar abscess, retropharyngeal abscess, infectious mononucleosis, bacterial tracheitis, and croup, are important causes of upper airway obstruction and are discussed in Chapter 12. Anaphylaxis causes acute upper airway obstruction and is addressed in Chapter 11. Other important causes of upper airway obstruction in older children are tonsillar and adenoidal hypertrophy and nasal polyps. Chronic obstructive conditions may manifest as **obstructive sleep apnea (OSA)** in the older child because the relaxed pharyngeal tone during sleep exacerbates the obstruction.

Obstructive Sleep Apnea

Patients with OSA develop periodic episodes of apnea during sleep. Despite normal communication along the brainstem-respiratory muscle pathways, total occlusion of the airway (because of low tone superimposed on anatomic abnormalities) prevents airflow. Symptoms of OSA in children include restless sleep, snoring or gasping, excessive daytime sleepiness, decreased growth velocity, behavioral problems, and poor school performance. In older children and adults, OSA associated with obesity and chronic hypercarbia is termed the *Pickwickian's syndrome*. Much more common in children, however, is obstruction caused by anatomic abnormalities (large tonsils and adenoids, macroglossia) or insufficient airway tone (tracheomalacia or laryngomalacia). **Polysomnography**, which measures respiratory effort, air flow, oxygenation, and heart rate, can be helpful in determining the type and severity of the apneic events. Symptoms may be relieved with removal of enlarged tonsils and/or adenoids. Otherwise, treatment involves overnight continuous positive airway pressure (CPAP) or, in refractory cases, tracheostomy. Severe untreated OSA can result in cor pulmonale (right-sided heart failure that results from chronic pulmonary hypertension) and eventual death.

🔨 20-1 KEY POINTS

1. Bilateral choanal atresia causes cyanosis in the delivery room and is a surgical emergency.
2. Obstructive sleep apnea (OSA) can lead to behavioral problems and poor school performance.
3. Polysomnography is the gold standard for diagnosis of OSA.

ASTHMA

PATHOGENESIS

Asthma is a chronic disease of reversible airway obstruction characterized by reversible airway obstruction, inflammation, and bronchial hyperresponsiveness. The diagnosis is based on recurrence of symptoms and symptoms responsiveness to bronchodilators and/or anti-inflammatory agents. **Bronchospasm**, which results from smooth muscle constriction, may occur after allergic, environmental, infectious, or emotional stimuli (the "*trigger*"). Common precipitants include cigarette smoke, URIs, pet dander, dust mites, weather changes, exercise, and seasonal or food allergens. Cellular mediators of inflammation are recruited to the lower airway surfaces, resulting in mucous production and further increasing airway hyperresponsiveness. The **inflammatory** response has both an immediate and late-phase response; it is the latter that results in the prolonged nature of an asthma exacerbation.

Asthma severity is classified based on the degree of impairment prior to initiation of appropriate therapy (Table 20-1).

EPIDEMIOLOGY

Asthma is the most frequently encountered pulmonary disease in children, and its prevalence is on the rise despite advances in therapy. It is the most common reason for hospitalization in pediatric practice. Ninety percent of patients present before 6 years of age.

■ **TABLE 20-1** Classification and Maintenance Treatment of Asthma

Severity	Symptoms	Maintenance Medications, Age ≤5 Yr		Maintenance Medications, Age >5 Yr	
		Preferred	Alternative	Preferred	Alternative
Mild intermittent	≤2 days/wk and/or ≤2 nights/mo	None	None	None	None
Mild persistent	>2 days/wk and/or >2 nights/mo	Low-dose inhaled corticosteroid	Cromolyn or leukotriene receptor antagonist	Low-dose inhaled corticosteroid	Cromolyn, leukotriene receptor antagonist, nedocromil, or sustained-release theophylline
Moderate persistent	Daily and/or >1 night/wk	Low-dose inhaled corticosteroid and long-acting inhaled β_2-agonist *or* medium-dose inhaled corticosteroid	Low-dose inhaled corticosteroid and either leukotriene receptor antagonist or theophylline	Low- to medium-dose inhaled corticosteroid and long-acting inhaled β_2-agonist	Low- to medium-dose inhaled corticosteroid and either leukotriene receptor antagonist or theophylline
Severe persistent	Continual daily, and frequent nighttime	High-dose inhaled corticosteroid and long-acting inhaled β_2-agonist *and* (if needed) oral corticosteroid	None accepted	High-dose inhaled corticosteroid and long-acting inhaled β_2-agonist *and* (if needed) oral corticosteroid	None accepted

Boys are affected twice as often as girls before adolescence, at which time the numbers become equal.

RISK FACTORS

Risk factors include genetic predisposition (parent(s) with reactive airways disease [RAD] or atopy), atopy, cigarette smoke exposure, living in urban areas, poverty, and African American race. RSV infection necessitating hospitalization is also associated with the development of asthma; this may represent an underlying increased propensity to wheeze rather than a cause.

DIFFERENTIAL DIAGNOSIS

When an infant presents with wheezing and respiratory distress, the differential diagnosis includes bronchiolitis, foreign body aspiration, gastroesophageal reflux, tracheoesophageal fistula, and vascular sling. Anaphylaxis and angioneurotic edema may cause wheezing at any age. Cough-variant asthma produces a chronic cough, which may be present during daily activities or at night during sleep. Wheezing may or may not be present. This symptom is similar to the cough accompanying postnasal drip, bronchitis, or cystic fibrosis.

CLINICAL MANIFESTATIONS

History and Physical Examination

The presentation of asthma is varied. The history may be positive for wheezing with viral respiratory infections. Other possible findings in the patient history include prolonged respiratory infections, decreased exercise tolerance, or persistent day or nighttime coughing. Children with acute exacerbations present in respiratory distress with dyspnea, wheezing, subcostal retractions, nasal flaring, tracheal tugging, and a prolonged expiratory phase as a result of obstruction of airflow. Cyanosis is uncommon. The absence of wheezing with poorly heard breath sounds is an ominous sign, indicating the child's respiratory system is too obstructed for air movement. **Mental status changes** suggest advanced hypercarbia and/or significant hypoxemia with impending respiratory failure.

DIAGNOSTIC EVALUATION

In older patients, PFTs can help delineate disease severity at baseline and during exacerbations. (Note: Other diagnostic methods that may be helpful in diagnosing asthma include the methacholine challenge test and exercise testing with spirometry.) Patients with persistent asthma (Table 20-1) should receive PFTs at least once or twice a year in order to tailor therapy. Baseline chest radiographs typically show at least mild hyperinflation and/or increased bronchial markings. Peak flow (PF) monitoring is especially important for patients with moderate to severe asthma. PF meters are small, portable, and easy to use. They measure how fast a patient can forcibly expire air after a maximal inhalation; decreased readings indicate increased obstruction to airflow. PF readings can begin to fall hours or even days before symptoms become evident. Reductions to 50% to 80% of predicted values indicate a mild-to-moderate exacerbation; readings less than 30% predicted are associated with severe obstruction.

During acute exacerbations, the chest radiograph demonstrates significant hyperinflation and occasionally focal or subsegmental atelectasis (Fig. 20-1). CO_2 retention can occur with fatigue and may be quite dramatic; hypoxemia is usually less pronounced.

TREATMENT

With appropriate therapy and good compliance, most patients with mild intermittent asthma can remain symptom free with few exacerbations. The most effective form of treatment consists of removing inciting agents (triggers) from the child's environment.

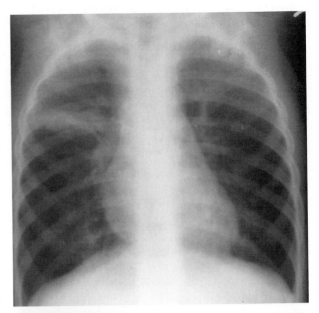
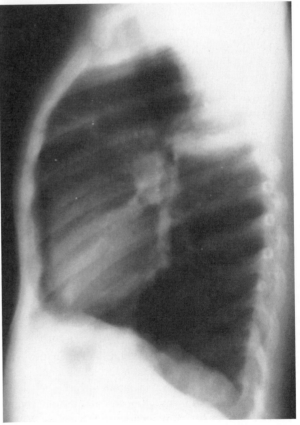

Figure 20-1 • Chest radiograph of a 3-year-old taken during an asthma exacerbation shows severe hyperinflation, increased anteroposterior diameter of the chest, a depressed diaphragm, and several areas of atelectasis.

Cigarette smoke should be strictly avoided. Limiting dust mite, mold, and pet exposure is beneficial to patients with an allergic component to their asthma.

The mainstays of medical maintenance therapy are **inhaled corticosteroids (ICS), β_2-agonists**, and **leukotriene receptor antagonists**. β_2-Agonists such as albuterol reduce smooth muscle constriction and can be administered via nebulization or metered-dose inhalation. Newer formulations of β_2-agonists such as levalbuterol offer a theoretical advantage with fewer side effects; however, research has yet to confirm this advantage. Longer-acting preparations (salbutamol, formoterol) are available for patients requiring daily β_2-agonist therapy. They may also be used in patients who require ICS therapy; the effect is additive, allowing for reduction of ICS dosing. β_2-agonists are effective in preventing exercise-induced asthma if used 15 to 30 minutes before vigorous activity. The abuse of bronchodilators may result in tolerance to their effects.

The introduction of ICS therapy has had a remarkable impact on the treatment of asthma. Aerosolized formulas are breathed directly into the lungs, with a substantial decrease in systemic side effects. Their use as a daily medication in persistent and severe asthma has become the standard of care. Increasing the dose of inhaled corticosteroids has become an important part of the initial response to an asthma exacerbation managed at home. Options include beclomethasone, budesonide, flunisolide, fluticasone, and triamcinolone. Concerns about possible growth suppression in children using daily inhaled corticosteroids have largely been put to rest. (Note: Early studies with beclomethasone, a first-generation inhaled corticosteroid, suggested small but measurable decreases in height growth. In long-term studies on second-generation steroids [budesonide and fluticasone], linear growth velocity declined initially but then rebounded, and all subjects obtained their expected adult height.) Oral steroid treatment is reserved for severe, persistent, poorly controlled RAD or acute exacerbations.

Leukotriene receptor antagonists (montelukast, zafirlukast, zileuton) are oral medications recommended for the treatment of chronic moderate to severe asthma and may allow some patients to reduce their dependence on β_2-agonist and daily inhaled steroid use. They are most effective in patients with exercise-induced asthma and asthma with a significant allergic component. Cromolyn sodium, another preventative medication, is being used less frequently since the advent of inhaled steroids. It works by stabilizing the mast cell membrane, preventing release of inflammatory mediators such as histamine. It is available in nebulized and metered-dose inhaler forms and is well tolerated, with no known adverse effects. It is not helpful during an acute attack but is a good form of prevention.

The use of theophylline, once a commonly prescribed oral bronchodilator, has fallen out of favor as a first-line treatment option. It has virtually no anti-inflammatory properties, is often poorly tolerated, and requires frequent drug-level monitoring. It is presently reserved for use as a chronic therapy in patients who do not respond to conventional medications.

Mild exacerbations are managed by the addition of short-acting inhaled bronchodilators to maintenance regimens. Additional steps may include doubling the dose of inhaled steroids for 7 to 10 days or initiating a 5-day pulse of oral steroids. Moderate to severe exacerbations usually require an emergency department visit, if not hospitalization.

Children who present to the emergency department in an acute asthma attack are initially assessed for airway patency and ability to aerate. Pulse oximetry measurement is a simple, rapid screen for hypoxemia. Patients in severe respiratory distress require ABG measurements to assess the need for supplemental oxygen and to recognize increasing $PaCO_2$, a sign of impending respiratory failure. A normal $PaCO_2$, in the face of tachypnea is an equally ominous sign because the $PaCO_2$ should be well below 40 with a rapid respiratory rate. Nebulized bronchodilators are administered continuously if needed. Subcutaneous epinephrine or terbutaline rapidly decreases airway reactivity. Corticosteroids, administered orally or intravenously, require 4 to 6 hours for a response but are indicated for treatment of inflammation and prevention of the late-phase response. Children who do not respond with complete resolution of symptoms after several hours (i.e., children in **status asthmaticus**) or those who require ongoing oxygen therapy should be hospitalized for continued treatment and close observation.

Despite advances in therapy, the mortality rate for asthma in children has continued to rise over the past two decades. Factors that increase the risk of death include noncompliance, poor recognition of symptoms, delay in treatment, history of intubation, black race, and steroid dependence.

20-2 KEY POINTS

1. The three main components of asthma are reversible airway obstruction, increased airway responsiveness (bronchospasm), and inflammation.
2. Disease severity is classified as mild intermittent, mild persistent, moderate persistent, and severe persistent.
3. Inhaled bronchodilators are the treatment of choice in an acute asthma exacerbation.
4. Inhaled corticosteroids and leukotriene inhibitors have improved symptom control for patients with moderate to severe asthma.
5. The disappearance of wheezing with increased respiratory distress signals increased obstruction rather than improvement.
6. The effects of oral or intravenous corticosteroids occur 4 to 6 hours after administration.

CYSTIC FIBROSIS

PATHOGENESIS

Cystic fibrosis (CF) is an inherited multisystem disease characterized by disordered exocrine gland function. The product of the cystic fibrosis transregulator (CFTR) gene is a cell membrane protein that functions as a cAMP-activated chloride channel on the epithelial cells of the respiratory tract, pancreas, sweat and salivary glands, intestines, and reproductive system. This channel is nonfunctional in patients with CF, so chloride remains sequestered inside the cell. Sodium and water are drawn into the cell to maintain ionic and osmotic balance, resulting in relative dehydration at the cell surface and abnormally viscid secretions. Other abnormalities resulting from the inactivity of this chloride channel include abnormal cell surface properties in the lung that facilitate binding of *Pseudomonas* and a decrease in nitrous oxide production, which mediates (decreases) inflammation and enhances bacterial killing.

EPIDEMIOLOGY

CF is acquired through **autosomal recessive** inheritance, with a disease frequency of 1 in 3,500 white births and 1 in 17,000 black births. The gene occurs with even lower frequency in other populations. More than 1,000 distinct gene mutations (mapped to a gene locus on chromosome 7) have been described;

70% of patients have the ΔF508 mutation. The median life expectancy is currently 33.4 years (in the United States) and has increased dramatically in the past decade.

CLINICAL MANIFESTATIONS

History and Physical Examination

Table 20-2 lists the most common presenting signs and symptoms of CF. All levels of the respiratory tract may be affected, including the nasal passages, sinuses, and lower airways. **Nasal polyps** in any pediatric patient should prompt further testing for CF. Opacification of the sinuses and sinusitis are extremely common. Mucus stasis and ineffective clearance lead to repeated bacterial colonization and frequent pneumonias. Typical early childhood pathogens include *Staphylococcus aureus* and *Haemophilus influenzae*. This is generally followed by colonization with *Pseudomonas aeruginosa* in late childhood and early adolescence. More than 90% of patients eventually acquire *P. aeruginosa*, and it is not eradicated. Colonization with *Burkholderia cepacia* is particularly ominous and associated with accelerated pulmonary deterioration and death.

Gastrointestinal manifestations include pancreatic insufficiency, bowel obstruction and rectal prolapse, diabetes, and hepatic cirrhosis. Interference with normal pancreatic enzyme secretion leads to decreased fat absorption; parents may notice that the child's stools are large, bulky, and foul smelling. Later, stool becomes extremely dense (rather than liquid), leading to possible distal intestinal obstruction. Failure to thrive is the most common manifestation of CF in infants and children. In the neonate, **meconium ileus** is virtually pathognomonic for CF.

DIAGNOSTIC EVALUATION

The classic diagnostic findings in CF include an elevated sweat chloride concentration, pancreatic insufficiency, and chronic pulmonary disease. Recurrent lower airway infection results in bronchiectasis, fibrosis, parenchymal loss, and the characteristic "bleb" formation found on chest radiographs (Fig. 20-2). Pulmonary function tests demonstrate mostly *obstructive* and some *restrictive* changes. The **sweat chloride level** remains the initial diagnostic test of choice. A level greater than 60 mEq per L is generally considered abnormal, but both false positives and false negatives occur, and occasionally a borderline test is hard to interpret. Genetic and prenatal testing are now available for the

TABLE 20-2 Clinical Manifestations of Cystic Fibrosis

Chronic Sinopulmonary Disease

Persistent colonization/infection with pathogens typical of CF lung disease, including:

Staphylococcus aureus

Pseudomonas aeruginosa (mucoid and nonmucoid)

Nontypeable *Haemophilus influenzae*

Burkholderia cepacia complex

Stenotrophomonas maltophilia

Endobronchial Disease Manifested by:

Cough and sputum production

Wheezing and air trapping

Radiographic abnormalities

Evidence of obstruction on PFTs

Digital clubbing

Chronic sinus disease:

    Nasal polyps

    Radiographic changes

Intestinal Abnormalities:

Meconium ileus

Exocrine pancreatic insufficiency

Distal intestinal obstruction

Rectal prolapse

Recurrent pancreatitis

Chronic hepatobiliary disease manifested by clinical and/or laboratory evidence of:

    Focal biliary cirrhosis

    Multilobular cirrhosis

Failure to thrive (protein–calorie malnutrition)

Hypoproteinemia–edema

Fat-soluble vitamin deficiencies

Genitourinary Abnormalities:

Obstructive azoospermia in males

Metabolic Abnormalities:

Salt-loss syndromes

Acute salt depletion

Chronic metabolic alkalosis

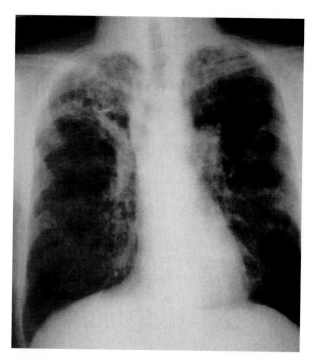

Figure 20-2 • Chest radiograph in this adolescent male with cystic fibrosis demonstrates marked chronic disease and bleb formation.

TREATMENT

Chest physical therapy, exercise, and frequent coughing are helpful in mobilizing secretions. Bronchodilators and anti-inflammatory medications relax smooth muscle walls, decrease airway reactivity, and curb tissue destruction. Recombinant human deoxyribonuclease, administered via nebulization, breaks down thick DNA complexes present in mucus as a result of cell destruction and bacterial infection. Alternate months of regular inhaled tobramycin may be indicated for patients infected with *Pseudomonas*. More recently azithromycin has proved effective as a possible immune modifier. Studies are underway to evaluate the use of anti-inflammatory drugs in CF to help preserve lung function.

Near-normal growth can often be achieved with pancreatic enzyme replacement, fat-soluble vitamin supplements, and high-calorie, high-protein diets. NG or gastrostomy tube feedings may be instituted if oral intake is inadequate. Children that maintain heights and weights above the 25th percentile have a better long-term prognosis.

Frequent disease exacerbations may be triggered by viral or bacterial infections and are treated by aggressive chest physical therapy, postural drainage, and antibiotics, which may be taken orally or inhaled if the exacerbation is mild and the organisms are

most common gene mutations, accounting for 85% of cases. A genotype with two abnormal alleles at the CFTR site confirms the diagnosis of CF.

not resistant. Usually, however, bacterial infections must be treated with an aminoglycoside (e.g., tobramycin) and a semisynthetic penicillin or cephalosporin, depending on organism sensitivities. Research aimed at the specific gene mutation is currently under way.

Prognosis continues to improve with aggressive treatment of pulmonary exacerbations and optimal nutritional support. Respiratory complications remain the major contributors to morbidity and mortality in CF.

Hemoptysis can be an alarming development that may occur during pulmonary exacerbations in long-standing disease. Frequent coughing and inflammation lead to erosion of the walls of bronchial arteries in areas of bronchiectasis, and expectorated sputum becomes streaked with blood. Frank blood loss of more than 500 mL in 24 hours (or more than 300 mL per day for 3 days) is considered an emergency, often treated by arterial embolization.

Spontaneous pneumothorax is another potentially life-threatening complication that may occur in CF. It is characterized by the sudden onset of severe chest pain and difficulty breathing. Placement of a chest tube results in rapid re-expansion, but approximately half of pneumothoraces recur unless sclerosis is performed. Sclerosis is avoided if at all possible because transplant becomes more difficult following this procedure.

Progressive obstruction and hypoxia in advanced disease can lead to chronic pulmonary hypertension and cor pulmonale. For CF patients with a life expectancy of 1 to 2 years, **lung transplantation** is a potentially viable option.

20-3 KEY POINTS

1. Cystic fibrosis (CF) is a disorder of exocrine gland function, affecting the lungs, sinuses, pancreas, sweat and salivary glands, intestines, and reproductive system.
2. Inheritance is autosomal recessive.
3. The disease is far more prevalent in whites than in other races.
4. Failure to thrive is the most common presentation of CF in children.
5. Meconium ileus in the neonate is virtually pathognomonic for CF.
6. Diagnosis is made by an elevated sweat chloride level in the presence of pulmonary disease/pancreatic insufficiency *or* by a genotype with two abnormal CFTR alleles.
7. Hemoptysis and spontaneous pneumothorax are two acute life-threatening complications of CF.

APNEA OF INFANCY

Apnea is defined as the cessation of breathing for longer than 20 seconds or pauses of any duration associated with color changes (cyanosis, pallor), hypotonia, decreased responsiveness, or bradycardia. It may be central (neurally mediated), obstructive, or mixed. Apnea is not a diagnosis but a potentially dangerous symptom, requiring aggressive workup to determine and treat the underlying cause. In contrast to apnea of prematurity, apnea of infancy occurs in full-term infants. Table 20-3 lists some of the potential causes.

■ **TABLE 20-3** Apnea of Infancy/Apparent Life-Threatening Events

Cause	Helpful Diagnostic Tests
Infectious	
Sepsis	CBC/Blood culture
Meningitis	LP
Pneumonia	Chest radiograph
Bronchiolitis (RSV)	RSV antigen test in season
Pertussis	PCR or fluorescent antibody staining
Neurologic	
Seizures	EEG
Central apnea	Polysomnography
Intraventricular hemorrhage	Cranial US
Respiratory	
Airway obstruction	Airway radiographs or bronchoscopy
Aspiration	Swallowing study
Cardiac	
Arrhythmias	ECG
Gastrointestinal	
Gastroesophageal reflux	Barium swallow or pH probe
Other	
Metabolic disorders	Tests for inborn errors of metabolism
Electrolyte disorders	Electrolyte panel/blood glucose
Abuse	Skeletal survey/funduscopic exam

CLINICAL MANIFESTATIONS AND DIAGNOSTIC EVALUATION

Apnea of infancy may come to medical attention after an **apparent life-threatening event (ALTE)**. ALTEs are very frightening to the caretaker; the infant either stops breathing or is found apneic and may be cyanotic or pale, hypotonic, difficult to rouse, or choking and gagging. The observer often believes that the child would have died without intervention (vigorous stimulation, cardiopulmonary resuscitation).

The goal of the diagnostic workup is to identify or rule out any life-threatening, treatable causes. Table 20-3 lists potential tests to be considered depending on the results of the history and physical examination. In approximately half the cases of apnea of infancy, no predisposing condition is ever found.

TREATMENT

Management involves treating the underlying disorder. When no treatable cause can be found, the infant may be placed on a home monitor that senses chest movement (breathing) and heart rate and sounds an alarm when the child becomes apneic or bradycardic. Apnea of infancy does not raise an infant's risk of dying of SIDS, which may be why home monitors have never been proven to decrease the likelihood of SIDS.

🔑 20-4 KEY POINTS

1. Apnea is a symptom, not a diagnosis.
2. Apnea of infancy does not increase the risk of SIDS, and home apnea monitors do not decrease the risk of SIDS.

RESTRICTIVE LUNG DISEASE

Restrictive lung diseases cause a decrease in most measurements of lung volume, including functional residual capacity, tidal volume, and vital capacity.

CHEST WALL ABNORMALITIES

Pectus excavatum refers to a depression in the sternum, and **pectus carinatum** refers to an outward deformity. Severe congenital forms of these malformations may result in restrictive lung disease as a result of mechanical interference with normal respiration.

Severe scoliosis can have the same effect. Marked obesity, in addition to being a risk for upper airway obstructive disease, may also be a cause of restrictive lung disease. Neuromuscular's disease may result in restrictive lung disease as a consequence of insufficient respiratory muscle strength (Guillain-Barré's syndrome, DMD).

SPACE-OCCUPYING LESIONS

Any lesion that occupies intrathoracic space will interfere with normal pulmonary expansion if large enough. Pleural effusion, pericardial effusion, chylothorax, hemothorax, pneumothorax, chest wall tumors, mediastinal masses, cystic adenomatous malformations, diaphragmatic hernias, and pulmonary sequestrations may all compete with normal lung for thoracic space.

INTERSTITIAL LUNG DISEASE

Recurrent aspiration typically leads to interstitial lung disease but may also result in obstructive lung disease. Acute chest syndrome in sickle cell disease is discussed in Chapter 10. A number of rare diseases can lead to interstitial changes, including chronic interstitial lung disease, desquamative interstitial pneumonitis, and sarcoidosis. **Pulmonary hemosiderosis** involves an abnormal accumulation of hemosiderin in the lungs as a result of diffuse alveolar hemorrhage. It may be associated with cow milk allergy in infants or Goodpasture syndrome in older children. Diagnosis is based on the presence of hemosiderin-laden macrophages (siderophages) in bronchial washings or gastric aspirates.

CLINICAL MANIFESTATIONS

Symptoms of restrictive lung disease typically reflect limited pulmonary reserve. Exercise intolerance, dyspnea, and shortness of breath are hallmarks. Space-occupying lesions can be detected by chest auscultation (noting decreased breath sounds over the affected area) and may be seen on chest radiograph or echocardiogram. The chronic nature of many restrictive lesions can put patients at risk for developing symptomatology of prolonged respiratory insufficiency. Pulmonary hypertension may develop and be detected by an accentuated second heart sound on exam. Clubbing of fingers and toes may be noted. Clinical manifestations of pulmonary hemosiderosis include hemoptysis/hematemesis and a microcytic hypochromic anemia.

VENTILATION-PERFUSION ABNORMALITIES

An important concept in many diseases affecting the respiratory system is ventilation and perfusion matching. Alveoli that are actively involved in respiration need to have adequate perfusion by local capillary blood flow. This is closely regulated by a number of local mediators. Most important, the arterioles that supply the alveolar capillaries are exquisitely sensitive to oxygen tension. When ventilation to an area of lung is compromised, local oxygen tension is reduced. As a result, the arterioles constrict, and blood is diverted to areas of lung engaged in active ventilation. When this system is disrupted, hypoxemia results. Conditions associated with diffusion defects include pulmonary embolus, some congenital vascular abnormalities, and prolonged atelectasis.

Additional Suggested Reading

Farrell PA, Weiner GM, Lemons JA. SIDS, ALTE, apnea, and the use of home monitors. *Pediatr Rev.* 2002;23:3–9.

Guill MF. Asthma update: epidemiology and pathophysiology. *Pediatr Rev.* 2004;25:299–305.

Guill MF. Asthma update: clinical aspects and management. *Pediatr Rev.* 2004;25:335–344.

Matiz AM, Roman EA. In brief: apnea. *Pediatr Rev.* 2003;24:32–34.

National Asthma Education and Prevention Program (United States Department of Health and Human Services). *Expert report: guidelines for the diagnosis and management of asthma. updated selected topics,* 2002.

Adolescent Medicine

Puberty is defined as the process of hormonal and physical changes whereby the body of a child matures into that of an adult, physiologically capable of sexual reproduction. **Adolescence**, in contrast, encompasses the physical changes of puberty as well as the cognitive, social, and psychological changes that mark the transition from youth to maturity. Some references further subdivide adolescence into an *early* period (middle school, 10 to 13 years of age); a *middle* period (high school, 14 to 17 years of age); and a *late* period (18 to 21 years of age). The psychosocial developmental tasks of adolescence may result in testing authority (to define the self and establish autonomy), high-risk behavior (because of poor impulse control, a preference for instant gratification, and a sense of immortality), and preoccupation with body image (related to the need to be attractive to peers).

Although adolescents are less likely than their younger counterparts to make use of health maintenance visits, regular contact with a primary care physician is particularly important for this age group because many of the diseases and injuries that occur in adolescence result from lifestyle choices that increase the risk of morbidity and mortality. Such behaviors include high-risk sexual activity, eating disorders, substance use and abuse, and actions resulting in accidental or intentional injury.

THE ADOLESCENT OFFICE VISIT

Observing the parent-and-child interaction is informative, and the parent should be encouraged to raise any concerns with the physician. However, it is important that *the majority of the interview and examination take place without the parent present*. Many adolescents will not be forthright about health-related issues when they believe their parents may find out about their responses. Although virtually all states mandate the reporting of suspected abuse, potential harm (violence or suicide), and certain infectious diseases (including some sexually transmitted diseases [STDs]), most also provide for **confidentiality** of information related to sexual activity and substance abuse. Some states allow all adolescents access to medical care without their parents' knowledge; in other states, only emancipated minors are permitted this right. Emergency treatment should never be withheld pending parental notification or approval.

Although studies show that adolescents are willing to discuss high-risk behaviors and preventative care issues with their physicians, most are uncomfortable initiating these conversations themselves. The acronym HEADSS (Table 21-1) is helpful in identifying pertinent areas in the adolescent social history. A nonjudgmental, indirect, empathetic method of questioning may be more effective in eliciting truthful answers.

Height, weight, and blood pressure should be recorded at every well care visit or at least every 2 years. Other recommended procedures include a hearing screen (once during adolescence), a vision screen (every 2 years), and hemoglobin/hematocrit and routine UA (at least once during adolescence). Tuberculosis testing and lipid screening are appropriate in some higher risk populations. The recommended examination and laboratory screening for sexually active patients is discussed in the following section.

Table 12-1 lists the immunizations recommended during adolescence.

TABLE 21-1 The Adolescent Psychosocial History: HEADSS[a]

Home (family members, relationships, and living arrangements)

Education (academic performance/educational goals)

Activities (peer relationships, work, and recreational activities)

Drugs (substance use/abuse, including tobacco, alcohol, steroids, inhalants, and illicit drugs)

Sexuality (dating, sexual activity, contraception, sexual orientation)

Suicide (depression, anxiety, other mental health concerns)

[a]Some experts suggest that a second "E" should be added to remind physicians to screen for behaviors associated with eating disorders, and that a third "S" should be included to prompt questions concerning safety (the potential for abuse or violent behavior [e.g., gang membership, owning a firearm]).

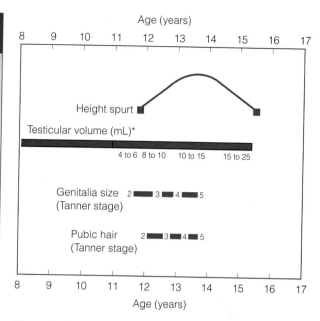

Figure 21-1 • Sequence of pubertal events in the average (American) boy.

🔑 21-1 KEY POINTS

1. It is important to know and understand state laws regarding access to care and confidentiality in the adolescent population. Emergency services should not be delayed or denied pending parental notification.
2. The acronym HEADSS denotes areas of the adolescent social history, which may identify issues and behaviors that are directly related to the patient's health and quality of life.
3. It is recommended that adolescents receive a hearing screen, UA, and hemoglobin/hematocrit at least once during adolescence, and height, weight, blood pressure, and vision screening at least every other year.

SEXUAL DEVELOPMENT/ REPRODUCTIVE HEALTH

As mentioned, **puberty** refers to those biologic changes that lead to reproductive capability. The events of puberty occur in a predictable sequence, but the timing of the initiation and the velocity of the changes are highly variable among individuals. The integration of the pubertal changes into the adolescent's self-concept is crucial to normal adolescence.

In boys, the initiation sequence of sexual development is testicular enlargement, followed by penile enlargement, height growth spurt, and pubic hair. This progression is shown in Figure 21-1.

In girls, the order of pubertal events in sexual development is thelarche (breast buds), followed by height growth spurt, pubic hair, and menarche. Figure 21-2 illustrates these changes.

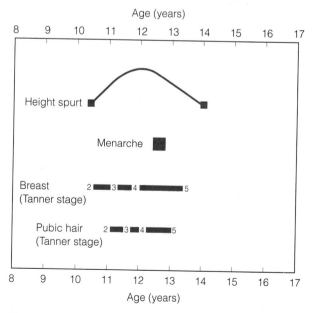

Figure 21-2 • Sequence of pubertal events in the average (American) girl.

The **Tanner staging system** is used to determine where a child is in the pubertal process. Table 21-2 shows the Tanner stages for the male genitalia, female breasts, and male and female pubic hair. Pubertal abnormalities are addressed in Chapter 6.

Preventative health care for sexually active adolescents includes additional elements on physical examination and laboratory screening. Annual pelvic exams are recommended for all sexually active young women. (Note: There is some debate about whether all women older than 18 years warrant annual pelvic exams as well.) Screening labs include Papanicolaou smear, cervical gonorrhea and chlamydia studies, and a wet mount of vaginal fluids. Adolescent males who are sexually active should have leukocyte esterase testing performed on first-void urine and should be offered urethral or urine-based nucleic acid amplification testing for gonorrhea and chlamydia. Screening for young men who report same-gender sexual contact includes anal and pharyngeal cultures for STDs as well as hepatitis B serology. Patients with evidence of an STD and/or self-report of high-risk behaviors should be offered contraception counseling and testing for syphilis and HIV.

■ TABLE 21-2 Secondary Sex Characteristics: Tanner

Breast development (females)

Stage I	Preadolescent; elevation of papilla only
Stage II	Breast bud; elevation of breast and papilla as small mound; enlargement of areolar diameter (11.15 ± 1.10)
Stage III	Further enlargement and elevation of breast and areola; no separation of their contours (12.15 ± 1.09)
Stage IV	Projection of areola and papilla to form secondary mound above level of breast (13.11 ± 1.15)
Stage V	Mature stage; projection of papilla only because of recession of areola to general contour of breast (15.33 ± 1.74)

NOTE: Stages IV and V may not be distinct in some patients.

Genital development (male)

Stage I	Preadolescent; testes, scrotum, and penis approximately same size and proportion as in early childhood
Stage II	Enlargement of scrotum and testes, skin of scrotum reddens and changes in texture; little or no enlargement of penis (11.64 ± 1.07)
Stage III	Enlargement of penis, first mainly in length; further growth of testes and scrotum (12.85 ± 1.04)
Stage IV	Increased size of penis with growth in breadth and development of glans; further enlargement of testes and scrotum and increased darkening of scrotal skin (13.77 ± 1.02)
Stage V	Genitalia adult in size and shape (14.92 ± 1.10)

Pubic hair (male and female)

Stage I	Preadolescent; vellus over pubes no further developed than that over abdominal wall (i.e., no pubic hair)
Stage II	Sparse growth of long, slightly pigmented downy hair, straight or only slightly curled, chiefly at base of penis or along labia (male: 13.44 ± 1.09; female: 11.69 ± 1.21)
Stage III	Considerably darker, coarser and more curled; hair spreads sparsely over junction of pubes (male: 13.9 ± 1.04; female: 12.36 ± 1.10)
Stage IV	Hair resembles adult in type; distribution still considerably smaller than in adult. No spread to medial surface of thighs (male: 14.36 ± 1.08; female: 12.95 ± 1.06)
Stage V	Adult in quantity and type with distribution of the horizontal pattern (male: 15.18 ± 1.07; female: 14.41 ± 1.12)
Stage VI	Spread up linea alba: "male escutcheon"

🔧 21-2 KEY POINTS

1. In boys, the initiation sequence of sexual development is testicular enlargement, followed by penile enlargement, height growth spurt, and pubic hair.
2. In girls, the order of pubertal events in sexual development is thelarche (breast buds), followed by height growth spurt, pubic hair, and menarche.
3. Annual pelvic exams are recommended for all sexually active young women. Adolescent males who are sexually active should be offered testing for gonorrhea and chlamydia.

EATING DISORDERS

PATHOGENESIS

Anorexia nervosa is an eating disorder characterized by impaired body image and intense fear of weight gain, culminating in the refusal to maintain a minimum normal body weight for age and height. External or internal psychological and/or social stressors superimposed on an inherited vulnerability lead to the development of anorexia.

Binge eating, followed by some compensatory behavior to rid the body of the ingested calories, is the hallmark of **bulimia nervosa**. Patients may purge (induce vomiting or take laxatives) or use other methods (fasting, intense exercise). Bulimics are usually aware that their behavior is abnormal.

EPIDEMIOLOGY

About 1 in 200 adolescent females meets the criteria for anorexia. Bulimia is more common, affecting 1% to 3% of young women. Approximately 10% of patients with eating disorders are male.

RISK FACTORS

Risk factors for eating disorders include positive family history and female gender. Both anorexia and bulimia are more common in whites. Personality risk factors associated with anorexia nervosa include intense preoccupation with appearance, low self-esteem, and obsessive traits.

CLINICAL MANIFESTATIONS

History

Patients with anorexia may present with secondary amenorrhea, constipation, syncope, upper or lower GI discomfort, and/or periodic episodes of cold, mottled hands and feet. If the chief complaint is weight loss, this invariably comes from the parents rather than the adolescent. Bulimia does not usually produce specific symptoms, although these patients are significantly more likely than their peers to suffer from major depression. Patients may be brought to the physician because they have been caught purging or because someone else has reported their behavior.

Physical Examination

Adolescents who suffer from anorexia are severely underweight (usually with a body mass index <17) and may appear cachectic. Vital signs often reveal hypothermia, bradycardia, and orthostasis or hypotension. The skin may be dry, yellowish, and hyperkeratotic. Thinning of scalp hair, increased lanugo hair, cool extremities, and nail pitting are additional signs. An estimated 30% to 40% of patients have a cardiac murmur consistent with mitral valve prolapse.

Patients with bulimia may be of normal weight or slightly overweight. Frequent self-induced vomiting (if present) results in calluses on the backs of the knuckles, eroded tooth enamel, and parotid gland enlargement.

DIFFERENTIAL DIAGNOSIS

Adolescents who participate in certain athletic activities (ballet, wrestling, gymnastics) in which weight gain is thought to negatively impact performance may manifest some of the behaviors associated with eating disorders such as purging and severe calorie restriction. However, most of these elite athletes have a normal body image.

The marked weight loss seen with anorexia may cause the clinician to consider malignancy, inflammatory bowel disease or malabsorption syndromes, and other chronic diseases (infections, endocrine disorders). The differential diagnosis for vomiting (bulimia) is discussed in Chapter 8.

DIAGNOSTIC EVALUATION

Anorexia and bulimia are both clinical diagnoses. Laboratory studies are used to assess the need for specific medical intervention rather than to confirm the disease. Table 21-3 lists diagnostic tests used to rule out or quantify certain conditions associated with anorexia and bulimia.

TABLE 21-3 Suggested Laboratory Tests for Adolescents with Eating Disorders

Study	Suspected Result
All patients:	
CBC	Neutropenia; also anemia and thrombocytopenia
Serum electrolytes	Hypokalemia/alkalosis (if purging)
	Hyponatremia (caused by manipulation of water intake)
BUN/creatinine	Increased BUN
Glucose	Normal or low
Calcium/ phosphate/ magnesium	Normal or low
ECG	Bradycardia, T-wave inversions, ST depression (anorexia)
	Prolonged QTc interval (bulimia, if hypokalemic)
Patients with anorexia:	
ESR[a]	Normal or low
UA	Decreased specific gravity
LFTs	Elevated
Cholesterol	Elevated
Serum protein/ albumin	Low
TSH/T$_4$[a]	Normal/normal to low
Bone density scan	Osteopenia (if amenorrheic >6 mo)
Patients with bulimia:	
Serum amylase	Elevated if vomiting

[a]Useful for ruling out other conditions in the differential.

TABLE 21-4 Anorexia and Bulimia: Indications for Hospitalization

Both conditions:

Failure to improve with outpatient therapy

Hypokalemia (serum potassium <3.2 mmol/L)

Hypochloremia (serum chloride <88 mmol/L)

Cardiac arrhythmias/prolonged QTc interval/bradycardia

Medical complications requiring inpatient intervention

Anorexia

Unstable vital signs

Severe weight loss

Need for enteral nutrition (food refusal)

Arrested pubertal development

TREATMENT

The treatment for eating disorders is multifactorial and includes nutritional support, behavioral therapy and psychotherapy, and correction of any medical complications resulting from the severe weight loss or purging. Table 21-4 notes the indications for hospitalization/inpatient therapy. Research is ongoing as to whether psychotropic medicines (particularly selective serotonin reuptake inhibitors) are useful in the treatment of these diseases. Full recovery can take up to several years and is more common in adolescents with bulimia. Published mortality rates for anorexia range as high as 4%.

21-3 KEY POINTS

1. Anorexia nervosa is an eating disorder characterized by severe weight loss, impaired body image, and intense fear of weight gain.
2. Bulimia nervosa involves binge eating followed by some compensatory behavior to rid the body of the ingested calories.
3. Mitral valve prolapse is not uncommon in patients with anorexia nervosa.
4. Eating disorders are clinical diagnoses. Certain characteristics of the history and physical examination and laboratory data may indicate the need for inpatient treatment.

SUBSTANCE USE AND ABUSE

Drug **use** is defined as the intentional use of any substance that results in alteration of the physical, psychological, cognitive, or mood state of the individual despite the potential for personal harm. Patients become addicted when they begin to **abuse** the drug in a compulsive, dependent manner despite significant functional impairment. This addiction may result from actual *physical dependence* (physiologic symptoms of withdrawal when the drug is removed) or *psychological dependence*. Table 21-5 details the effects of intoxication with alcohol and several other substances which may be used and abused by the adolescent.

EPIDEMIOLOGY

Unfortunately, substance use among adolescents is not uncommon. Estimates (based on anonymous self-reports) are that approximately half of 18-year-olds have tried an illegal drug. One in three has used an illicit drug other than marijuana. At least 30% admit to binge drinking within the previous month. One in four high school students reports daily tobacco use.

RISK FACTORS

Table 21-6 lists the risk factors and protective factors related to substance use in adolescents.

CLINICAL MANIFESTATIONS

The clinical manifestations of acute intoxication with the substances of interest are listed in Table 21-5, along with specific treatments for each drug.

All adolescents should be questioned at every maintenance visit regarding tobacco, alcohol, and substance use.

DIAGNOSTIC EVALUATION

Although drug testing is easily available through most laboratories, testing an adolescent at the request of the parents without the patient's knowledge is generally discouraged. Attempts should be made to involve the suspected user in the discussion and obtain consent for any recommended diagnostic studies.

MANAGEMENT

Patients suspected of drug/alcohol dependence should be referred to an addiction specialist and may require intensive inpatient or outpatient therapy. Adolescents who admit to tobacco use must be encouraged to stop. If the patient is interested in quitting, nicotine replacement therapy ("the patch," gums, etc.) should be offered. Some adolescents may require more intensive behavioral therapy or bupropion.

🔑 21-4 KEY POINTS

1. Addiction is defined as the habitual, compulsive use of a drug despite significant functional impairment and undesirable consequences.
2. Patients who are smokers should be encouraged to quit at each health visit. Those who express interest in doing so should be offered replacement therapy, behavioral therapy, social support, and in some cases bupropion.

VIOLENCE IN THE ADOLESCENT POPULATION

EPIDEMIOLOGY

Traumatic injury is the leading cause of death in the adolescent population (Chapter 2). Homicide and suicide are second and third on this list, respectively. Adolescents may be victims of violence, perpetrators of violence against others, and/or intentionally harmful to themselves.

RISK FACTORS

Individual risk factors for violent behavior include previous arrest for juvenile crime, early exposure to violence (firsthand and in the media), being a victim of abuse, and drug and alcohol use. Although young women are more likely than young men to experience sexual abuse, adolescent males are far more likely to be the victims and perpetrators of violent acts. Other factors associated with an increased likelihood of violent behavior include low socioeconomic status and easy access to guns.

The strongest risk factor associated with attempted suicide is **a prior attempt**. Other factors that increase the likelihood of attempted suicide include an existing psychiatric disorder (depression, etc.), substance abuse, a history of being abused, a family history of a major affective disorder and/or suicide, and a recent

■ TABLE 21-5 Clinical Manifestations and Managements of Drug Intoxication in Adolescents

Substance	Symptoms of Acute Use	Signs of Acute Use	Specific Treatment
Alcohol	Decreased inhibition, impaired coordination, poor judgment; progressing to slurred speech, ataxia, confusion, coma, and respiratory depression	Nausea/vomiting, flushed skin, sluggish pupils, decreased reflexes, hypoglycemia	Respiratory support; gastric lavage/charcoal; thiamine, glucose administration as indicated
Marijuana	Euphoria, relaxation, impaired cognition; progressing to mood instability and hallucinations	Drowsiness, slowed reaction times, tachycardia, orthostatic hypotension, injected conjunctiva, dry mouth	Benzodiazepines if severe agitation present
MDMA (Ecstasy)	Sense of happiness, enhanced well-being; progression to agitation, confusion, shock	Hyperthermia, hypertension, tachycardia, tachypnea, dilated pupils, agitation, hyponatremia	Activated charcoal; benzodiazepines for agitation/hypertension; fluid and electrolyte management; cooling blanket if needed
Cocaine/amphetamines	Elation, increased alertness, insomnia, anxiety; progressing to delirium, chest pain, psychosis, seizures, coma	Delirium, hyperthermia, tachycardia, hypertension, dilated pupils, hyperreflexia, tremor	Benzodiazepines/haloperidol; cooling blanket if needed; treatment for hypertension, arrhythmias as indicated[a]
Phencyclidine (PCP)	Euphoria or anxiety, impaired cognition, ataxia, hallucinations; progressing to psychosis, respiratory depression, coma, death	Restlessness, labile affect, hyperthermia, tachycardia, hypertension, flushing, nystagmus, small pupils, impaired coordination, seizures	Respiratory support, gastric lavage/charcoal, benzodiazepines/ haloperidol, treatment of hypertension, seizures if indicated
Hallucinogens (including LSD)	Euphoria, increased alertness; progressing to nausea, anxiety, paranoia, hallucinations, seizures, coma	Restlessness, labile affect, hyperthermia, tachycardia, hypertension, flushing, dilated pupils with injected conjunctiva, hyperreflexia	"Talking down" in a calm environment with minimal stimulation; benzodiazepines; cooling blanket if hyperthermic; treatment of hypertension, seizures as indicated
Heroin	Euphoria followed by sedation, impaired cognition, nausea/vomiting, stupor, respiratory depression, coma	Altered (depressed) mental status, hypothermia, decreased respiratory rate, hypotension; pinpoint, unresponsive pupils	Cardiorespiratory support; gastric lavage, charcoal (if ingested); naloxone
Inhalants	Euphoria, impaired judgment; progressing to hallucinations, psychosis, seizures, coma	Agitation or stupor, slurred speech, nystagmus/eye watering, rhinorrhea, increased salivation	Cardiorespiratory support if needed

[a]Lidocaine should not be used to treat arrhythmias in patients with cocaine intoxication because it can precipitate seizures in this population.

life stressor. *Adolescents who live in a home with a firearm have a tenfold greater risk of suicide than their peers.*

CLINICAL MANIFESTATIONS

Physicians and other health care personnel who interact regularly with adolescents are in a position to question them about whether they feel safe and whether they have witnessed or been the victims of aggression. Asking how patients deal with anger, if they have ever been in a fight, and whether there is a gun in the home may also open avenues of discussion. All adolescent patients should be subjected to screening questions for depression (sadness, despair, hopelessness)

TABLE 21-6 Risk Factors for Substance Use

Illicit drugs

Genetic predisposition (for addiction)

Use of drugs by family and friends

Easy access to drugs

Low levels of parental involvement and support

Poverty

Academic failure

Alcohol

Genetic predisposition (for alcoholism)

Use and abuse of alcohol by parents, peers

Low levels of parental involvement

Tobacco

Parental smoking and tobacco use

Easy access to cigarettes, other tobacco products

No restrictions on smoking in the home

Protective factors

Stable home environment

Parental supervision

Membership in positive social organizations

Academic achievement

Association with abstinent peers

MANAGEMENT

Encouraging parents to limit exposure to violence in media should be part of preventive health counseling beginning by the toddler years. Securing mental health services for the affected adolescent (and social services for the family) may provide the support needed to make the transition to a productive adulthood and avoid involvement with the juvenile justice system.

As previously mentioned, doctor–patient confidentiality does not extend to information that suggests the potential for immediate harm. Any patient who attempts suicide, even if the attempt is interpreted as merely a "gesture," should be hospitalized and undergo psychiatric evaluation.

21-5 KEY POINTS

1. Traumatic injury is the leading cause of death in the adolescent population.
2. The strongest risk factor associated with attempted suicide is a prior attempt.
3. Adolescents who live in a home with a firearm have a tenfold greater risk of suicide than their peers.
4. Any patient who attempts suicide should be hospitalized and undergo psychiatric evaluation.

and, if these are positive, suicidal ideation. Those patients who admit to having a plan for suicide are at particular risk.

Additional Suggested Reading

Anderson SL, Schaechter J, Brosco JP. Adolescent patients and their confidentiality: staying within legal bounds. *Contemp Pediatr.* 2005;22:143–152.

Barangan CJ, Alderman EM. Management of substance abuse. *Pediatr Rev.* 2002;23:123–131.

Goldenring JM, Rosen DS. Getting into adolescent heads: an essential update. *Contemp Pediatr.* 2004;21:64–90.

Hatcher-Kay C, King CA. Depression and suicide. *Pediatr Rev.* 2003;24:363–371.

Klein JD, Camenga DR. Tobacco prevention and cessation in pediatric patients. *Pediatr Rev.* 2004; 25:17–26.

Sieving RE, Oliphant JA, Blum RW. Adolescent sexual behavior and sexual health. *Pediatr Rev.* 2002; 23:407–416.

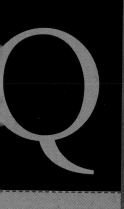

Questions

1. Trisomy 21 is associated with:
   a. malrotation
   b. endocardial cushion defects
   c. cleft palate
   d. renal disease
   e. sensorineural hearing loss

2. An adolescent comes to you with a chief complaint of painless urethral discharge. You note normal enlargement of the penis with a well-developed glans, enlarged testes with reddened, textured skin over the scrotum, and pubic hair of adult texture and color with no spread to the medial surface of the thighs. This patient's examination is most consistent with which Tanner stage of development?
   a. stage I
   b. stage II
   c. stage III
   d. stage IV
   e. stage V

3. Which of the following history and injury patterns is most likely to be the result of child abuse?
   a. A toddler with widespread splash burns and a history of being placed in bath water that was too hot.
   b. A 4-year-old with a spiral fracture of the femur and a history of a bike accident in which his lower leg was wedged in between the frame and the pedal.
   c. An infant with a scalp contusion and a history of falling off a counter onto a wood floor.
   d. A 10-month-old with posterior rib fractures in various stages of healing and a history of falling down the stairs.
   e. A 20-month-old who presents with acute acetaminophen ingestion.

4. Which of the following statements about neuroblastoma is *true*?
   a. Neuroblastoma is a benign tumor of the neural crest cells that form the adrenal cortex and the paraspinal parasympathetic ganglion.
   b. The majority of neuroblastoma tumors occur in the thoracic cavity.
   c. Neuroblastoma is the most common malignant tumor in infancy.
   d. In neuroblastoma of the abdomen, displacement of the kidney and distortion of the calyceal system often occur.
   e. Most patients are treated with surgery alone because distant metastases are rare.

5. A 5-year-old boy is brought to your office complaining of progressive fatigue, weakness, and nausea over the past few months. He was a model student, but he is now having trouble in school and displaying frequent outbursts, the last of which resulted in him being sent home for hitting another child. Initial laboratory results show mild hypoglycemia, hyponatremia, and hyperkalemia. The child is diagnosed with adrenal insufficiency and treated appropriately; however, his behavior continues to worsen, and he begins to have difficulty walking and speaking. Which of the following is the most likely etiology of his behavior problems?
   a. Tay-Sachs disease
   b. Gaucher disease
   c. Niemann-Pick disease
   d. adrenoleukodystrophy
   e. Rett syndrome

6. The laboratory workup of a 7-year-old patient with a chief complaint of decreased growth velocity reveals hyperchloremic metabolic acidosis with a normal anion gap and a urine pH of 5.0. Which of the following is the most useful test in distinguishing which type of renal tubular acidosis she is likely to have?
   a. serum potassium
   b. serum chloride
   c. serum sodium
   d. urine chloride
   e. urine sodium

7. Peripheral pulmonic stenosis, atrial septal defect, ventricular septal defect, chorioretinitis, hepatosplenomegaly, jaundice, and "blueberry muffin spots" are the clinical manifestations typically associated with which congenital infection?
   a. toxoplasmosis
   b. syphilis
   c. rubella
   d. cytomegalovirus
   e. herpes simplex virus 2
   f. HIV

8. A child in the emergency department has point tenderness over the proximal tibia and an appropriate history of trauma. The radiograph shows a fracture through the growth plate that extends into the epiphysis and joint space. This type of fracture would be characterized as:
   a. Salter-Harris type I
   b. Salter-Harris type II
   c. Salter-Harris type III
   d. Salter-Harris type IV
   e. Salter-Harris type V

9. An overweight 7-year-old presents for laboratory assessment prior to beginning an intense treatment program including dietary modification, regular physical activity, and behavior modification. Which of the following clinical values is not part of the metabolic syndrome X?
   a. body mass index >95th percentile for age
   b. a mutation in prohormone convertase I
   c. elevated blood pressure on three separate occasions
   d. increased low-density lipoprotein levels
   e. glucose resistance, suggested by a low fasting glucose-to-insulin ratio

10. What is the most significant serious complication arising from Kawasaki disease?
    a. coronary aneurysms
    b. kidney failure
    c. arthritis
    d. GI bleeding
    e. hypertension

11. A 1,500-g 29-week-old Asian male neonate was born prematurely to a 28-year-old Gravida 2, Para1 (G2P1001) serology-negative woman by normal spontaneous vaginal delivery. Apgar scores were 5 and 7 at 1 and 5 minutes, respectively. The neonate is in significant respiratory distress, with poor air movement. The neonate is intubated, given surfactant, and taken to the newborn intensive care unit (NICU) for further management. A blood culture is sent soon after arrival in the NICU. No abnormalities are noted on CSF evaluation. Ampicillin and gentamicin are started empirically until the blood culture result is known. Over the next

12 hours, the child is noted to have poor perfusion, hypotension, decreased urine output, coagulation tests consistent with DIC, and bilateral pulmonary infiltrates. Results of maternal vaginal and rectal cultures for group B streptococci are unknown. Which of the following bacteria is most likely to be responsible for the child's sepsis?
   a. group B streptococci
   b. *Streptococcus pneumoniae*
   c. *Chlamydia trachomatis*
   d. *Staphylococcus epidermis*
   e. *Staphylococcus aureus*

12. No red reflex is seen on funduscopic examination of a newborn. Which of the following is the most likely diagnosis?
    a. retinoblastoma
    b. leukocoria
    c. congenital cataract
    d. congenital glaucoma
    e. toxocariasis

13. An 18-month-old toddler is referred in by the local poison center after ingesting an unknown but "significant" amount of his father's amitriptyline (Elavil) within the last 2 hours. The child arrives awake, alert, and in no distress. Vital signs are stable. An ECG is obtained prior to initiating activated charcoal. Which of the following results are specific for tricyclic antidepressant ingestion and, if present, increase the risk of cardiac arrhythmias?
    a. premature atrial beats
    b. premature ventricular contractions
    c. small spiked P waves in leads II and III
    d. shortened PR interval
    e. QRS widening (duration >160 msec)

14. Which of the following medication groupings is most appropriate for a patient older than 5 years with moderate persistent asthma?
    a. none
    b. a daily low-dose inhaled corticosteroid
    c. a daily medium-dose inhaled corticosteroid and a long-acting inhaled β_2-agonist
    d. a daily medium-dose inhaled corticosteroid and theophylline
    e. a daily medium-dose inhaled corticosteroid and nedocromil

15. A 3-year-old boy presents to the pediatrician with fever, pallor, anorexia, joint pain, petechiae, and hepatosplenomegaly. Which of the following is the *most* likely diagnosis?
    a. acute lymphoblastic leukemia
    b. acute myelogenous leukemia
    c. juvenile chronic myelogenous leukemia
    d. aplastic anemia
    e. osteosarcoma

16. A neonate born at 28 weeks' gestation is now 2 weeks of age. Nasogastric feeds are started. Forty-eight hours after starting feeds, the neonate develops a distended abdomen, bloody stool, pneumatosis intestinalis, and free air on abdominal radiograph. Laboratory studies reveal thrombocytopenia. The child becomes persistently hypotensive despite maximal medical therapy. The most likely diagnosis is:
    a. sepsis
    b. aspiration pneumonia
    c. malrotation
    d. necrotizing enterocolitis
    e. jejunal atresia

17. A 15-month-old African American infant with Down syndrome is seen for a well child visit. His weight and height are at the 5th percentile for age. A nutritional history reveals that the child was exclusively breast-fed until 8 months of age when iron-fortified cereal was added. He has stubbornly refused all foods except pasta and canned spaghetti with red sauce. Which of the following is not directly supportive of a diagnosis of rickets?
    a. palpable enlargement of the costochondral junctions
    b. a "Ping-Pong ball" springiness to pressure on the skull
    c. a large, open anterior fontanelle
    d. inability to walk
    e. genu valgum

18. An 11-year-old girl is referred to your office following an "abnormal" screen for scoliosis. You diagnose idiopathic scoliosis on examination using the Adam forward bending test. Subsequent radiographs reveal a lateral curvature of 35 degrees. The patient is premenarchal. You refer the patient to an orthopedic surgeon and counsel the parent that the specialist will probably recommend:
    a. external bracing
    b. follow-up radiographs every 6 months
    c. stretching exercises
    d. surgical fixation
    e. no intervention

19. You see a 4-year-old child for declining school performance and behavior problems. His mother notes that he is a poor sleeper. He snores loudly and often gasps in his sleep. Sometimes she sleeps with him because she is afraid he will stop breathing. You note a slight fall off the growth curve and very large tonsils. A neck film demonstrates large adenoids as well. The child's insurance company will not pay to have the tonsils and adenoids removed unless you can prove they are causing him significant health problems. Which test is the most likely to give you that information?
    a. bronchoscopy
    b. overnight pulse oximetry monitoring
    c. polysomnography
    d. fluoroscopy
    e. overnight EEG monitoring

20. An adolescent boy is wheeled into the emergency department following a motor vehicle accident. The paramedics report that he was initially confused and could not give his name. However, his mental status improved during the ambulance ride, and he is able to tell you his name and today's date, although he has amnesia regarding the event. His head CT shows a biconcave area of hemorrhage. When he returns from radiology, he is somnolent and difficult to arouse. His right pupil is dilated, and he appears to have developed left-sided paralysis. What is the most likely etiology of this patient's rapidly deteriorating mental status?
    a. subdural hemorrhage
    b. epidural hemorrhage
    c. subarachnoid hemorrhage
    d. generalized cerebral hypoxia
    e. generalized cerebral edema

21. You are asked to assess a small for gestational age infant. The infant's mother admits to frequent cocaine use and unprotected sexual intercourse before and during her pregnancy. On physical examination, the newborn is noted to have a large liver and spleen, marked lymphadenopathy, and nasal discharge that your attending physician labels the "snuffles." Which test on the infant is most likely to reveal the diagnosis?
    a. blood culture
    b. CBC
    c. hepatitis B antigen
    d. urine for cytomegalovirus
    e. FTA-ABS

22. A woman with a seizure disorder under medical management wants to conceive a child. Her risk of having a child with a neural tube defect is greatest if her current medical regimen includes which of the following?
    a. phenobarbital
    b. phenytoin
    c. ethosuximide
    d. carbamazepine
    e. primidone

23. You are called to the delivery room for a routine birth. The infant cries when the cord is cut. You examine the child under the warmer and notice that when he stops crying, his chest heaves and he turns blue. You are unable to pass the NG tube through the nose for suctioning. Which condition is most likely causing this infant's respiratory distress?
    a. choanal atresia
    b. vocal cord paralysis
    c. subglottic stenosis

d. recurrent laryngeal nerve damage

e. laryngeal web

24. Regarding attention deficit hyperactivity disorder, which of the following is not considered a common possible co-morbid condition?

a. tic disorders

b. aggression disorders

c. oppositional defiant disorder

d. conduct disorder

e. mood disorders

25. An adolescent boy comes to your office with a complaint of progressive scrotal enlargement associated with mild discomfort. When the patient is supine, no abnormalities are palpated in the scrotal sacs. Both testes are of appropriate size, nontender, and without masses. When you examine the patient standing, however, you can feel a characteristic "bag of worms" in the left scrotal sac. What is the patient's most likely condition?

a. testicular torsion

b. hydrocele

c. varicocele

d. epididymitis

e. hypospadias

26. A 27-kg child with a history of vomiting for 36 hours is judged to be 10% dehydrated based on vital signs and physical examination. The serum sodium measurement is 134 mEq/L. An initial 540-mL bolus of normal saline results in stabilization of the heart rate and improved capillary refill. Which of the following is the most appropriate par-enteral fluid choice for the next 8 hours?

a. D5 0.2 normal saline with 20 mEq/L KCl (added after urination) at 220 mL/hour

b. D5 0.2 normal saline with 20 mEq/L KCl (added after urination) at 180 mL/hour

c. D5 0.2 normal saline with 20 mEq/L KCl (added after urination) at 120 mL/hour

d. D5 0.45 normal saline with 20 mEq/L KCl (added after urination) at 220 mL/hour

e. D5 0.45 normal saline with 20 mEq/L KCl (added after urination) at 180 mL/hour

27. You are called to evaluate a newborn girl for intrauterine growth retardation. You notice on examination that she is below the fifth percentile for weight, length, and head cir-cumference. She also has hepatosplenomegaly. You obtain a head US that demonstrates periventricular calci-fications. Which of the following is the most likely cause of these findings?

a. herpes simplex virus

b. placental insufficiency

c. chorioamnionitis

d. trisomy 13

e. cytomegalovirus

28. A 12-year-old male adolescent presents with a 1-month history of fever, weight loss, fatigue, and pain and localized swelling of the midproximal femur. Which of the following is the most likely diagnosis?

a. Ewing sarcoma

b. osteosarcoma

c. chronic osteomyelitis

d. benign bone tumor

e. eosinophilic granuloma

29. Your supervising physician's young son arrives with her husband to pick her up from work. He walks confidently up and down the clinic steps while waiting. When you engage him in conversation, you can understand approx-imately half of what he says. He is able to "get Mommy's stethoscope and put it in the bag." Which of the following most closely approximates his developmental age?

a. 15 months

b. 18 months

c. 24 months

d. 30 months

e. 36 months

30. A 3-month-old infant presents with a history of abnormal movements that his parents think might be seizures. You observe an episode of recurrent rhythmic flexor-extensor spasms that repeat approximately 30 times before subsid-ing. The EEG shows hypsarrhythmia, and a Wood lamp examination is positive for several flat hypopigmented macules scattered over the skin surface. This child's infan-tile spasms are most likely a result of which of the follow-ing underlying disorders?

a. von Recklinghausen disease

b. tuberous sclerosis

c. von Hippel-Lindau disease

d. Sturge-Weber disease

e. bilateral acoustic neurofibromatosis

31. An afebrile 4-year-old child with a limp has discomfort with rotation and flexion at the left hip joint. The WBC count is 9,000/mm³ and the ESR is 15 mm/hour. He has an antalgic gait (a gait clearly affected by pain) but does not refuse to walk. Which of the following is the most likely cause of this child's limp?

a. Staphylococcus aureus septic arthritis

b. S. aureus osteomyelitis

c. toxic synovitis

d. Kingella kingae septic arthritis

e. K. kingae osteomyelitis

32. A 16-year-old girl comes to your adolescent clinic with a chief complaint of the recent onset of pain with sexual intercourse, increased vaginal secretions, and general malaise. She is tolerating oral intake. She has a fever of 101°F; otherwise her vitals are stable. On physical examination, she exhibits adnexal and cervical motion tenderness, and gram-negative intracellular diplococci are seen on Gram stain of an endocervical sample. A pregnancy test is negative. What is the most appropriate next step in management of this patient?
    a. release to home with good contact information and treatment of any organisms found by nucleic acid amplification testing
    b. one dose of IM ceftriaxone and one dose of oral azithromycin
    c. one dose of IM ceftriaxone and 14 days of oral doxycycline
    d. one dose of IM ceftriaxone and 7 days of oral metronidazole
    e. admission to the hospital for intravenous cefotetan and doxycycline

33. A 5-year-old boy who returned from a trip to his grandparents' farm in South Carolina develops a fever of 103.5°F, a headache, vomiting, and an erythematous macular rash on his wrists and ankles. On physical examination, he is moderately tachycardic with otherwise stable vital signs and no focal signs of infection. A CBC reveals a normal WBC count and differential and normal hemoglobin. However, the patient's platelet count is 75,000/μL. Serum electrolytes are normal. Blood cultures and immunofluorescent studies are sent. What is the most appropriate next course of action?
    a. discharge home on tetracycline with close follow-up and reliable caregivers
    b. discharge home on doxycycline with close follow-up and reliable caregivers
    c. hospitalization for observation pending further test results
    d. hospitalization for intravenous doxycycline and cefotaxime
    e. hospitalization for intravenous doxycycline

34. A 6-month-old male infant presents to the pediatrician with a resting heart rate of 50. Physical examination reveals no rash, and there is no history of rash. On chest radiograph, there is no cardiomegaly. ECG revealed D-looped ventricles. The family history reveals maternal systemic lupus erythematosus. Which of the following diagnoses is the most likely cause for the bradycardia?
    a. Lyme disease
    b. congenital complete heart block
    c. sinus node dysfunction
    d. cardiomyopathy
    e. sinus bradycardia

35. An 8-year-old boy arrives at the emergency department via ambulance in respiratory distress. His past medical history is unremarkable for chronic illness, and he has no known risk factors for contracting tuberculosis. He is hypoxic and requires oxygen. A STAT portable chest radiograph reveals a large right-sided pleural effusion, which shifts in the decubitus position. Fluid is obtained via thoracentesis for Gram stain and culture. In considering empirical antibiotic treatment, what of the following is the most likely pathogen responsible for this patient's disease?
    a. *Mycoplasma pneumoniae*
    b. *Klebsiella pneumoniae*
    c. *Staphylococcus aureus*
    d. Nontypeable *Haemophilus influenzae*
    e. *Neisseria meningitidis*

36. A 20-month-old who was treated with high-dose amoxicillin for acute otitis media 3 weeks ago now presents with bulging erythematous tympanic membrane, acute-onset ear pain, and decreased mobility on pneumatic otoscopy examination. Which of the following is not an appropriate antibiotic choice for this child?
    a. oral azithromycin
    b. oral amoxicillin/clavulanic acid
    c. IM ceftriaxone
    d. oral cefprozil
    e. oral cefdinir

37. An afebrile 5-year-old girl presents with tachycardia at 220 beats per minute. On ECG, a regular narrow-complex tachycardia is seen. The rhythm converts with one dose of adenosine intravenously to normal sinus rhythm with pre-excitation (delta waves) noted throughout the precordial leads. There is no cardiomegaly on chest radiograph. The narrow-complex tachycardia is *most* likely consistent with which of the following?
    a. Wolff-Parkinson-White syndrome
    b. idiopathic concealed bypass tract
    c. sinus tachycardia
    d. atrial flutter
    e. atrial fibrillation

38. An 11-year-old girl comes to your office complaining of progressive fatigue and pain in her knees and elbows. She has a red rash spread over both cheeks below her eyes. A UA is positive for RBCs. You suspect systemic lupus erythematosus (SLE) and order a CBC, ANA test, and other immuno serologies. Which of the following, if positive, is the most specific for SLE?
    a. Anti-Smith antibodies
    b. Anti–double-stranded DNA antibodies
    c. Antiphospholipid antibodies

d. Anticardiolipin antibodies

e. Antinuclear antibodies

39. An 8-month-old infant presents with an itchy, erythematous, weeping, papulovesicular rash on the face and the extensor surfaces of the arms and legs. His mother notes that the rash got better (but did not go away) when she used hydrocortisone cream for 2 weeks. The family history is positive for seasonal allergies in the father and "wheezing" in the mother as a child. What is this child's most likely diagnosis?

a. psoriasis

b. eczema

c. contact dermatitis

d. seborrhea

e. urticaria

40. A 5-year-old boy presents to the pediatrician with fever and new 3/6 systolic ejection murmur heard best at the right upper sternal border. On extremity examination, splinter hemorrhages and petechiae are noted. Which of the following is the most likely diagnosis based on the clinical description?

a. endocarditis

b. rheumatic heart disease

c. Kawasaki disease

d. pericardial effusion

e. dilated cardiomyopathy

41. Which of the following statements is true regarding children with sickle cell disease?

a. Vaccinations are not required because they receive penicillin prophylaxis.

b. Gallstones typically develop before 3 years of age.

c. Episodes of dactylitis should be treated with antibiotics.

d. Hydroxyurea maintenance therapy decreases the number and severity of vasoocclusive crises.

e. Acute chest syndrome requires only supportive care.

42. A 4-year-old male child presents with abrupt-onset petechiae and ecchymoses. Other than the skin findings, the child appears well and is hemodynamically stable. No splenomegaly is noted. A CBC reveals a normal WBC count, a normal hematocrit, and a platelet count of 30,000. Large platelets are seen on the peripheral smear. No premature white cell forms are seen on peripheral smear. The parent reports that the child had a viral illness 2 weeks before presentation. Which of the following is the most likely diagnosis?

a. isoimmune thrombocytopenia

b. leukemia

c. sepsis

d. immune thrombocytopenic purpura

e. hypersplenism

43. A 3-year-old boy presents with an elbow hemarthrosis after falling on his elbow. There is no history of spontaneous bleeding. There is no history of epistaxis, gingival bleeding, or cutaneous bruising. The child's maternal grandfather had frequent spontaneous bleeding and hemarthroses after trauma on multiple occasions. Laboratory results revealed a prolonged PTT, normal PT, and a platelet count of 150,000. The factor VIII coagulant activity (VIII:c) is low, and the factor IX level is normal. What is the most likely diagnosis?

a. idiopathic thrombocytopenic purpura

b. von Willebrand disease

c. vitamin K deficiency

d. hemophilia A

e. liver disease

44. A 12-month-old male infant presents with a hemoglobin of 7.5 and a hematocrit of 22%. The mean corpuscular volume is 65 and the adjusted reticulocyte count is 1.0%. What is the most likely cause of anemia in this child?

a. iron deficiency anemia

b. anemia of chronic disease

c. transient erythrocytopenia of childhood

d. thalassemia syndrome

e. parvovirus B19 aplastic crisis

45. Galactosemia, a disorder of carbohydrate metabolism, is inherited in an autosomal recessive fashion. What is the risk of galactosemia in a child whose parents are both carriers for the disorder?

a. 100%

b. 75%

c. 50%

d. 25%

e. 0%

46. You are performing an admission examination on a 15-year-old patient with a diagnosis of anorexia nervosa who has failed outpatient therapy. On cardiac examination, you hear a mid-systolic click followed by a murmur. What is the most likely cardiac abnormality resulting in this examination?

a. mitral valve prolapse

b. prolonged QTc syndrome

c. Wolff-Parkinson-White syndrome

d. sinus node dysfunction

e. sinus bradycardia

47. A newborn male child has a flat facial profile, upward slanted palpebral fissures, epicanthal folds, a small mouth with a protruding tongue, small genitalia, and simian creases on his hands. What of the following chromosomal disorders is most likely in this child?

a. trisomy 21

b. trisomy 18

c. trisomy 13

d. Klinefelter syndrome

e. Turner syndrome

48. A 12-year-old boy with Crohn disease is admitted with an acute exacerbation. He is complaining of abdominal pain and diarrhea. The most effective management in this acute setting is which of the following?
   a. TNF-α inhibitor
   b. corticosteroids
   c. metronidazole
   d. sulfasalazine
   e. azathioprine

49. You are called to evaluate a full-term newborn at 30 hours of age because she is jaundiced. Her unconjugated bilirubin level is 15 mg/dL, and her hematocrit is 48. Which of the following is the most likely cause?
   a. echovirus hepatitis
   b. physiologic jaundice
   c. polycythemia
   d. ABO incompatibility
   e. biliary atresia

50. Which of the following statements is true?
   a. Ulcerative colitis typically is characterized by rectal sparing.
   b. Ulcerative colitis typically is characterized by skip lesions.
   c. Crohn disease typically is characterized by transmural disease.
   d. Crohn disease typically is characterized by crypt abscesses.
   e. Having Crohn disease dramatically increases the risk of carcinoma of the colon.

51. A 5-year-old boy presents pulseless, with ventricular tachycardia at 280 beats per minute on ECG. Immediately the child is intubated, ventilated, and successfully defibrillated. After defibrillation, an ECG reveals a corrected QT interval of 500 msec. Which of the following therapies is the *most* appropriate chronic therapy for long QT syndrome?
   a. nadolol
   b. digoxin
   c. verapamil
   d. lidocaine
   e. furosemide (Lasix)

52. A 3-year-old boy presents with violent episodes of intermittent colicky pain, emesis, and blood per rectum. A tubular mass is palpated in the right-lower quadrant. The abdominal radiograph reveals a dearth of air in the right lower quadrant and air-fluid levels consistent with ileus. Which of the following procedures will best assist in diagnosis and treatment?
   a. esophagogastroduodenoscopy
   b. rectal biopsy
   c. air contrast or barium enema
   d. stool culture
   e. colonoscopy

53. A 6-week-old breast-fed infant presents to your office one morning appearing quite well. The mother states that for the last week, the infant has had numerous periods of inconsolable crying lasting several hours each. Nothing seems to help. You find that most of the spells occur in the late afternoon and evening; between the episodes, the baby looks and feeds quite well. What is the most likely diagnosis?
   a. otitis media
   b. intussusception
   c. milk protein intolerance
   d. colic
   e. malabsorption

54. An 18-month-old female child presents with blood-streaked stool. The stool is grossly positive on Hemoccult testing. Which of the following diagnoses is most likely?
   a. anal fissure
   b. peptic ulcer disease
   c. Mallory-Weiss tear
   d. inflammatory bowel disease
   e. necrotizing enterocolitis

55. During a male newborn examination, the testes are not palpable in the scrotal sacs. One testis is palpable high in the right inguinal canal and cannot be gently manipulated into the anatomically correct position. The left testis is not palpable but is discovered in the abdomen after consultation with a pediatric urologist and abdominal US. In preparation for counseling the parents, you note that infants with cryptorchidism have an increased risk of all of the following except:
   a. ultrastructural changes
   b. impaired sperm production
   c. malignant degeneration
   d. inguinal hernia
   e. microphallus

56. A 3-month-old is brought to your office with a history of failure to thrive and poor feeding. He occasionally vomits small amounts of formula. His birth weight, length, and head circumference were at the 50th percentile; however, his weight has dropped to the 5th percentile and his height to the 10th percentile. His vital signs are normal, and the physical examination is otherwise unrevealing. Venous blood gas and electrolyte study results include pH 7.32; sodium 134 mEq/L; potassium 4.5 mEq/L, chloride 106 mEq/L, and bicarbonate 10 mEq/L. Which of the following diagnoses is the most likely?
   a. chronic diarrhea
   b. renal tubular acidosis

c. pyloric stenosis
d. inborn error of metabolism
e. cystic fibrosis

57. A 16-year-old female patient presents with short stature and no secondary sexual characteristics. What diagnosis must be considered?
    a. Turner syndrome
    b. isolated growth hormone deficiency
    c. Cushing disease
    d. familial short stature
    e. Addison disease

58. A 3-year-old girl is diagnosed with new-onset insulin-dependent diabetes mellitus. Which of the following laboratory findings is consistent with diabetic ketoacidosis?
    a. hypoglycemia
    b. hypercarbia
    c. ketones in urine
    d. increased venous blood pH
    e. decreased BUN

59. Crops of papular, vesicular, pustular lesions starting on the trunk and spreading to the extremities, in addition to small, irregular red spots with central gray or bluish white specks that appear on the buccal mucosa, is the classic description of which of the following infections?
    a. measles
    b. erythema infectiosum (fifth disease)
    c. roseola infantum
    d. zoster (shingles)
    e. rubella
    f. hand-foot-mouth disease
    g. chickenpox

60. A mildly febrile 6-year-old patient presents to your office with dysuria and urinary frequency and urgency. She has a history of one prior urinary tract infection approximately 8 months ago. You obtain a dipstick urinalysis and send a urine culture. The dipstick is positive for nitrites and leukocyte esterase. The most appropriate course of action is:
    a. Await culture results and tailor therapy based on bacterial sensitivities.
    b. Begin empirical amoxicillin.
    c. Begin empirical amoxicillin and schedule the child for a renal US within the next 6 weeks.
    d. Begin empirical amoxicillin and schedule the child for a renal US and voiding cystourethrogram within the next 6 weeks.
    e. Admit the child to the hospital for intravenous ampicillin and gentamicin and schedule a DMSA scan.

61. Which of the following clinical pictures is most likely to indicate a speech or language disorder?

a. whole-word repetition in a 3-year-old
b. 50% of speech intelligible to strangers in a 2-year-old
c. 75% of speech intelligible to strangers in a 3-year-old
d. inability to produce the "s" sound correctly at the beginning of words in a 6-year-old
e. no single words in a 15-month-old

62. An infant who was discharged from the hospital on day 2 of life presents to your office 3 days later for follow-up. The mother did not receive prenatal care. You notice bilateral purulent discharge from the eyes. There is marked eyelid edema and conjunctival swelling (chemosis). What is the most likely pathologic agent?
    a. *Chlamydia trachomatis*
    b. *Neisseria gonorrhoeae*
    c. group B streptococcus
    d. *Toxoplasma gondii*
    e. *Treponema pallidum*

63. You are called to evaluate a newborn with an apparent foot deformity. On close examination, you note adduction of the forefoot, inversion of the foot, and plantar flexion at the ankle that is relatively fixed. Which of the following is true of this patient's condition?
    a. This clinical picture is most consistent with metatarsus adductus.
    b. This deformity will respond to stretching exercises.
    c. This deformity will correct spontaneously when the child is able to bear weight.
    d. This deformity will require surgical repair.
    e. This deformity may be associated with other congenital malformations.

64. A 4-week-old male infant born at full term presents with emesis, dehydration, and poor weight gain. The pediatrician evaluating the child palpates an olive-sized mass in the child's epigastrium. She believes the infant may have pyloric stenosis. Which of the following clinical presentations is most consistent with pyloric stenosis?
    a. projectile nonbilious emesis
    b. bilious emesis
    c. bloody diarrhea
    d. violent episodes of intermittent colicky pain and emesis
    e. right-lower-quadrant abdominal pain

65. A 5-year-old migrant child arrives at your clinic in early summer with a vaccination record that indicates she has received three DTaP doses, three Hib doses, three IPV doses, three PCV doses, and three HepB doses. Which of the following vaccinations should be administered at this visit?
    a. DTap, Hib, IPV, MMR, varicella, PCV
    b. DTap, IPV, MMR, varicella
    c. DTap, Hib, IPV, varicella, PCV

d. DTap, Hib, IPV, MMR, PCV

e. HepB, DTap, Hib, IPV, MMR, varicella, PCV

66. You are seeing a 4-month-old former 30-week premature infant for well child care in late October. Referral for administration of which of the following would be most appropriate to limit her risk of severe bronchiolitis?

a. a portable home oxygen machine

b. influenza vaccine

c. nebulized racemic epinephrine

d. IM palivizumab

e. ribavirin

67. A new patient, a 3-year-old boy, comes to your office with a chief complaint of "swollen bumps" on his neck. His mother notes that he has been diagnosed with infections in his "lymph nodes" many times over the past few years. All episodes resolved with antibiotic therapy but have recurred. A nitroblue tetrazolium test reveals that the patient's phagocytes are unable to reduce tetrazolium. What is this child's most likely diagnosis?

a. X-linked (Bruton) agammaglobulinemia

b. chromosome 22q11.2 deletion syndrome

c. severe combined immunodeficiency syndrome

d. aplastic anemia

e. chronic granulomatous disease

68. A 3-month-old female infant presents to your emergency department unresponsive and with fever, tachypnea, bradycardia, and hypotension. What order should you follow in your initial assessment?

a. airway, breathing, circulation, disability, exposure

b. breathing, airway, circulation, disability, exposure

c. circulation, airway, breathing, exposure, disability

d. exposure, breathing, airway, circulation, disability

e. exposure, airway, breathing, circulation, disability

69. A 1-month-old female infant, born at full term, is noted to have a harsh holosystolic 3/6 heart murmur heard best at the left lower sternal border. The child is not cyanotic and does not have hepatomegaly or tachypnea at rest. The child feeds without tachypnea or diaphoresis, and weight gain is appropriate. There is no cardiomegaly on chest radiograph. Which of the following is the *most* likely diagnosis?

a. ventricular septal defect

b. atrial septal defect

c. patent ductus arteriosus

d. pulmonary stenosis

e. aortic stenosis

70. At a 2-year well child visit, you collect information that your patient lives in a very old rented home with peeling paint. Both the capillary (screening) and venous blood lead measurements are 50 μg/dL. Which of the following courses of action is most appropriate?

a. d-Penicillamine 30 mg/kg/day by mouth for 1 month

b. blood alcohol level, 75 mg/m^2 IM every 4 hours for 5 days

c. edetic acid, 1,000 mg/m^2/day IV for 5 days

d. Repeat the blood lead level in 1 week and test all siblings.

e. Repeat the blood lead level in 1 month and optimize calcium and iron intake.

71. You are examining a 3-year-old girl at her well child visit. While she is staring at her stuffed cow in your hands, you quickly cover her right eye with an index card. When the index card is removed seconds later, you notice that the right eye "drifts" back toward the center. This reaction in response to the cover test indicates what abnormal condition?

a. strabismus

b. amblyopia

c. leukocoria

d. retinoblastoma

e. nasolacrimal duct obstruction

72. At the health maintenance visit for a 12-year-old girl, you note that she has entered her pubertal height growth spurt. The patient's mother asks about what changes the child should be expecting in her body over the next few years. As part of your review, you mention that the most typical sequence of pubertal events in girls is which of the following?

a. height growth spurt, thelarche, pubic hair, menarche

b. height growth spurt, pubic hair, thelarche, menarche

c. thelarche, height growth spurt, pubic hair, menarche

d. thelarche, pubic hair, height growth spurt, menarche

e. thelarche, height growth spurt, menarche, pubic hair

73. Which of the following statements regarding injury in the pediatric population is false?

a. Scald injuries account for the majority of accidental burn injuries in toddlers.

b. 95% of intracranial injuries in infants are caused by abuse.

c. The Back-to-Sleep campaign, which recommends placing infants in the prone position for sleeping, has been credited with a significant reduction in the incidence of SIDS.

d. Home apnea monitor use has been shown to reduce the incidence of SIDS significantly.

e. The American Academy of Pediatrics no longer recommends that parents keep syrup of ipecac in the home for use in acute ingestions.

74. What is the most appropriate indication for using intravenous epinephrine (1:10,000)?
   a. ventricular ectopy
   b. asystole
   c. severe refractory metabolic acidosis and/or hyperkalemia
   d. bradycardia caused by atrioventricular block
   e. supraventricular tachycardia

75. A full-term 4,000-g male infant is noted to be cyanotic 6 hours after birth. He has increased pulmonary vascular markings on chest radiograph without cardiomegaly. He is tachypneic with good pulses and perfusion. There is no heart murmur, but there is a loud single S_2. The ECG is normal for a newborn. The preductal and postductal oxygen saturation levels are 65%. A hyperoxia test reveals a preductal right radial ABG while breathing 100% O_2 of 7.33/35/35/21/–1.5. Which of the following congenital heart defects is *most* likely?
   a. D-transposition of the great arteries with intact ventricular septum
   b. Ebstein anomaly
   c. total anomalous pulmonary venous return with obstruction
   d. tricuspid atresia with normally related great arteries
   e. tetralogy of Fallot

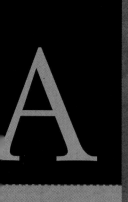

Answers

1. b (Chapter 9)

Functional and structural abnormalities in children with trisomy 21 include generalized hypotonia (obstructive sleep apnea); cardiac defects (endocardial cushion defects and septal defects are seen in 50% of cases); GI anomalies (duodenal atresia and Hirschsprung disease); atlantoaxial instability; developmental delay; moderate mental retardation; and hypothyroidism. There is a higher frequency of leukemia in children with trisomy 21 than in the general population.

2. d (Chapter 21) (See Table 21-2)

The examination described is most consistent with Tanner stage IV development. Stage III is characterized by lengthening of the penis but little change in the diameter or glans; pubic hair becomes darker and curled and spreads over the pubis. In stage V, the penis is adult in size and appearance, and the pubic hair has spread to the medial thighs.

3. d (Chapter 2)

Abuse should be considered in a nonambulatory child with fractures. Posterior rib fractures are common in abused patients, and the evidence of fractures in different stages of healing suggests ongoing injuries over time. Splash burns are consistent with accidental scald injuries. Spiral fractures can occur with torsion injuries that are not abusive. In the case of the infant with the head contusion, the injury is consistent with the history. Accidental ingestions are common in toddlers.

4. c (Chapter 17)

Neuroblastoma is the most common malignant tumor in infancy. Neuroblastoma is a malignant tumor of the neural crest cells that form the adrenal medulla and the paraspinal sympathetic ganglion. Abdominal tumors account for 75% of the neuroblastoma tumors (two thirds, adrenal medulla; one third, retroperitoneal sympathetic ganglion). Thoracic tumors account for 20% of neuroblastoma tumors and tend to arise from paraspinal ganglion in the posterior mediastinum.

Neuroblastoma of the neck (5% of neuroblastoma tumors) involves the cervical sympathetic ganglion. In neuroblastoma of the abdomen, there is often displacement of the kidney and minimal distortion of the calyceal system. This is in contrast to Wilms tumor, in which there is significant distortion of the calyceal system. Because 70% of children with neuroblastoma have distant metastases, treatment generally involves surgery (for tumor debulking) and chemotherapy.

5. d (Chapter 15)

The child in the vignette is initially diagnosed with adrenal insufficiency, which can be associated with adrenoleukodystrophy. Treatment of the insufficiency does not help with the personality changes and declining cognitive faculties. His difficulty with walking is likely because of increasing spasticity. The first three disorders listed are all gray matter degenerative diseases that present earlier in life with hypotonia, mental retardation, and seizures. Rett syndrome is a disease of general cerebral atrophy that presents almost exclusively in girls early in the second year of life.

6. a (Chapter 14)

Type 4 distal renal tubular acidosis is the most common renal tubular acidosis (RTA) in both adults and children. Ammonia production is impaired by high serum potassium levels resulting from hypoaldosteronism or pseudo-hyperaldosteronism. The other types of RTA are all associated with low serum potassium levels. It is important to calculate the urine anion gap in patients with hyperchloremic metabolic acidosis; it should be positive in types 1 and 4 distal RTA and negative in cases of proximal RTA. The serum chloride is high in all types of RTA.

7. c (Chapter 13)

Congenital rubella is caused by rubella virus. Clinical manifestations of congenital rubella include peripheral pulmonic stenosis, atrial septal defect, ventricular septal defect, ophthalmologic defects (cataracts, microphthalmia, glaucoma, chorioretinitis), hepatosplenomegaly, jaundice, "blueberry muffin spots," and failure to thrive. Toxoplasmosis is caused by *Toxoplasma gondii*, an intracellular protozoan parasite found in mammals and birds, in particular cats. Feline stool and undercooked meat are how transmission occurs. Infected infants suffer from intrauterine meningoencephalitis and present with microcephaly, hydrocephalus, microphthalmia, chorioretinitis, intracerebral calcifications, and seizures. Congenital syphilis results from *Treponema pallidum*. Syphilis in the untreated pregnant woman may be transmitted to the fetus at any time, but fetal transfer is most common during the first year of maternal infection. Neonates symptomatic at birth may exhibit nonimmune hydrops, thrombocytopenia, leukopenia, pneumonitis, hepatitis, rash, and osteochondritis. In the first year of life, affected infants have intermittent fever, osteochondritis, persistent rhinitis (snuffles), hepatosplenomegaly, lymphadenopathy, jaundice, and failure to thrive. Congenital cytomegalovirus (CMV) infection is the most common congenital infection in the newborn in developed countries. Most cases are clinically inapparent. Late sequelae such as nerve deafness and learning disabilities may develop in 10% of clinically inapparent infections. The syndrome of congenital CMV (cytomegalic inclusion disease) is uncommon, occurring in 5% of infants with CMV infection. Clinical manifestations include intrauterine growth retardation, intracerebral (usually periventricular) calcifications, chorioretinitis, microcephaly, jaundice, hepatosplenomegaly, and purpura. Neonatal herpes simplex virus (HSV) infection generally occurs during the infant's transit through the vaginal canal. Asymptomatic infection is rare. HSV infection manifests itself in three distinct constellations of symptoms: Infants may have localized infection of skin, eye, mouth (SEM disease); disseminated infection; or localized CNS infection. Infants infected with HIV are, in the vast majority of cases, asymptomatic at birth. During the first few months, infants develop thrush, lymphadenopathy, and hepatosplenomegaly. During the first year of life, common symptoms include recurrent refractory infection, severe intractable diarrhea, and failure to thrive.

8. c (Chapter 19)

A fracture through the growth plate that extends into the epiphysis and into the joint space is consistent with a Salter-Harris type III fracture. If the fracture extended into the metaphysis only, this would constitute a type II fracture. Fractures through both the metaphysis and epiphysis into the joint space are type IV. Type I fractures occur along the growth plate only, whereas type V fractures result form compression of the growth plate. Type III fractures such as the one described in the vignette may require open reduction and fixation but have a relatively good prognosis.

9. b (Chapter 16)

Metabolic syndrome X consists of obesity (body mass index greater than the 95th percentile for age), hypertension, dyslipidemia, and insulin resistance. This syndrome is associated with an increased risk for type 2 diabetes and coronary disease. Mutations in prohormone convertase 1 have been identified in obese patients and may be contributory, but genetic mutations are not part of the syndrome described.

10. a (Chapter 3)

The primary serious complications of Kawasaki disease are cardiac, including coronary vasculitis and aneurysm formation. Prognosis is tied to cardiac involvement; cardiac instability can produce arrhythmias, infarction, or congestive heart failure within days of presentation. Aneurysms and coronary artery disease persist and may result in death months to years later. Patients with Kawasaki disease may manifest sterile pyuria; however, they are not at risk for kidney failure. Arthritis, GI bleeding, and hypertension are also neither early nor late complications of Kawasaki disease.

11. a (Chapter 13)

Neonatal sepsis is generally divided into early-onset sepsis, late-onset sepsis, and nosocomial sepsis. *Staphylococcus aureus* is typically a nosocomial infection found in preterm infants in the neonatal intensive care unit from 7 days of life to discharge. It is not a typical pathogen of early-onset sepsis. The neonate described has early-onset sepsis (birth to 7 days of life), which occurs after colonization with bacteria from the mother's genitourinary tract. The bacteria responsible for early-onset sepsis include group B streptococci, *Escherichia coli*, *Klebsiella pneumoniae*, and *Listeria* monocytogenes. Group B streptococci are the most common cause of neonatal sepsis; sepsis caused by these organisms classically occurs with a bimodal distribution, early onset and late onset. *Streptococcus pneumoniae* sepsis typically occurs in infants and school-age children rather than neonates. *Chlamydia trachomatis* classically causes conjunctivitis and afebrile pneumonia, whereas *Staphylococcus epidermidis* causes bloodstream infections in neonates with central venous catheters; neither causes fulminant neonatal sepsis.

12. c (Chapter 18)

The absence of a red reflex on funduscopic examination (also called leukocoria, for "white" pupil) calls for immediate consultation with a pediatric ophthalmologist. The most common cause is a congenital cataract, which may occur spontaneously, secondary to a genetic predisposition, or as a result of metabolic disease or intrauterine infection. Retinoblastoma, congenital glaucoma, and toxocariasis may also cause leukocoria but are much less common than congenital cataracts.

13. e (Chapter 2)

When the QRS complex is widened, the risk of convulsions and cardiac dysrhythmias increased. Other ominous ECG findings include a prolonged PR interval, QTc prolongation, and rightward axis shifting of the terminal 40 msec of the QRS complex. Premature atrial and ventricular beats are not associated with tricyclic ingestion. Small spiked P waves may be seen with digitalis intoxication but are not seen with tricyclics.

14. c (Chapter 20)

The preferred therapy regimen for a patient older than 5 years with persistent asthma (symptoms daily before treatment or waking with symptoms more than 1 night per week) is daily medium-dose inhaled corticosteroid and a long-acting inhaled β_2-agonist. Answer A is most appropriate for patients with mild intermittent asthma, who can control their sporadic symptoms with an inhaled β_2-agonist as needed. Answer B is the preferred therapy for a patient with mild persistent asthma. Theophylline is an older medication that works well in some patients but requires frequent monitoring and has no anti-inflammatory properties. Nedocromil is a mast cell membrane stabilizer that may be an alternative to low-dose inhaled corticosteroids in patients with mild persistent asthma.

15. a (Chapter 17)

The leukemias account for the greatest percentage of childhood malignancies. Acute leukemias constitute 97% of all childhood leukemias and are divided into acute lymphocytic leukemia (ALL) and acute myelogenous leukemia (AML). ALL accounts for 75% of all childhood acute leukemias. A history of fever, pallor, anorexia, bone pain, lymphadenopathy, petechiae, and hepatosplenomegaly is consistent with ALL. Leukemic cell dissemination results in bone marrow failure, reticuloendothelial system infiltration, and penetration of sanctuary sites (CNS and testicles). Marrow infiltration results in crowding out of normal marrow blood cell precursors, which then results in anemia (pallor) and thrombocytopenia (petechiae). Infiltration of the reticuloendothelial system results in lymphadenopathy and hepatosplenomegaly. Bone pain is caused by expansion of the marrow cavity, destruction of cortical bone by leukemic cells, or metastatic tumor. Although fever and petechiae are consistent with aplastic anemia, bone pain, lymphadenopathy, and hepatosplenomegaly are not.

16. d (Chapter 13)

Necrotizing enterocolitis (NEC) refers to a process of acute intestinal necrosis after ischemic injury to the bowel and secondary bacterial invasion of the intestinal wall. Bowel ischemia as a result of respiratory compromise in the preterm infant causes bowel injury. The introduction of enteral feeding provides the substrate for bacterial overgrowth. Bacterial invasion of the bowel wall leads to tissue necrosis and perforation. Pneumatosis intestinalis results from gas production in the bowel wall and is pathognomonic for NEC. Premature infants with birth weights less than 2,000 g who have been asphyxiated are the population

at highest risk. Prenatal factors associated with NEC include maternal age older than 35 years, maternal infection requiring antibiotics, premature rupture of membranes, and cocaine exposure. Perinatal factors include maternal anesthesia, depressed Apgar score at 5 minutes, birth asphyxia, respiratory distress syndrome, and hypotension. Postnatal factors include patent ductus arteriosus, congestive heart failure, umbilical vessel catheterization, polycythemia, and exchange transfusion.

17. e (Chapter 16)

Rickets in the clinical condition results from a deficiency of 1, 25-dihydroxycholecalciferol, a metabolite of vitamin D. Enlargement of the costochondral junctions (rachitic rosary); craniotabes (thinning of the outer skull layers resulting in a "Ping-Pong ball" feel on skull examination); delayed closure of an enlarged anterior fontanelle; and delayed walking (which usually occurs by 14 months) are all possible manifestations of rickets. Genu valgum ("knock-knee" deformity) is not found in rickets; in fact, patients are likely to be bowlegged instead.

18. a (Chapter 19)

Scoliosis in a premenarchal female is likely to progress and should be treated aggressively. Curvature of 25 to 45 degrees requires bracing to halt progression of the curve. If external bracing is not successful and the curve progresses to greater than 40 to 50 degrees, surgery is required. Stretching exercises are not effective in the treatment of scoliosis.

19. c (Chapter 20)

Polysomnography is not always necessary to diagnose obstructive sleep apnea, but it is the gold standard. This test is performed in the hospital overnight and includes monitoring of the respiratory effort, airflow, oxygenation, and heart rate. Bronchoscopy would show enlarged adenoids but does not measure airflow. Overnight EEG monitoring may be done in children who have central sleep apnea or are suspected of having certain types of seizures (nocturnal seizures). Pulse oximetry monitoring is performed as part of polysomnography. Fluoroscopy has no role in the diagnosis of obstructive sleep apnea.

20. b (Chapter 15)

The pattern of impaired-lucid-impaired mental status is typical for epidural hemorrhages. The biconcave bleed seen on head CT, asymmetric pupils, and hemiparesis point to a right-sided epidural bleed. Patients with subdural bleeds typically have impaired but intact mental status throughout. The CT shows a crescent-shaped area of bleeding. Subarachnoid bleeds are seen in severe injuries; the CT shows bleeding into the ventricular spaces. These patients are often unconscious. Patients with generalized cerebral hypoxia and edema may also be unconscious, with seizing or posturing.

21. e (Chapter 13)

The newborn described in this scenario demonstrates signs and symptoms of congenital syphilis, characterized by hepatomegaly, splenomegaly, mucocutaneous lesions, jaundice, lymphadenopathy, and the characteristic snuffles, a clear, copious nasal discharge. The mother's high-risk behaviors suggest that multiple sexually transmitted diseases may be present. Both RPR and Venereal Disease Research Laboratory (VDRL) tests are very likely to be positive, but the fluorescent treponemal antibody absorption (FTA-ABS) test is a true treponemal test and is less likely to result in a false positive. A CBC may suggest infection but will not give the specific diagnosis. A blood culture will be negative in this case. Newborns infected with hepatitis B have a high likelihood of developing chronic disease but generally appear unaffected at birth. Most cases of congenital cytomegalovirus are also clinically inapparent; however, 5% of those infected present with some constellation of intrauterine growth retardation, purpura, jaundice, hepatosplenomegaly, microcephaly, intracerebral calcifications, and chorioretinitis.

22. d (Chapter 15)

Women who are taking carbamazepine or valproic acid are at an increased risk of producing a child with a neural tube defect if they are treated with this drug during their pregnancies. The mechanism for this is unclear. The other anticonvulsants listed do not increase the risk for neural tube defects specifically, although they may be associated with a higher risk for other birth defects. Other drugs that do increase the risk of neural tube defects include aminopterin, pyrimethamine, trimethoprim, sulfasalazine, methotrexate, phenothiazine, and cyclophosphamide.

23. a (Chapter 20)

Upper airway obstruction in the neonate can result from all the conditions listed. However, the child does not turn blue when crying (mouth breathing). The inability to pass the NG tube in this clinical setting is virtually diagnostic of bilateral choanal atresia. There is no communication between the nose and pharynx, and thus no air flow. Bilateral choanal atresia is an emergency. This patient will likely require endotracheal intubation and surgery to correct the defect. Vocal cord paralysis may result from recurrent laryngeal nerve damage during delivery. If this were the case, the infant should have a hoarse cry, and stridor might be noted. Subglottic stenosis and laryngeal web would also result in stridor. In all three of these conditions, passage of the NG tube would not be impeded.

24. a (Chapter 4)

Patients with attention deficit hyperactivity disorder (ADHD) should always be screened for comorbid conditions because they are not uncommon. Examples include problems with aggression, oppositional defiant disorder, conduct disorder, and mood disorders (i.e., depression). The development of tics and/or dyskinesias is more closely associated with the use of stimulant medication such as methylphenidate, dextroamphetamine, or mixed amphetamine salts to ameliorate the symptoms of the ADHD itself.

25. c (Chapter 14)

This patient's clinical condition is most consistent with a varicocele, an enlarged vein with associated enlargement of the pampiniform plexus caused by the absence of the venous valves responsible for advancing blood flow toward the heart. Varicoceles become detectable in boys during adolescence, occur more commonly on the left, and are usually nontender. They are generally not visible when the patient is supine but become evident upon standing when the veins distend and produce the characteristic "bag of worms" within the scrotum. Testicular torsion and epididymitis are both extremely painful and have a rapid onset. Hydroceles are fluid-filled sacs in the scrotal cavity that may communicate with the peritoneal cavity and are usually diagnosed in infancy or early childhood. Hypospadias is a disorder of the penis that is evident from birth.

26. a (Chapter 7)

A 27-kg child judged to be 10% dehydrated is 3,000 mL behind on fluids (3 kg). So 540 mL is subtracted from the deficit, leaving 2,460 mL left to be given over the next 24 hours (because the child has isotonic dehydration). Half of this is provided over the first 8 hours (1,230 mL at 153 mL/hour) along with maintenance fluids (67 mL/hour). The most appropriate fluid choice for a child this age is D5 0.2 normal saline (with 20 mEq/L KCl to be added after the patient has urinated).

27. e (Chapter 13)

Cytomegalovirus is likely responsible for this syndrome of intrauterine growth retardation, hepatosplenomegaly, and periventricular calcifications. Chorioretinitis, "blueberry muffin" rash, anemia, thrombocytopenia, and jaundice may also be seen. It is diagnosed by rapid antigen detection or viral culture from the infant's urine. Herpes simplex virus is more likely to be acquired perinatally rather than as a congenital infection syndrome, and growth retardation is not a likely feature. Placental insufficiency is a much more common cause of intrauterine growth retardation, but it is not associated with the other findings described in this infant. Chorioamnionitis is a risk factor for early sepsis. Trisomy 13 is associated with a number of physical findings not seen in this infant, including cleft lip or palate, polydactyly, hypotelorism, microphthalmos, and overlapping fingers.

28. a (Chapter 17)

The clinical description is most consistent with Ewing sarcoma. Unlike osteosarcoma, Ewing sarcoma tends to involve systemic symptoms, such as fever, weight loss, and fatigue. Ewing sarcoma usually involves the diaphyseal portion of the long bones. The most common sites for Ewing sarcoma are the midproximal femur and the bones of the pelvis. The most common sites of osteosarcoma are the distal femur, proximal tibia, and proximal humerus. Benign bone tumors and eosinophilic granuloma are generally not painful. Chronic osteomyelitis may present with fever, pain, and localized swelling, but weight loss is unlikely.

29. c (Chapter 4)

The child in question can walk up and down steps (gross motor) and follow two-step commands (language). A stranger can understand approximately half of what he says (language). These skills are typically achieved at 24 months. Other observations would be the presence of parallel play (social) and the ability to remove clothing (fine motor).

30. b (Chapter 15)

Infantile spasms typically present between 2 and 7 months of age and may be idiopathic or associated with other neurologic or developmental diseases. Hypsarrhythmia, characterized by widespread random, high-voltage slow waves and spikes that spread to all cortical areas, is the characteristic EEG finding in infantile seizures. All children with infantile seizures should receive a Wood lamp examination to determine whether ash-leaf spots, the lesions described here, are present. Ash-leaf spots are the earliest manifestation of tuberous sclerosis, a neurocutaneous disease that may present with infantile spasms. Von Recklinghausen disease and bilateral acoustic neurofibromatosis are forms of neurofibromatosis. Café-au-lait spots, which are hyperpigmented, are seen in these diseases. Von Hippel-Lindau disease presents in adolescence. Infants with Sturge-Weber may have seizures, but the port-wine stain is present at birth and the primary skin lesion.

31. c (Chapter 19)

The patient most likely has toxic synovitis. His symptoms are localized to the hip joint on examination; point tenderness would be more suggestive of osteomyelitis. The relatively low WBC count and ESR are consistent with toxic synovitis rather than septic arthritis. In addition, the patient will bear weight on the extremity (albeit with a limp), something most patients with septic arthritis refuse to do. *Staphylococcus aureus* and *Kingella kingae* are both common pathogens causing septic arthritis and osteomyelitis in this age group.

32. c (Chapter 12)

This patient has a clinical picture consistent with pelvic inflammatory disease (PID). Patients with suspected PID should be treated with antibiotics that have activity against *Neisseria gonorrhoeae* and *Chlamydia trachomatis*. Metronidazole would

ideally be added for coverage of anaerobic and gram-negative organisms; however, this may decrease compliance and is not required. One dose of azithromycin was thought to eradicate *C. trachomatis* for the upper genital tract; this is no longer considered adequate treatment for PID. This patient is stable, tolerating oral intact, and not pregnant, so hospitalization is unnecessary.

33. d (Chapter 12)

This patient's history and clinical picture are most consistent with Rocky Mountain spotted fever or ehrlichiosis. He is significantly ill (and vomiting) and should be admitted to the hospital. Both Rocky Mountain spotted fever and ehrlichiosis are rapidly progressive; treatment should be initiated immediately when these diseases are suspected. Delay in treatment can be fatal. Because this patient has no history of a tick bite and is sufficiently ill, empirical antibiotic treatment should include coverage for Rocky Mountain spotted fever and ehrlichiosis (doxycycline) and meningococcemia (cefotaxime or ceftriaxone).

34. b (Chapter 3)

Congenital complete heart block is most likely given the maternal history of systemic lupus erythematosus. Because there is no history of rash, Lyme disease causing complete heart block is unlikely. Tick exposure at this age is also unlikely. Cardiomyopathy is an unlikely cause of the complete heart block, given the lack of cardiomegaly on chest radiograph. Sinus node dysfunction occurs usually secondary to atrial suture lines or atrial dilation. This child has no history of surgery, and there is no evidence of atrial dilation on chest radiograph or ECG. Sinus bradycardia is a normal variant common among athletes.

35. c (Chapter 12)

Cases of suspected bacterial pneumonia that are complicated by large (compromising) pleural effusions (or pleural abscesses) are most likely caused by *Staphylococcus aureus*. *Streptococcus pneumoniae* is the most common cause of bacterial pneumonia after infancy and can result in an effusion; however, the effusions seen with *S. pneumoniae* (and the other pathogens listed) are usually small. An appropriate initial antibiotic choice for this patient is ampicillin/sulbactam. Vancomycin may be considered if there is significant risk of methicillin-resistant *S. aureus*.

36. a (Chapter 12)

High-dose amoxicillin is appropriate first-line therapy for most patients with acute otitis media. However, this patient should not be treated with first-line therapy because he received antibiotics for acute otitis media less than 1 month ago. Appropriate choices for second-line therapy include oral amoxicillin/clavulanic acid, oral cefprozil (a second-generation cephalosporin), oral cefdinir (a third-generation cephalosporin), and IM ceftriaxone. Azithromycin, a macrolide, is not recommended for acute otitis media.

37. a (Chapter 3)

The regular narrow-complex rhythm during tachycardia excludes atrial fibrillation, which is an irregular narrow-complex rhythm. Flutter waves were not noted when adenosine was given, making a diagnosis of atrial flutter unlikely. The preexcitation noted after conversion with adenosine is consistent with Wolff-Parkinson-White (WPW) syndrome. The fact that the tachycardia was narrow complex makes the tachycardia "orthodromic"—re-entrant tachycardia that travels down the atrioventricular node and up the bypass tract. If no pre-excitation was noted after conversion with adenosine, then an idiopathic bypass tract would be more likely. Sinus tachycardia is unlikely given the very fast rate, the fact that the child is afebrile, and the fact that there is no evidence of cardiomyopathy.

38. a (Chapter 11)

Anti-Smith antibodies are very specific for systemic lupus erythematosus (SLE) (although not very sensitive; they are only present in approximately 30% of patients). A positive ANA test is very sensitive for SLE but not very specific; other rheumatologic conditions may result in a positive ANA titer (including some classifications of JRA). Levels of anti–double-stranded DNA antibodies parallel (especially renal) disease severity. Antiphospholipid and anticardiolipin antibodies are often present but are not as specific as anti-Smith antibodies.

39. b (Chapter 11)

This clinical picture, including the age of the child, the appearance of the rash, the response to treatment, and the family history, is most consistent with eczema (also called atopic dermatitis). In children younger than 2 years, the rash described usually appears on the extensor surfaces of the arms and legs, the wrists, ankles, neck, and face. The diaper area is spared. Atopic dermatitis responds to treatment with topical steroids (such as hydrocortisone cream). There is an increased incidence of atopic disease in a child when either or both parents have a history of atopic disease.

40. a (Chapter 3)

Fever and new murmur may be consistent with rheumatic heart disease or endocarditis. The splinter hemorrhages and petechiae make endocarditis highly likely and rheumatic heart disease unlikely. Dilated cardiomyopathy may present with new murmur, but the murmur is generally caused by atrioventricular valve regurgitation, which has a blowing quality and is heard best at the left lower sternal border or apex. If ventricular thrombus is associated with the dilated cardiomyopathy, splinter hemorrhages and petechiae may be noted. Patients with Kawasaki disease present with high fever, but murmur and splinter hemorrhages are not commonly noted.

41. d (Chapter 10)

Hydroxyurea maintenance therapy reduces the number and severity of vasoocclusive crises in individuals with sickle cell disease. Children with sickle cell disease, like all children, require all routine childhood vaccinations. Despite penicillin prophylaxis, children with sickle cell disease are still at high risk of sepsis caused by *Streptococcus pneumoniae*. These children require both the pneumococcal conjugate vaccine (7-valent) during infancy and the pneumococcal polysaccharide vaccine (23-valent) at 4 to 6 years of age. Gallstones typically develop during adolescence as a result of chronic hemolysis. Dactylitis, or hand-foot syndrome, is the earliest manifestation of vaso-occlusive disease. It is caused by avascular necrosis of the metacarpal and metatarsal bones and requires analgesics, not antibiotics. Acute chest syndrome requires both supportive care (supplemental oxygen, RBC transfusions) and antibiotics.

42. d (Chapter 10)

The most likely diagnosis is immune thrombocytopenic purpura. Isoimmune thrombocytopenia is noted in newborns, not in children. Isoimmune IgG antibodies are produced against the fetal platelet when the fetal platelet crosses the placenta and has antigens that are not found on the maternal platelet. The maternal antibodies cross the placenta and attack the fetal platelets. Leukemia, sepsis, and hypersplenism may all cause thrombocytopenia in the child's age group but are unlikely in this case. The WBC count is normal, and no immature white cells are seen on the peripheral smear. Sepsis is unlikely, given that the child appears well and is hemodynamically stable. Hypersplenism is unlikely when the spleen is normal on palpation.

43. d (Chapter 10)

The most likely diagnosis is hemophilia A. Hemophilia A is an X-linked disorder caused by a deficiency of factor VIII. Hemophilia B is also an X-linked disorder and caused by factor IX deficiency. Hemophilias A and B are characterized by spontaneous or traumatic hemorrhages, which can be subcutaneous, intramuscular, or within joints (hemarthroses). Life-threatening internal hemorrhages may follow trauma or surgery. The PTT is prolonged, the PT is normal, and in hemophilia A the factor VIII coagulant activity (VIII:c) is decreased. Other than their factor replacement regimens, there is no distinguishable difference between hemophilias A and B. Idiopathic thrombocytopenic purpura is unlikely in this patient because the platelet count is normal at 150,000. With no history of epistaxis, gingival bleeding, or cutaneous bruising, von Willebrand disease is unlikely. Hemarthroses are not typical for von Willebrand disease. Vitamin K deficiency occurs in the neonate who is exclusively breast-fed and has not received prophylactic vitamin K injection after birth or in the child with significant fat malabsorption. In vitamin K deficiency and in liver disease, there is a prolonged PT and normal factor VIII coagulant activity. The most appropriate therapy for complications of hemophilia A is to infuse factor VIII concentrate.

44. a (Chapter 10)

The adjusted reticulocyte count (ARC) = [(measured hematocrit)/(normal hematocrit for age)] × reticulocyte count. An ARC less than 2.0 suggests ineffective erythropoiesis, whereas an ARC greater than 2.0 signifies effective erythropoiesis. Anemia caused by a lack of production of RBCs therefore has an ARC less than 2.0, whereas anemias resulting from hemolysis or chronic blood loss have an ARC greater than 2.0. The mean corpuscular volume (MCV) is used to describe the anemia as microcytic, macrocytic, or normocytic. All of the anemias noted in the question result from decreased red cell production and have an inadequate reticulocytosis (ARC < 2.0). Decreased red cell production is caused by either deficiency of hematopoietic precursors or bone marrow failure. The microcytic anemia described in the question is most likely because of iron deficiency, which is not only the most common microcytic anemia but also the most common cause of anemia during childhood. It is most often seen between 6 and 24 months of age. Thalassemia syndromes are also microcytic anemias but are less common than iron deficiency anemia. Anemia of chronic disease may be microcytic or normocytic. Transient erythrocytopenia of childhood is a normocytic anemia that is an acquired red cell aplasia. Parvovirus B19 aplastic crisis is a normocytic anemia that results from parvovirus B19 marrow suppression of erythropoietic precursors.

45. d (Chapter 9)

The child has a 25% chance of acquiring the autosomal recessive disorder. Because each parent is a carrier for the disorder, each parent has one normal allele and one mutant allele. The probability of the child receiving an affected allele is 0.5 from each parent. Therefore, the child has a 25% risk (0.5 × 0.5).

46. a (Chapter 21)

Up to a third of patients with anorexia nervosa develop mitral valve prolapse, evidenced by a midsystolic click and/or murmur. Other cardiac abnormalities (arrhythmias) can occur as a complication of anorexia but are less common. Anorexic patients often present with bradycardia; however, bradycardia alone does not result in a click or murmur. A prolonged QTc interval may develop in patients who purge by vomiting (which is more common in bulimia) because of hypokalemia. Sinus node dysfunction and Wolff-Parkinson-White syndrome are not known complications of eating disorders.

47. a (Chapter 9)

The clinical description is that of a patient with trisomy 21, or Down syndrome. Common dysmorphic facial features include flat facial profile, upward slanted palpebral fissures, a flat nasal bridge with epicanthal folds, a small mouth with a protruding tongue, micrognathia, and short ears with downward folding earlobes. Other dysmorphic features are excess skin on the back of the neck, microcephaly, a flat occiput (brachycephaly), short stature, a short sternum, small genitalia, and a gap between the first and second toes ("sandal gap toe"). Anomalies of the hand include single palmar creases (simian creases) and short, broad hands (brachydactyly) with fingers marked by an inward curved fifth finger and a hypoplastic middle phalanx (clinodactyly). Features of trisomy 18 include hypertonia, microcephaly, corneal opacities, micrognathia, and rocker-bottom feet. Features of trisomy 13 include microcephaly, occipital scalp defects, iris coloboma, microphthalmia, cleft lip and palate, and clenched hands. Boys with Klinefelter syndrome do not have physical features identifiable at birth that could lead to suspicion of the disorder. Girls with Turner syndrome have a webbed neck, low posterior hairline, wide-spaced nipples, cubitus valgus (wide carrying angle), and edema of the hands and feet.

48. b (Chapter 8)

Corticosteroids remain the mainstay of therapy for acute exacerbations of inflammatory bowel disease. Tumor necrosis factor (TNF)-α inhibitors are new medications for control of significant disease. The antibiotic metronidazole is an effective adjunct for Crohn disease. Sulfasalazine is the most commonly used maintenance medication for inflammatory bowel disease. Azathioprine is an immunosuppressive medication used for control of chronic symptoms as a steroid-sparing agent.

49. d (Chapter 8)

This infant's bilirubin is rising faster than 5 mg/dL/24 hours and is therefore likely pathologic rather than physiologic. Hepatitis usually gives conjugated hyperbilirubinemia secondary to hepatocyte injury, and echovirus generally presents with other symptoms in addition to hyperbilirubinemia. The hematocrit of 48 rules out polycythemia. Biliary atresia is a disorder of biliary secretion and therefore causes conjugated hyperbilirubinemia. Maternal antibodies to the infant's RBCs, as seen in ABO incompatibility, are a relatively common cause of unconjugated hyperbilirubinemia. This infant requires phototherapy and close monitoring of the hemolytic process.

50. c (Chapter 8)

Crohn disease typically is associated with ileal and/or colonic involvement with skip lesions, rectal sparing, segmental narrowing of the ileum (string sign), granuloma, intestinal fistula, and transmural disease. The presence of Crohn disease increases the risk of colon cancer only slightly. Ulcerative colitis typically is characterized by rectal involvement, rectal bleeding, crypt

ANSWERS

abscesses, and diffuse superficial mucosal ulceration, and its presence significantly increases the risk of colon cancer.

51. a (Chapter 3)

β-Blocker therapy is the most appropriate chronic therapy for long QT syndrome. Nadolol minimizes the number of premature ventricular contractions (PVCs). Fewer PVCs decreases the risk of PVC R-wave depolarization on the vulnerable part of the T wave, thereby decreasing the risk of ventricular tachycardia and ventricular fibrillation seen in long QT syndrome. Lidocaine would be an appropriate acute therapy at the time of the ventricular tachycardia to stabilize the myocardium.

52. c (Chapter 8)

The history, physical examination, and abdominal radiograph are classic for a diagnosis of intussusception, the "telescoping" of a proximal segment of bowel into a more distal segment. In cases of intussusception, barium enema demonstrates a "coiled spring" appearance to the bowel in the right lower quadrant. The barium or air enema results in hydrostatic reduction of the intussusception in 75% of cases.

53. d (Chapter 8)

The infant in this question most likely has colic, although significant disease should be ruled out with a good history and physical examination. Colic begins at approximately 3 weeks of age and can last up to 3 months of age. It is characterized by an infant who seems generally well during most of the day but develops crying spells that last several hours at a time up to three times a week. These tend to be in the evening hours. The infant is generally inconsolable during these spells. Formula changes have not been found to ameliorate true colic. A 6-week-old breast-fed infant is a little young for both otitis media and intussusception; no fever is present, and the symptoms have been going on for too long to be either of these conditions. Malabsorption presents with diarrhea and often failure to thrive, neither of which is present here. Milk protein intolerance is extremely unlikely in a breast-fed infant.

54. a (Chapter 8)

The most common cause of rectal bleeding in toddlers is an anal fissure. If there were significant upper GI tract bleeding from peptic ulcer disease or a Mallory-Weiss tear, the child would have melena instead of blood-streaked stool. Inflammatory bowel disease and necrotizing enterocolitis could both cause lower GI tract bleeding (hematochezia or blood-streaked stool) but are unlikely in an 18-month-old.

55. e (Chapter 14)

Testes that remain outside the scrotum develop ultrastructural changes and impaired sperm production, resulting in possible infertility. There is also an increased risk of malignancy, even after the testis is surgically relocated (and even in the contralateral testis). Ninety percent of patients with cryptorchidism also have inguinal hernias. Cryptorchidism may occur as an isolated defect or be part of a genetic syndrome; however, there is no known increase in the risk of microphallus in these patients.

56. d (Chapter 7)

The child in the vignette has a metabolic acidosis (pH ≤ 7.4) with an increased anion gap. Such a clinical picture is usually caused by increased acid production (such as diabetic ketoacidosis), decreased acid excretion (renal failure), or inborn errors of metabolism. Chronic diarrhea usually causes either normal anion gap acidosis or, if it is chloride wasting, metabolic alkalosis. Pyloric acidosis also results in metabolic alkalosis because of HCl loss via vomiting. Children with cystic fibrosis may exhibit alkalosis. Renal tubular acidosis results in a metabolic acidosis with a normal anion gap. In this case, the anion gap is $(134 + 4.5) - (106 + 10) = 22.5$, outside the normal range of 12 ± 4.

57. a (Chapter 6)

Turner syndrome is relatively common, with an incidence of 1 in 2,500. Female patients present with short stature and delayed puberty caused by primary ovarian failure. Other stigmata, including webbed neck, a low hairline, and increased carrying angle, may not be present. Patients with Cushing syndrome present with other physical characteristics, including moon facies, buffalo hump, and abdominal striae. In isolated growth hormone deficiency and familial short stature, patients do not have delayed puberty. Patients with Addison disease present with fatigue, weakness, nausea, and vomiting. In the acute setting, they may present with cardiovascular shock.

58. c (Chapter 6)

The child with diabetic ketoacidosis (DKA) usually exhibits some combination of polyuria, polydipsia, fatigue, headache, nausea, emesis, and abdominal pain. When DKA occurs, ketones are formed in the blood and cleared in the urine. Hyperglycemia, and not hypoglycemia, is typical. Primary metabolic acidosis with secondary respiratory alkalosis is noted (decreased venous blood pH and hypocarbia). Dehydration results in an elevated BUN level. When DKA is present, the patient is total body potassium depleted from significant potassium loss in the osmotic diuresis. However, serum potassium measurements at presentation may appear high, low, or normal.

59. a (Chapter 5)

Measles is caused by a paramyxovirus and characterized by malaise, high fever, cough, coryza, conjunctivitis, Koplik spots, and an erythematous maculopapular rash. Koplik spots are small, irregular red spots with central gray or bluish white specks that appear on the buccal mucosa. Rubella is caused by rubella virus and characterized by mild fever and erythematous maculopapular rash, with generalized lymphadenopathy, especially of the posterior auricular, cervical, and suboccipital nodes. Roseola infantum is caused by herpesvirus 6 and characterized by high fever followed by a maculopapular rash that starts on the trunk and spreads to the periphery. The fever typically resolves as the rash appears. Erythema infectiosum is caused by parvovirus B19 and characterized by marked erythema of the cheeks ("slapped cheek" appearance) and an erythematous, pruritic, maculopapular rash starting on the arms and spreading to the trunk and legs. Hand-foot-and-mouth disease is caused by coxsackie A virus and characterized by ulcers on the tongue and oral mucosa and a maculopapular vesicular rash on the hands and feet. Chickenpox is caused by varicella-zoster virus and characterized by fever and a pruritic papular, vesicular, pustular rash starting on the trunk and spreading to the extremities. The infected child is infectious until the last lesion is crusted over. Zoster, or shingles, is caused by reactivation of varicella-zoster virus from the dorsal root ganglion and characterized by fever and painful pruritic crops of vesicles along a dermatomal distribution in an individual with previous varicella-zoster infection.

60. d (Chapter 14)

A child with a suspected urinary tract infection (UTI) and positive leukocyte esterase on dipstick urinalysis should be treated for presumptive UTI until culture results become available. Children older than 5 years with a recurrent UTI warrant further workup to rule out anatomic abnormalities (renal US) and vesicoureteral reflux (VCUG). A non-toxic-appearing child of this age does not need to be admitted to the hospital for treatment. But empirical treatment should never be withheld in a febrile child with a suspected UTI and a dipstick UA that is positive for leukocyte esterase.

61. e (Chapter 4)

A 15-month-old with no single words requires a formal hearing assessment and referral to a speech therapist. Children who are 12 months of age should be using "ma-ma" and "da-da" as well as one other word. By contrast, all the other scenarios listed are developmentally normal for age. Whole-word repetition is consistent with developmental disfluency in 3- and 4-year-olds. A stranger should be able to understand 50% of a typical 2-year-old's speech and 75% of a typical 3-year-old's speech. The inability to pronounce certain sounds correctly is normal until 7 years of age.

62. b (Chapter 18)

Gonococcal ophthalmia neonatorum has an onset of symptoms at 2 to 4 days of age. Characteristic features include bilateral involvement, purulent discharge, marked eyelid edema, and chemosis. Diagnosis is suggested by Gram stain and confirmed on conjunctival culture plated on chocolate or Thayer-Martin agar. The infant must be treated with parenteral antibiotics to prevent blindness and other complications. The great majority of gonococcal eye infections are prevented by the instillation of silver nitrate or erythromycin in the neonatal nursery. Chlamydial infections of the eye may usually present at 4 to 10 days of life with unilateral or bilateral mucopurulent discharge and conjunctival injection. Group B streptococcus does not typically cause of ophthalmia neonatorum, although it can cause sepsis and other complications in the neonatal period. Congenital toxoplasmosis can cause chorioretinitis that persists long term. Congenital syphilis does not have any characteristic findings on eye examination.

63. e (Chapter 19)

This clinical picture is most consistent with idiopathic talipes equinovarus. Dorsiflexion at the ankle is not possible in patients with this disorder. Metatarsus adductus, or in-toeing of the forefoot, is a less severe condition that often responds to regular passive stretching. Talipes equinovarus results in a severe limp and foot ulcerations if correction is not achieved by the time the child begins to ambulate. Many but not all cases do require surgical repair; serial bracing or casting has enjoyed a revival of sorts in recent years. One in 7 patients with talipes equinovarus has an associated congenital malformation.

64. a (Chapter 8)

Projectile nonbilious vomiting is the cardinal feature seen in virtually all patients with pyloric stenosis. Physical findings vary with the severity of the obstruction. The classic finding of an olive-sized, muscular, mobile, nontender mass in the epigastric area occurs in most cases. Dehydration and poor weight gain are common when the diagnosis is delayed. Hypokalemic, hypochloremic metabolic alkalosis with dehydration is seen secondary to persistent emesis in the most severe cases.

65. b (Chapter 12)

This child has received vaccinations through the typical 6-month-old visit. She requires another DTaP, which, since it was given after her fourth birthday, will make her current until she requires a booster Td 10 years from now. She also requires an IPV, which, because it will be administered after her fourth birthday, will make her current for that vaccine without requiring any other doses. She needs an initial MMR, with a second to follow 4 weeks later. She needs a single varicella vaccine unless there is a reliable history that she has contracted the disease. The risk of serious *Haemophilus influenzae* is very low in this age group, so the Hib is not indicated. Most pediatricians would not administer the PCV or PPV unless there is a specific health condition that increases the likelihood of invasive pneumococcal disease. She has already completed the required hepatitis B vaccination course.

66. d (Chapter 12)

Palivizumab is an RSV monoclonal antibody approved for monthly injection during the winter months in children at high risk for severe RSV disease. These include children younger than 24 months who are former premature infants or have chronic pulmonary disease (bronchopulmonary dysplasia) requiring oxygen therapy within the last 6 months. A portable home oxygen machine would not decrease the child's risk for contracting RSV or any of the other viral pathogens responsible for bronchiolitis. The influenza vaccine is not approved for children younger than 6 months of age. Nebulized racemic epinephrine and ribavirin may be administered in a hospital setting once the patient is already significantly affected; they are not appropriate for prophylactic use.

67. e (Chapter 11)

Any patient with recurrent or resistant generalized lymphadenopathy should be tested for chronic granulomatous disease (CGD). Children with CGD have phagocytes that can engulf but not kill catalase-positive organisms. The cells cannot produce the oxidative burst needed to generate hydrogen peroxide. The nitroblue tetrazolium test and the dihydrorhodamine reduction test both detect this inability.

68. a (Chapter 1)

The primary survey is the initial evaluation of the critically ill or injured child when life-threatening problems are identified and prioritized. The proper order of the primary survey or initial assessment is airway, breathing, circulation, disability, and exposure. After the primary survey is complete, resuscitation should occur if the condition is life-threatening. Once the life-threatening issues are addressed, the secondary survey should be performed.

69. a (Chapter 3)

A harsh holosystolic murmur heard best at the left lower sternal border is most consistent with a ventricular septal defect. The child does not have symptoms of congestive heart failure (no cardiomegaly on chest radiograph, tachypnea or diaphoresis with feeds, or hepatomegaly); therefore, the defect is likely restrictive. A systolic ejection murmur at the left upper sternal border is consistent with either an atrial septal defect or pulmonic stenosis. A systolic ejection murmur at the right upper sternal border is consistent with aortic stenosis. A continuous "machinery-type" murmur heard best at the left upper sternal border radiating to the left axilla is consistent with a left patent ductus arteriosus.

70. c (Chapter 2)

EDTA is an appropriate treatment for asymptomatic patients with blood lead levels between 45 and 69 µg/dL. It is administered in the hospital. In- or outpatient oral succimer is also an option, depending on the patient's lead level and the home/social situation; d-penicillamine is reserved for patients who have complications from EDTA or succimer. BAL is only added to inpatient therapy when the patient's level reaches 70 µg/dL or greater. Siblings of any patient with elevated lead levels should be tested, and nutritional therapy is certainly not contraindicated; however, patients with levels exceeding 45 µg/dL require chelation treatment per American Academy of Pediatrics and Environmental Protection Agency recommendations.

71. a (Chapter 18)

A positive cover test is consistent with strabismus, or misalignment of the eyes. This child is at risk for amblyopia (reduced vision in the affected eye) and loss of depth perception. She should be referred to a pediatric ophthalmologist for evaluation and treatment, which may include surgical realignment. Leukocoria describes a "white" pupil (that is, absence of the red reflex). Retinoblastoma is a potential cause of leukocoria. Nasolacrimal duct obstruction occurs in infancy and presents with tearing.

72. c (Chapter 21)

The typical sequence of pubertal events in the female begins with thelarche (breast budding). The height growth spurt follows soon thereafter. Pubic hair generally begins to develop during Tanner stage II, but it becomes more pronounced and typical in character in stage III. Menarche is the final event in pubertal development.

73. c (Chapter 2)

As recommended by the Back-to-Sleep campaign initiated by the National Institutes of Health, infants should be placed in the supine position (on their backs) for sleeping. The majority accidental burn injuries in toddlers are scald injuries; usually slash marks are evident. Burns with a stocking or glove distribution are consistent with intentional injury. Intracranial injuries in an infant without a history of severe, substantiated injury (such as a motor vehicle accident or fall from a window) should be considered abusive. Home apnea use does not decrease the risk for SIDS. Syrup of ipecac is no longer recommended for home use in cases of acute poisoning.

74. b (Chapter 1)

Epinephrine is used for asystole, bradycardia, and/or ventricular fibrillation. Low-dose epinephrine increases systemic vascular resistance, chronotropy, and inotropy, thereby increasing cardiac output and systolic and diastolic blood pressure. By increasing systolic blood pressure, cerebral blood flow is increased; by increasing diastolic blood pressure, coronary perfusion is increased. Low-dose epinephrine may change fine ventricular fibrillation to coarse ventricular fibrillation and promote successful defibrillation.

75. a (Chapter 3)

The most likely congenital heart defect is D-transposition of the great arteries with intact ventricular septum. Typically, there is increased pulmonary vascularity on chest radiograph, a single S_2, and no heart murmur. To differentiate among cyanotic congenital heart defects that present with a Pao_2 less than 50 mm Hg on the hyperoxia test, the clinician should first examine the chest radiograph. If massive cardiomegaly is noted, Ebstein anomaly is the most likely diagnosis. If massive cardiomegaly is ruled out, the pulmonary vascularity should be evaluated. Increased pulmonary blood flow suggests the presence of D-transposition of the great arteries with intact ventricular septum, whereas pulmonary edema may indicate the presence of total anomalous pulmonary venous return with obstruction. The remaining possible diagnoses (tetralogy of Fallot, tetralogy of Fallot with pulmonary atresia, pulmonary atresia with intact ventricular septum, critical pulmonary stenosis, tricuspid atresia with normally related great arteries) all have decreased pulmonary vascularity and normal or slightly enlarged cardiac silhouette on chest radiograph. These defects are differentiated by their axis of ventricular depolarization and the presence or absence of a heart murmur. Tricuspid atresia with normally related great arteries has a superior axis, lying in the 270- to 0-degree quadrant. Critical pulmonic stenosis and pulmonary atresia with intact ventricular septum both have axes in the 0- to 90-degree quadrant. They are differentiated by the presence of the loud pulmonary ejection murmur heard in critical pulmonic stenosis. Similarly, tetralogy of Fallot and tetralogy of Fallot with pulmonic atresia both have axes in the 90- to 180-degree quadrant, and they are distinguished from each other by the pulmonic stenosis murmur noted in tetralogy of Fallot.

ANSWERS

Index

Page numbers followed by *f* refer to illustrations; page numbers followed by *t* refer to tables.